ALL IN HER HEAD

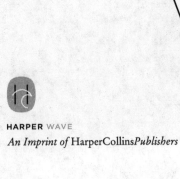

HARPER WAVE

An Imprint of HarperCollins*Publishers*

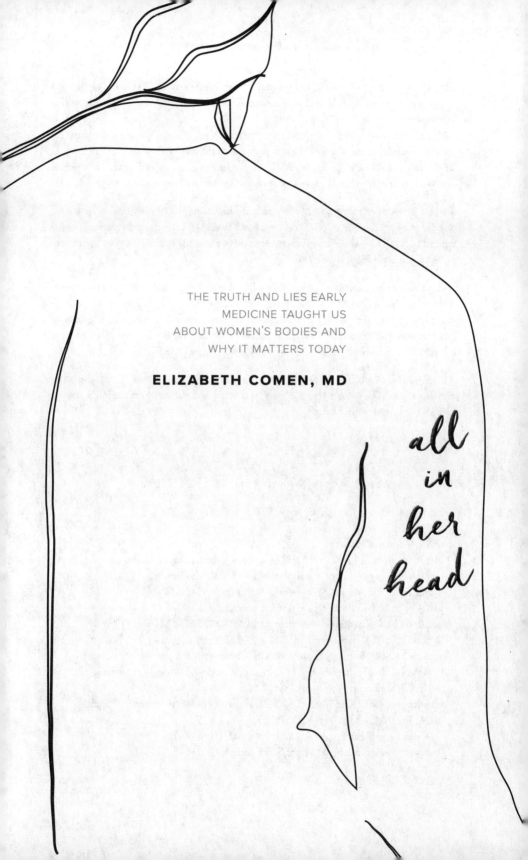

THE TRUTH AND LIES EARLY
MEDICINE TAUGHT US
ABOUT WOMEN'S BODIES AND
WHY IT MATTERS TODAY

ELIZABETH COMEN, MD

*all
in
her
head*

FIRST EDITION

Designed by Elina Cohen
Title and dedication art courtesy of Shutterstock / Olga S L

Library of Congress Cataloging-in-Publication Data

Names: Comen, Elizabeth, author.
Title: All in her head : the truth and lies early medicine taught us about
  women's bodies and why it matters today / Elizabeth Comen.
Description: First edition. | New York, NY : HarperCollins Publishers,
  [2024] | Includes bibliographical references and index.
Identifiers: LCCN 2023045471 (print) | LCCN 2023045472 (ebook) | ISBN
  9780063293014 (hardcover) | ISBN 9780063293021 (ebook)
Subjects: LCSH: Women's health services—History | Women—Health and
  hygiene—History. | Women—Health and hygiene—Sociological aspects. |
  Sexism in medicine.
Classification: LCC RA564.85 .C625 2024 (print) | LCC RA564.85 (ebook) |
  DDC 362.1082—dc23/eng/20231215
LC record available at https://lccn.loc.gov/2023045471
LC ebook record available at https://lccn.loc.gov/2023045472

24 25 26 27 28 LBC 9 8 7 6 5

FOR MY PEARLS: PAST, PRESENT, AND FUTURE

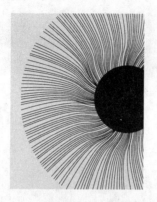

CONTENTS

Each day, I walk—and work—in the shadow of death. It is a constant presence: lurking in the background of every conversation, darkening the scans where a cancerous mass has settled and spread, following me into the exam rooms where I meet with patients in twenty-minute increments. The rooms are designed to be sterile but serene, brightly lit with cream linoleum floors and a peaceful nature scene—a field of wildflowers, a bubbling brook—hung on the wall where a patient lying on the exam table can turn her head to see it. Even the medical gowns, made of seersucker in shades of pink and white, are designed to soothe, to engender a sense of calm. As if the woman on the table could imagine she's somewhere else, somewhere nicer, like a spa.

As if she could forget why she's here.

As if the shadowy presence of death, creeping and terrible, were something that could be ignored.

◆ ◆ ◆

On this August morning in 2018, that shadow was darker and closer than ever, the fantasy of spa-like serenity nowhere to be found. The hospital's breast cancer ward was busy, and noisy, with the whooshing and beeping of machines, the shuffling of doctors and nurses, and the low voices and occasional sobs that the drab brown privacy curtains hung around each patient's bed did nothing to muffle.

I took a deep breath, bracing myself for the conversation to come. Patients often fear, as death approaches, that their doctor will give up on them—that we'll have nothing more to offer when we can no longer offer the hope of a cure. But while the time may come when a patient's targeted therapies stop working, an oncologist never stops caring. And this visit, one of the last I would ever have with my patient, was perhaps the most important. Instead of a hopeful prognosis or a new treatment plan, I was offering something more simple: my presence. Today I would make a series of promises: I will not leave you. I will manage your pain and ease your suffering. I will help you and your family face what's coming. I will be with you until the end.

Ellen looked at me apologetically as I stepped around the curtain beside her bed. Her breathing was labored, and a series of tubes protruded from her abdomen and chest, a final, fruitless effort to drain the fluid that was filling her body, compressing her organs to the point of failure. Her eyes were tinged yellow with jaundice, and the skin of her sunken cheeks was as colorless as the flat, beige wall behind her bed. Her hair, which she'd always worn in a short, stylish pixie cut even before chemotherapy made her temporarily bald, was damply matted to her forehead.

Ellen's downturn had come just four weeks earlier, six years after she first walked into my office with a metastatic, incurable breast cancer that had spread to her bones, liver, and lungs. For most of those years, I had prided myself on plotting a course of treatment that allowed her to not just survive but truly live: working for a nonprofit, mothering four teenage girls, and traveling extensively with her husband and family. Every smiling photo from one of Ellen's adventures—standing with her girls at the top of a mountain or laughing with her husband at the base of a waterfall—was a victory for me, too. Her treatment had worked so well, for so long.

But today, Ellen's adventures were at an end. The room itself felt like a liminal space, a place where my patient survived from ragged breath to ragged breath, the inevitability of her death weighing heavy in the silences between. I held her hand as she asked questions to which there were no easy answers: What it would feel like as she slipped away? Would she be scared? Would there be pain? When our conversation was finished, she squeezed my hand, and I lingered for a few moments longer, holding space for the unspoken.

Finally, I leaned in to hug her goodbye, one last time. I pressed my cheek to hers. I felt the dampness of her skin, the jangle of her fragile bones. I thought about how brave she had been, how wonderful, how alive, and wished I could have given her more time.

And then she said it. Not her last words, but the ones I'll never forget.

"I'm so sorry for sweating on you."

◆ ◆ ◆

Ellen was not the first patient to say these words to me. As an oncologist specializing in the care of breast cancer, I have sat with thousands of women at the moment of diagnosis with this life-threatening disease. And in those first moments after I tell a patient she has cancer, no matter who she is, her responses almost invariably follow the same trajectory:

Am I going to die?
Why did this happen to me?
I'm so sorry for sweating.

Sweating is, of course, a normal physical response to stress—and nothing causes stress like a visit to the oncologist. No other illness stokes our fears the way that cancer does, and the women I see in my practice every day are invariably frightened: of suffering, of dying, of living in remission for years only to have their cancer recur. But the emotion I encounter most in the examination room, more potent and insidious than fear, is shame. The list of things for which patients have apologized to me over the years is both endless and obscene: these women are sorry not just for sweating, but for being sick, for having to seek treatment at all. They blame themselves for missed mammogram appointments, for failing to see their own symptoms, for not accurately diagnosing themselves with cancer amid the mad rush of full-time work, motherhood, caring for elderly parents, running a household. They are even ashamed of the side effects of the treatments and surgeries that allow them to survive. One of my most remarkable patients, a tough, no-nonsense woman of seventy-five who had raised thirteen children and worked all her life on a cattle farm, turned up at her postsurgery follow-up with something I'd never seen before: a flesh-colored adhesive nipple pasted over her mastectomy scar. When I asked her about it, she said she'd ordered it on the internet—for me.

"It's so disgusting," she said, referring to the scar. "I didn't want to make you uncomfortable."

In all my years of both training and practice in internal medicine and oncology, I cannot recall a male patient ever expressing this sort of shame. As a physician aiming to partner with women in their return to good health, I find this difference baffling.

As a student of medical history, I know that the discrepancy is far less mysterious.

The women who apologize to me for being sick are part of a medical legacy, passed down over hundreds of years and still visible today. From that legacy, a story has emerged. It's a story about what a woman's body should look like and how it should feel, in work, in play, in learning and thought, in sex, in motherhood, in sickness and in health—and yes, even on her deathbed. It is a story whose authors have long since left us, although their names and likenesses can still be seen in museums, on plaques, in textbooks that guide today's medical students on their journey to becoming practicing physicians. And while the authors of this story were indeed men, that's not the problem with it.

The problem is, the story is not true.

◆ ◆ ◆

The physicians whose work shaped the world of medicine and women's experience therein were like any of us: products of their own time and experiences, subject to influence not just by the mores of the moment but by their own emotional and social experiences with women, and the expectations of society vis-à-vis a doctor's relationship with his female patients. On the former front, one finds a familiar litany of patriarchal concerns about women: their sexuality, their work, their reproductive abilities, the dangerous possibilities were they to ever become fully liberated architects of their own destinies. But on the latter, separate and apart from the physician's own feelings about these threats, is the fact that any doctor who encouraged a daughter or wife to flout the proscriptions of polite society risked the wrath of the patient's angry father or husband (who would, of course, refuse to pay the bill). Everyone has a master, after all, and the fault lies less with the individual men than with the system in which they lived and labored. Western medical storytelling has largely eschewed the discussion of women's bodies, let alone elevated them as powerful, capable, or of equal worth to men's. In the medical history that defines women's "normal" bodily functions—as well as their pain, pleasure, strength, and intellectual capacity—the voices of women themselves are notably absent.

This was true two hundred years ago. It is still true today. We may have left behind the politics, economics, and emotions that shaped the lives of women throughout history—and particularly during the nineteenth-century period of medical discovery, which continues to define the practice of medicine two hundred years later—but they have not left us. This past is a presence in every doctor's office and every research institution; in medical exam rooms, anatomy cadaver labs, hospital hallways, and operating rooms. It haunts our footsteps as we navigate the medical maze of women's health that was built by men whose ideas about women, while sometimes well-intentioned, were limited at best, paranoid, misogynist, and abusive at worst. It was with me that day in Ellen's room, as shadowy and omnipresent as death itself, lurking beside her as she lay dying. And sweating. And apologizing.

When women come to me for treatment, one of the most important questions I ask is this: What brings you joy? It's a question that many patients find surprising; in our collective understanding of medicine, a doctor's role is to treat disease and prevent death, not to express curiosity about what kind of life you wish to live. But seeing the full humanity of my patients is intrinsic to the practice of medicine. If I prescribe chemotherapy likely to cause nerve damage to a woman whose passion is playing the piano, if I assume that an elderly woman won't be bothered by a cancer-suppressing medication that causes sexual side effects, if I focus on my patient's survival at the expense of her living a joyful life thereafter—then I've failed.

This book is an extension of that same sacred duty: To lift the veil on hidden information. To shine a light into the shadows of this lurking, insidious legacy. To empower women with the tools they need not just to survive but to thrive.

When a woman thinks alone she thinks evil.

—*Malleus Maleficarum*, 1487

In the late fifteenth century, Catholic clergymen authored a remarkable document titled *Malleus Maleficarum*, or *The Hammer of the Witches*. Over the next several centuries, this document was used to hunt down and systematically murder tens of thousands of women who were accused of practicing witchcraft. These killings were a moral atrocity; they were also the start of a long-term movement to sideline women from medicine by making it dangerous, even deadly, to practice it. At this time, the rising power of the church was transforming all aspects of life, including healthcare, ushering in a vogue for faith-based healing in which the real cure for illness was confession and prayer. Generations of healers, mainly women trained in practical methods like botany, midwifery, and herbal therapies, were subject to torture and death. *The Hammer of Witches* was particularly explicit as to the threat presented by female healers who attended to reproductive care, pregnancy, and childbirth: "Witches who are Midwives in Various Ways Kill the Child Conceived in the Womb, and Procure an Abortion; or if they do not this, Offer New-born Children to the Devil." (Perhaps unsurprisingly, the clergymen's fear of midwives offering herbal abortions was second to another, more pressing concern: that witches had the power to "deprive man of his virile member.")

While medical and scientific advances progressed for the next several centuries (and both faith-based healing and burning women at the stake fell out of style), the field of medicine would continue to be haunted by the misogyny and superstition that fueled the witch hunts of the 1600s. The scientific revolution buttressed a series of forward leaps in medical knowledge—germ theory, laboratory science, the burgeoning fields of statistics and epidemiology, and the rise of professional medical societies and schools, including the founding of the American Medical Association in 1847—but at the same time, women were increasingly sidelined from not just the practice of medicine but the study of it. American medical schools, modeled after their European counterparts, created a path to a new, prominent societal status for physicians; they also by and large explicitly forbid female applicants. By the turn of the twentieth century, women had been systematically shut out, including from the fields in which they had once been traditional knowledge bearers. It wasn't just germ theory, laboratory medicine, and science; the field of midwifery, subsumed into the new specialization of gynecology, was now the exclusive purview of men.

From this moment, male doctors became unique, powerful shareholders and experts on women's bodies—while women's healing and knowledge were downgraded and dismissed as old wives' tales. And in the coming years, the professional field of medicine would stratify along gendered lines into doctors on one side, nurses on the other: a world where male superstars performed miracles while female supporting actors mopped up the mess. The role of women was proscribed in medicine as in society, bolstered by the stereotype of the female nurturer: Doctors cured. Nurses cared.

Today's medical schools do not exclude women—indeed, female medical students now matriculate in greater numbers than men—but the elevation of a masculine ethos in medicine persists even as the gender parity of those practicing it has improved. Academic medicine still celebrates authorship of scientific papers as the pinnacle of achievement; merely caring for patients conveys neither glory nor glamour. Women remain underrepresented and overlooked in medical research, even though many treatments interact differently in a female body than in a male one. And when controversies arise within medicine, they still break down along gendered lines in a way that invariably elevates a rational, traditional, masculine-coded approach over the squishy, feminine woo-woo: "Eastern vs. Western," "natural vs. science-based," "alternative vs. conventional."

In the pages ahead, we will acquaint ourselves with the female body the way that doctors in training do—and the way that they have done since the dawn of medical specialization in the late nineteenth century. Physiology textbooks divide the body into eleven discrete organ systems: Integumentary, Skeletal, Muscular, Circulatory, Respiratory, Digestive, Urinary, Immune, Nervous, Endocrine, and Reproductive. In medical school, I learned that these systems taken together encompass the entirety of the human body—but experience has taught me that when it comes to women, the literature overlooks as much as it reveals. (For instance, an education in the female reproductive system leaves unspoken the matter of sexuality, and the sexual health of women as it exists apart from having a baby, as will become apparent in our chapter devoted to reproduction and sexuality.)

Together, we will shine a light on the female medicalized body—and illuminate the myths and blind spots we've unwittingly inherited through generations. We will go back in time to meet the legendary—and sometimes infamous—doctors who shaped the field of medicine, as well as the patients they cared for (or in some cases, didn't). We will explore the sanitoriums of eighteenth-century Europe, the anatomy labs of Victorian New York City, the makeshift hospitals of the antebellum South. We will witness the dawn of women's medicine in all its glory, and sometimes brutality, and rediscover the moments at which rapid advancements in medicine left crucial questions unasked, crucial knowledge undiscovered. And as we walk together through the past, I will draw upon my own experience treating thousands of women, as well as the testimony of expert leading physicians and scientists in their respective fields, to connect the dots whereby our medical past commands women's medical present. Today, we are burdened not only by the legacy of ignorance, indifference, oppression, and subjugation toward women's medical issues but also an entire system built around it: electronic medical records, insurance bottlenecks, and specialization have fragmented our understanding and treatment of the body, with women impacted most. In too many fields, the pathologies specific to women remain underfunded, under-researched, and frequently misdiagnosed.

◆ ◆ ◆

The bias in medicine extends to female physicians as well as patients. Like so many women, my path into the medical profession has been littered with obstacles specific to my sex; I have been undermined, underestimated, and held to standards that my male colleagues are not. Even as medical schools boast graduating classes that are predominantly female, women lag far behind in leadership roles, and are paid millions of dollars less than men over the course of their careers. Female physicians are more likely to take on volunteer "peace-making" roles in academic institutions, and be pushed toward caretaking as opposed to leadership. Yet evidence shows that women also spend more time with patients, embrace more empathic roles, and connect with their patients better (resulting in better outcomes). One recent study revealed that women operated on by men have significantly worse outcomes, including death, than when operated on by women. (As for the men, their outcomes were the same whether a man or woman operated on them.) What such research reveals is not the inherent superiority of female physicians, but the way that gendered cultural norms may allow women to meet the needs of their patients more effectively than their male counterparts. Why is it that male physicians are more likely to interrupt their patients sooner than female physicians? Is it that women are expected to be better listeners, to interrupt less, to demonstrate emotion and empathy? What would happen if we built those expectations into every medical education, for every doctor, from the very beginning? What would medicine look like if all the female energy that was squeezed out and sidelined from it over the course of two millennia was allowed back in?

This is not to imagine a power struggle between healers and scientists, or suggest that modern medicine need incorporate moonlight chanting sessions and herbal therapies to achieve true equality for the sexes. Rather, it is to ask for a medical world that is more human, more holistic, more capable of seeing the patient as a whole person and not just a series of broken parts.

◆ ◆ ◆

Thousands of years ago, a Viking warrior was laid to rest in a grave adorned with a sword, an axe, a spear, armor-piercing arrows, a battle knife, two shields, and two horses, all suggestive of a professional, high-ranking commander. When the grave was discovered in the late nineteenth century, experts agreed that this must be the burial site of an esteemed male warrior. It wasn't until the 1970s that some scientists looked more closely at the remains and asked: Could these small, gracile bones be the remains of a woman?

The greater scientific community balked; the very idea of a female warrior was too ridiculous to entertain. And yet, fifty years later, a

DNA analysis of the Viking skeleton by Stockholm University osteologist Anna Kjellström conclusively proved it accurate. It only took so long, and required so much, because the bones told a different story than the medical institutions and experts of the 1800s did. The skeleton was clearly female—but the men only saw what they wished to see, what they'd been taught to see.

History is also watching us. When the remains of today's medical system are scrutinized by students centuries down the line, what will they understand about how we cared for women? Will we be curled up with our spoils, recognized for our strength, valued warriors in the fight against suffering and illness? Or will we be buried in the ruins of a broken system out of which we never found the strength to dig? I will not be alive to know the answer—but I feel compelled to try.

In Ukraine in 1919, my great-grandmother Pearl watched, clutching her children, as Cossacks murdered her husband in front of her. But when the soldiers turned back and reached for her son, she flung her body in between them, fighting tooth and nail. Her son was saved. Pearl was not so lucky.

The injuries she had sustained at the hands of the soldiers eventually proved fatal—but for the few months she survived after the assault, they were something worse. They were shameful. When my grandmother, her daughter, recounted the story decades later, she would not speak of them except to say that death was a blessing by comparison.

I think often of my great-grandmother, as I think of the patients I've known, and lost. I think of Ellen, apologizing on her deathbed. I think of how she wasn't the first woman to do this, and won't be the last.

But our last moments on Earth should not be imbued with fear, with stigma and shame—nor should the moments we live before. We need to stop apologizing for our medical needs, and start asking the questions that lead to better knowledge, better health, and better lives. We need to ask how to cultivate a relationship with our bodies that is not just comfortable, but joyful; how to know when something isn't right and to advocate, not apologize, for our needs; how to navigate a healthcare system that will never be perfect but could be better; how to be as assertive, as informed, and as confident in the care we deserve in a doctor's office as we are in the rest of our lives.

I have had too many women first ask these questions when they had months to live. I want us all to ask them now, unapologetically—and keep asking until we have the answers. This book is a tribute to women's lives: the ones they lived, the ones they've lost, and the ones they deserve.

Let's begin.

CHAPTER 1

skin

INTEGUMENTARY
IT'S WHAT'S INSIDE THAT COUNTS

The year is 1962. Timmie Jean Lindsey is twenty-nine years old, with bright blue eyes and dark hair styled in a short bouffant. Sophia Loren had the same haircut when she was photographed by Loomis Dean in the late 1950s: cropped close at the nape of her neck, curly and voluminous on top. On Loren, the cut was glamorous, tousled, and sexy. On Timmie, it's practical: the cut hides her ears, which have always stuck out, and doesn't get in the way when she's at work, which is all the time. Her life story is short but already full of dead ends and missed opportunities: an impulsive marriage at fifteen, a divorce at twenty-six. She works at a factory now, on an assembly line. Most of her coworkers are women—the work, assembling circuit boards made of tiny, intricate parts, is easier if you have small hands—and most are like her, struggling to make ends meet. Six children, a factory job, a paycheck that simply can't be stretched far enough to pay for everything they need.

It's poverty that brings Timmie to the Jefferson Davis Hospital in Houston—poverty and shame. She's been dating since her divorce, or trying to, but all she has to show for it are a series of broken hearts and two crummy tattoos, a red rose on each breast. Her last boyfriend, Fred, had encouraged her to get them while the two of them were on vacation, and Timmie impulsively agreed. Now, Fred is in the wind, but the tattoos are still there, reminding her every day of the failed relationship, the mistakes she made. The tattoos can be removed via microdermabrasion, but she can't afford to pay for that, which is why she's sitting in an examination room at the city hospital, where she qualifies as a charity patient.

Timmie wants the red roses gone. She wants the skin of her breasts unmarked, unblemished; she wants to scour all evidence—of the tattoo, the vacation, or Fred himself—from her life, and start fresh, as if it never happened.

She does not want breast implants.

She's going to get them anyway.

◆ ◆ ◆

The integumentary system is the body's largest: its surface. Skin, hair, teeth, fingernails: all form a barrier between your vulnerable organs and the harsh, dangerous world, a system whose sole purpose is to protect what's inside from the outside. As a result, integumentary medicine has a uniquely superficial component, comprising not only the treatment of rashes, lesions, and other malignancies but also the cosmetic, the aesthetic. Doctors primarily preoccupied with beauty are free, if they wish, to focus more on style than substance, on nipping and tucking and taking apart perfectly healthy bodies in the hopes that nature itself might be improved upon.

Unlike other chapters in this book, this is not a history of women's health issues going overlooked, ignored, or misdiagnosed for lack of interest. Indeed, it's a physician's preoccupation with women's bodies, women's beauty, that has driven many of the advancements in the field—and sometimes without much concern for what the women themselves think about it. In the field's infancy, male doctors found themselves empowered to act as both enablers and enforcers of women's beauty, putting the stamp of medical legitimacy on the social pressure to be pretty. Today, the practice of cosmetic medicine is one that walks the line between empowering women to control their bodies and trapping them in a gilded cage of punishing beauty standards.

Despite its posh present-day connotations as a leisure activity for upper-class women, plastic surgery has its roots on the battlefield, and among men. The early patients were soldiers, and the field's first and most dramatic advancements began as a quest to address the facial injuries resulting from trench warfare. The weaponry of the era—grenades, mortars, and machine guns—was unprecedented in its impact on a human body, both capable of inflicting massive injuries and more likely to blow up in a man's face, literally. Many survivors were brutally disfigured, with missing eyes, shattered jaws, skin and bone sheared away, leaving a gaping black hole where a nose and cheek used to be. The legitimization of plastic surgery as a medical field coincides almost exactly with the return to society of injured veterans from World War I. The American Association of Plastic Surgeons was founded in 1921, the American Society of Plastic and Reconstructive Surgeons in 1931, and the American Board of Plastic Surgery in 1937. That latter institution signified a breakthrough: the following year, in 1938, the American Board of Plastic Surgery was officially recognized as a subsidiary of the American Board of Surgery.

At the same time, the advent of modern anesthesiology completely changed the nature of surgery itself as well as the patients who arrived in search of it. Before general anesthesia, the only way to have surgery was fully conscious (or, at best, in a stupor brought on by the use of alcohol or opium as a painkiller), and patients were strapped or held down so that they couldn't flinch away when the cutting began. The notion of elective surgery was inconceivable; given the pain and horror involved, few people went under the knife unless absolutely necessary, and doctors confined themselves to operations that aimed at restoring normal function—chewing, swallowing, breathing—rather than physical appearance. But now, doctors could operate on pliant, unconscious patients who neither flinched, wriggled, nor screamed, and the promise of being able to sleep through the worst of the operation enticed an entirely new sort of person to the plastic surgeon's office. The possibility of surgery as self-improvement emerged.

As the field evolved, surgeons began to divide into two camps: those who did reconstructive surgeries on damaged faces and bodies, and those who performed cosmetic procedures on otherwise healthy people. And here, the line between medical and moral authority began to blur. Doctors, long valued for their expertise in matters of health and healing, were now the arbiters of aesthetics, too. Beauty, as always, was in the eye of the beholder—but now, the beholder was holding a scalpel.

If soldiers whose faces had been torn away by bursting shell on the battlefield could come back into an almost normal life with new faces created by the wizardry of the new science of plastic surgery, why couldn't women whose faces had been ravaged by nothing more explosive than the hand of the years find again the firm clear contours of youth?

—Max Thorek, MD, plastic surgeon, 1943

The patients for reconstructive versus cosmetic surgeries split noticeably along gender lines. Reconstruction was mainly the purview of men with facial disfigurements, and treated as a medical necessity even when the reason for the surgery was, in fact, social in nature: looking like a monster made a man unemployable, even if he was functionally capable of living and working normally. But the cosmetic surgeons, who mainly treated women, were seen as lacking legitimacy by the larger medical establishment: the reconstructive surgeons were doctors practicing medicine, while the aesthetic ones were quacks hawking shoddy and unnecessary procedures to ugly, gullible ladies.

And yet, an unattractive woman who improved her appearance did experience social and economic benefits, not unlike a man who'd had his broken face put back together again. For men, looking normal (if not explicitly handsome) was the key to remaining visible, employed, productive members of society. But for women, whose access to society was even more closely tied not just to looking normal but to being sexually desirable, cosmetic surgery promised to make the difference between a lonely, unhappy life on the fringes and a full, productive one as a wife and a mother. Men could have surgery and get a job; women could do the same and get a man.

The question was how to pathologize the plight of the unpretty woman, how to make a surgical intervention to improve her appearance seem like a matter of medical necessity, with all the same urgency and legitimacy of restoring the looks of a soldier whose nose had been sheared off by shrapnel.

◆ ◆ ◆

It's the spring of 1932, and a standing-room-only crowd has pushed its way into the Grand Ballroom at New York City's Pennsylvania Hotel. The room is huge and ornate, lit by a massive crystal chandelier that hangs from a ceiling painted with a decorative art nouveau motif of interlocking circles. The open floor is flanked by thick columns that support a second-floor gallery area; between each column stretches a waist-high marble balcony decorated with intricate relief sculptures and an iron handrail on top. Every seat on the ballroom floor is filled, and so it is in this gallery where the remaining onlookers have clustered, pressing up against the handrails, all hot breath and warm bodies, clamoring for a view of the spectacle below. On a platform at the center of the room, blinking in the glow of two enormous klieg lights, stands J. Howard Crum, bespectacled and clad in a surgical smock with his sleeves rolled up above the elbow—but all eyes are on his patient, who reclines on a chair beside him. We know Crum's name but not hers, and she is not just anonymous but shapeless: a white sheet drapes her body; a white turban covers her hair. The upper half of her face is hidden behind a paper mask with small, diamond-shaped cutouts that don't quite line up with her eyes: only one is clearly visible, dark brown and staring out at the crowd that stares raptly back at her.

Crum has performed this operation for an audience before, in this same ballroom, as more than a thousand people looked on in amazement. His patient the first time was a sixty-year-old actress named Martha Petelle, a former beauty whose good looks were restored over the course of two days with a face-lifting procedure Crum calls the "Hollywood." But this operation is something more, something special. The masked woman on his table today isn't an actress, but a murderer, recently released from the prison where she served twenty years for killing her husband.

◆ ◆ ◆

Years from now, Crum will write about this patient, remembering the day she arrived at his office: "Could anyone mistake the type shown so clearly and definitely in her face? On it the marks of her mental activities are carved as exactly as a sculptor would have chiseled them in stone." To his mind, the connection between ugliness and criminality is obvious, even organic: when a woman so clearly looked like a bad person, how could she help but become one? And if an ugly face begat ugly character, then surely redemption could be found in beauty—and so, too, could the legitimacy of Crum himself as a practitioner of medicine. Someday, he believes, the gatekeepers of medical society will finally open their doors to doctors like him. They'll see how wrong they were to shun him, dismiss him, call him a quack and a scoundrel. Someday, Crum is certain, the whole world will come to realize what the awestruck audience in front of him so intuitively understands: that some of the cruelest pathologies are the ones that only go skin-deep.

Crum's patient sits, awaiting her transformation. Her expression, what little can be seen of it behind the mask, is placid. Her face has been numbed with novocaine. She's ready: to be made new, made whole, to erase all traces of the person who took a man's life and spent the past twenty years in a cage. To look like a woman who deserves a better life, and then, perhaps, to have one.

When the scalpel descends, when he begins to cut, she doesn't make a sound.

Though plastic surgery cannot, of course, eradicate the inward signs and scars from the heart, there is no doubt that such a removal of the outward signs may do much to heal and restore a broken heart.

—J. Howard Crum, MD, 1933

J. Howard Crum became one of the most renowned and sought-after plastic surgeons of his era—and arguably the first celebrity plastic surgeon, decades before the idea became commonplace. He was the first to pioneer plastic surgery as a sort of spectator sport, and his public demonstrations seem an obvious harbinger of the social media accounts or extreme makeover shows where celebrity plastic surgeons advertise their transformative services today.

When the *New Yorker* wrote about his face-lifting procedure in July 1932, it was with amusement, admiration, and only the tiniest hint of snark: "He won't do fat women, and does very few men," the writer observed, going on to add that "a whole lot of lifted women have never admitted the fact even to their closest friends. They tell their snoopy husbands that they got cut in a taxicab."

Perhaps because he was so far ahead of his time, Crum's persona, practice, and philosophy proved just a little too wild for the folks at the American Medical Association; he never did gain admittance, or the respect granted to doctors in more "serious" medical disciplines. No doubt, he would have been fascinated to see how his showmanship eventually caught on with contemporary audiences: it's impossible not to see the parallels between Crum's belief that he could rehabilitate a murderer by making her beautiful, and the premise of shows like *Extreme Makeover* or the short-lived, sadistic reality TV freak show called *The Swan*. In the latter, "ugly" women spent three months in a mirrorless house undergoing not just multiple plastic surgeries but also coaching, dental work, and intensive therapy, until they reemerged transformed. The reveal would inevitably be preceded by the house therapist gushing about the contestant's new lease on life, how her surgically sculpted face and body allowed her to begin the healing within.

And yet, Crum was also onto something when it came to the pathological nature of ugliness and its impact on women's lives, a topic he remarked on in the 1930s in language that feels eerily (and maybe depressingly) contemporary: despite the "present world-wide emancipation of woman . . . a beautiful face is still reckoned as one of woman's most valuable assets."

The idea of a medical link between health, well-being, and beauty—a broken heart on the inside, a busted face to match—soon became central to the practice of elective cosmetic interventions on otherwise healthy women. Plastic surgeons sought science-based legitimacy for their field, and to distance themselves from squishy, subjective notions of aesthetics, by reimagining their work as something akin to psychiatry—only here, the mental problem had a surgical solution.

Suddenly, ugliness was no longer an aesthetic matter but a pathological one, a disease whose symptoms manifested as the psychological condition known as an inferiority complex. Unattractive features (or the effects of age) were increasingly reimagined as "deformities" that rendered the patient functionally incapable of living a normal life. The effort to lend scientific legitimacy to cosmetic surgeries resulted in some truly remarkable, and often racist, lines of reasoning: at one point, the criteria for diagnosing deformity was rife with racial stereotypes about the undesirability of "ethnic" features, as plastic surgeons claimed that remaking patients to look more generic (read: white) would save them from persecution, discrimination, and other psychological harms. Amusingly, doctors also argued that a patient need not actually be a member of an ethnic minority to derive psychological benefits from these procedures; medically speaking, they said, it was just as bad to look like a Jewish or Asian person as it was to actually be one. One of these physicians, Maxwell Maltz, even went so far as to suggest that a college student who had committed suicide might have been saved—if only he'd done something about his unattractively oversized nose.

In 1943, plastic surgeon Max Thorek waxed poetic on the life-saving boon to mental health offered by the availability of cosmetic surgery: "the sudden hope, surging through feminine—and sometimes masculine—hearts, that where nature had been niggardly in her gifts of pulchritude, the knife of the surgeon could remedy the lack."

Of course, it was always women who were seen to be at the greatest disadvantage for having been overlooked when nature was handing out pulchritude. The equation of female ugliness with the type of life-altering disfigurement that left former soldiers requiring surgery just to live normally only works in a world where a woman's social value is inextricably tied to her physical appearance—and not only that, but to her sex appeal. And so perhaps it was inevitable that the plastic surgeon's gaze, and scalpel, would eventually be aimed below the neck.

Frank was a very qualified physician, but he liked big breasts.

—Bernard Patten, MD, retired neurologist and friend of Dr. Frank Gerow, 2007

It's 1962, and Dr. Frank Gerow has successfully installed the first silicone breast implant in an adult female patient named Esmeralda. It's been three weeks since the surgery, with no complications . . . except, of course, that the bitch keeps trying to remove the implant by chewing through her stitches.

That's the problem: Esmeralda is a dog. If Gerow is going to advance the practice of breast augmentation—and, perhaps more importantly, show up his colleagues at Jefferson Davis, who are currently at work on creating an artificial heart—he needs a human subject on whom to test his invention.

As luck would have it, Timmie Jean Lindsey and her tattooed breasts are waiting for him in an examination room right down the hall.

Gerow, along with friend and colleague Dr. Thomas Cronin, is working at the cutting edge of a new—and entirely unregulated—area within the field of plastic surgery. Breast enlargement is a procedure still in its infancy, and Gerow is sure he can improve upon the current available options, which look unnatural and feel even less so. It's a trip to a blood bank that sparks his eureka moment: taking a bag full of blood in his hand, Gerow can't help noticing that the tactile sensation is not unlike grabbing a woman's breast.

Struck by the notion of filling actual breasts with bags full of, if not blood, then a bloodlike substance that would increase their size without looking or feeling unnatural, the next breakthrough comes when Gerow and Cronin learn about the existence of silicone. Silicone has the proper density, the right feel. Prior to this, doctors have tried injecting syringes full of silicone directly into a patient's breast tissue, often using the young wives of medical students as guinea pigs. But the results have not been great; the silicone settles unevenly and then gathers scar tissue, causing painful hardening, even disfigurement. It's the containment of the silicone within a sleeve that proves to be key. It's this type of implant that Gerow and Cronin install in Esmeralda the dog—and then, not long after, in twenty-nine-year-old Timmie Jean Lindsey.

Gerow has already met Timmie once, when she came in to get her tattoos removed. Although she has no notions of enhancing her breasts, he can't help noticing that she's the perfect candidate: she's young, she's healthy, and she has a B-cup bosom that looks . . . well, the way breasts tend to look after a woman has had, and nursed, six children. But when Gerow asks his patient if she'd like a set of breast implants, she's decidedly reluctant. Her breasts don't bother her, and anyway, she's heard the horror stories about women who've tried to have their breasts enlarged, through sponge implants or silicone injections. She even knows one of them, a cousin, who underwent the procedure only to report that her new breasts didn't retain their shape and tended to migrate while she slept.

But it just doesn't matter, not really, that Timmie Jean Lindsey doesn't want implants. Her doctors want her to want them. They need her to. And when she demurs again, telling them that she would prefer to have her ears pinned back than her breasts enhanced, Gerow and Cronin counter that they'll fix those, too—if she agrees to the surgery.

In the end, Timmie leaves the hospital looking quite different from the way she did when she came in: Her ears no longer stick out. Her tattoos are gone. Instead, she has a pair of subtle twin scars where they put the implants in—and a pair of not-so-subtle C-cups.

◆ ◆ ◆

To the doctors involved in Timmie Jean Lindsey's transformation, this was a happy ending: a successful surgery on a willing, though admittedly coerced, patient. When journalists at the *Houston Chronicle* hunted down Dr. Thomas Biggs, the sole surviving member of the surgical team, decades later, his recollection was rosy: "She trusted us without any hesitation," he said. And perhaps by the time Lindsey was on the operating table, this was true—but the fact that the procedure was not her idea, that she indeed expressed her preference not to have it, seems to have gone overlooked.

Then again, Timmie Jean Lindsey was an atypical patient. Most plastic surgeons are accustomed to seeing patients who not only want to be there but who have sought their services independently. When the patient walks through the door of a plastic surgery practice, she is there with a purpose, a problem: a hooked nose, a drooping eyelid, a receding chin. There's no medical mystery, no puzzling symptoms in search of an explanation. The patient brings their own diagnosis; the surgeon steps in with the scalpel.

This doctor-patient dynamic is not just unique but frequently gendered: most plastic surgery patients are women, and the majority of these receive treatment from male doctors. Other areas of medicine have seen great advancements in gender parity; this one, despite some incremental change, remains largely dominated by men. A 2017 study found that male plastic surgeons outnumber female ones at a ratio of five to one; the ASPS did not have its first female president until 2007.

As a result, the history of plastic surgery is primarily a story about male doctors operating on female patients. But perhaps more importantly, it's a story about men with the power to make women beautiful, and the authority to decide what "beautiful" looked like. The development of new and improved plastic surgical techniques often finds advancements driven by the personal taste of a male doctor, not by what women wanted themselves, and female patients treated more like guinea pigs than consumers driving demand. For a given procedure to be developed, refined, and made ubiquitous has always depended on a man finding it interesting enough to pursue.

This is true of not just cosmetic procedures, but reconstructive ones—where the patient has been ravaged by something much more brutal than the simple passing of time. As late as the mid-1970s, many doctors believed that reconstructing the breasts of post-mastectomy cancer patients was a frivolous, unnecessary endeavor. The notion that women who had undergone radical mastectomy might be traumatized by the permanent disfigurement of their bodies was scoffed at, including by some of the most respected physicians at the time. T.A. Watson, a leading radiation oncologist treating breast cancer patients, wrote in 1966 that suggestible women were only professing to be devastated by the loss of their breasts because doctors insisted on asking about it: "We are frequently amazed at the therapeutic passions aroused by what is . . . an affliction of a superficial easily disposable utilitarian appendage."

Watson's attitude toward reconstruction, and to the women who wanted it, speaks not only to a serious dearth of compassion ("easily disposable utilitarian appendage"!!!) but a one-track mindset bent on aggressively eradicating disease, no matter the cost. Doctors were there to keep women from dying, not to ensure their quality of life thereafter—indeed, the reluctance to reconstruct a breast post-mastectomy stemmed in part from a fear among physicians that doing so would cause them to miss the recurrence of more cancer—and so their patients were simply expected to make peace with their breastless bodies; after all, per Watson, they hadn't lost anything of value.

To be sure, Watson had critics among oncologists and surgeons at the time, and some doctors not only recoiled at his callousness but worked hard to advance less disruptive treatments—lumpectomy and radiation, for instance, rather than the total amputation of the breast. But the major advancement of breast implants as a reconstructive solution for women who'd undergone mastectomy was ultimately developed not by a doctor who treated cancer, but by a plastic surgeon who had a thing for big tits.

I'm so proud that it's available to so many women. It's not vanity getting reconstruction. I think it's necessary. It puts them back whole again. I'm so happy if Dr. Gerow's silicone implants are what started it all.

—Timmie Jean Lindsey, *New York Daily News*, 2012

Over the years, Timmie Jean Lindsey has often been sought out by journalists to reminisce about her role as Gerow's guinea pig. The general wisdom and government regulations surrounding silicone implants have continued to evolve since Lindsey received the surgery; thousands of women ultimately filed lawsuits against Dow Corning, the manufacturer, claiming that their implants had caused connective tissue diseases and cancer, and the FDA hastily banned silicone implants from the market in 1992 (the moratorium would be lifted fourteen years later). But although Lindsey's implants calcified over the years, she never had them removed. And when asked what she thinks about the surgery now, the thrust of her comments has been ambivalent. In one case, she said she saw it as a privilege to have been offered the surgery, seemingly un-aware that she was giving the doctors something, too. And while she testified to the increased attention from men that her new breasts garnered, the interviews she gave as an older woman found her more comforted, and more proud, that her participation in this experimental surgery might have helped normalize the procedure for post-mastectomy patients.

Arguably, Gerow's silicone implants did play a big role in recon-structive surgeries for women who'd lost their breasts to cancer. But Gerow himself never conceived of implants in such an altruistic ca-pacity; he was just a guy who liked breasts, and especially liked the idea of making breasts bigger. The population he had in mind for his surgery wasn't cancer patients but rather women whose bosoms sagged after childbirth.

Like so many of the men in this book, Gerow managed to pos-itively impact his field not as a result of good intentions, but de-spite some deeply questionable ones. After he and Cronin finished patenting their implant technology, the men embarked on a quest to legitimize breast enhancement surgeries using the now-familiar logic that having small breasts was a life-limiting deformity. Gerow's remarks from the Third International Congress of Plastic Surgery in 1963 leave no doubt as to where his priorities lay:

"For some years now, at least in the United States, women have been bosom conscious. Perhaps this is due in large measure to the tremendous amount of publicity which has been given to some movie actresses blessed with generous sized breasts. Many women with limited development of the breasts are extremely sensitive about it, apparently feeling that they are less womanly and therefore, less at-tractive. While most such women are satisfied, or at least put up with 'falsies,' probably all of them would be happier if, somehow, they could have a pleasing enlargement from within."

If the notion that small breasts were a deformity in need of sur-gical correction seems absurd, it did not register as such within the field of plastic surgery. Doctors re-christened the condition of small-breastedness with the scary-sounding medical term "micromastia," which quickly became ubiquitous in medical reference books and textbooks. Twenty years after Gerow and Cronin persuaded Timmie Jean Lindsey to let them place implants in her chest, the American

Society of Plastic and Reconstructive Surgeons petitioned the FDA to deregulate silicone implants as a matter of medical necessity, describing small breasts as not just a deformity but a disease: "There is a substantial and enlarging body of medical information and opinion, however, to the effect that these deformities are really a disease which in most patients result in feelings of inadequacy, lack of self-confidence, distortion of body image and a total lack of wellbeing due to a lack of self-perceived femininity. The enlargement of the female breast, is, therefore, often very necessary to insure an improved quality of life for the patient."

And so, while doctors like T.A. Watson were still decrying the selfish narcissism of women who grieved the loss of their "superficial, easily disposable utilitarian appendages"—even as he saved their lives—Frank Gerow not only pioneered the practice of breast augmentation but also instilled in the public consciousness the idea that it was a vital, even medically necessary procedure. He didn't just enhance women's breasts. He gave them permission to care about how their breasts looked, to believe that they were not easily disposable appendages but a valuable and vital asset to their womanhood, their health, their happiness.

Many people, not unreasonably, thought that the triumph of feminism would relegate beauty to a back seat so far as its importance in a woman's life was concerned. But the power of beauty is unconquerable as love or death.

—J. Howard Crum, MD, 1929

There's a Talmudic proverb that was once popularized by Anaïs Nin, the world-famous French diarist and bon vivant: "We do not see things as they are, we see them as we are." But when Nin looked in the mirror, she saw something else: physical imperfections that were already holding her back, and would only further decrease her value to society as she got older. In fact, Nin underwent cosmetic surgery twice: a rhinoplasty in her thirties, a facelift sometime later. The nose job, which she had in the early to mid-1930s, was still quite uncommon at the time, and Nin was fully aware that she risked permanently marring her face in her quest to make it a little bit prettier; she wrote in her diary that she planned to cut ties with virtually everyone and withdraw from public life if the surgery went awry. And yet, waking up and looking in the mirror, her reaction was pure elation: "Then came the moment when I saw my nose in the mirror, bloodstained and straight—Greek!"

Long before casually nipping and tucking oneself came into vogue, Nin had the same intuitive understanding as Crum did as to the location of her social value: not in her heart or her pen, but on the surface of her skin. Also crucial to Nin's understanding was that beauty was hers to pursue but not define—because beauty was not only about beauty, but desirability. And who decided what was desirable?

Men, of course.

A hundred years of advancement, both in feminism and medicine alike, has done nothing to resolve the tension surrounding cosmetic surgery. On the one hand, we imagine that women are empowered by the ability to change the way they look—except that this "empowerment" takes the form of complete and utter submission, the woman lying unconscious on a table while a person she barely knows with a blade slices into her pliant flesh. And what are we to make of the competing notions that beauty is the most superficial and shallow of pursuits, while at the same time being the greatest asset a woman can have?

Today, this paradox is best exemplified by the rise of the medical spa, a facility which fully inhabits the tension between medicine and aesthetics, health and beauty. But the medspa is just the latest iteration of a long tradition whereby a physician's stamp of approval serves to lend a seriousness, a legitimacy, to beauty treatments: Palmolive, for instance, ran ads from 1946 to 1953 promoting it as a doctor-approved product, promising a "lovelier complexion" couched in the idea that clear skin was a sign of good health. It's a pattern found throughout history. In 1962, a woman is talked by a breast-obsessed doctor into the implants she never knew she wanted; in 1983, the medical establishment evangelizes about the medical necessity of enhanced breasts; and by 2010, breast implants are the single most popular cosmetic surgery in the United States.

Plastic surgery is far more regulated today than it was when Dr. Gerow installed untested implants in Timmie Jean Lindsey's chest in 1962. But the legacy of those early days is still with us—including in the process whereby a woman's normal, healthy body is pathologized as a deformity in need of a surgical fix, and where the "ideal" is based as much as on what men desire as what women want.

This curves doll came in for a full tummy tuck and BBL with Liposuction360. She is only One Month post op and she is living for these results 🔥🔥 Dr. Curves understood exactly what she was looking for 😌

—Andrew Jimerson II, MD, Instagram, 2022

His name is Andrew Jimerson, but everyone calls him "Dr. Curves"; it's his handle on Instagram, where he promotes butt lifts, breast implants, and other cosmetic surgeries to more than half a million followers. The posts are playful, cheeky, unabashedly provocative. One video shows a patient sitting in an examination chair, looking ruefully at the camera above overlaid text that reads, *I would never dance for a BBL*. She shakes her head and slices her hand through the air in the universal gesture for "nope." But then the video cuts to a photograph of Jimerson, smiling and handsome in his medical scrubs. The text overlay reads, *What if I'm the doctor?*

The video cuts back to the patient: she's standing on the chair, her paper gown thrown open to reveal a black surgical thong and bra, gyrating and shaking, laughing and sticking her tongue out. The caption reads: *Nowww you see if it's by Dr. Curves that's another story*.

The post has thousands and thousands of likes, and hundreds of approving comments, most of them from women. A representative reply reads, *Shit I'll do more than dance for a bbl*, followed by three laugh-crying emojis.

In any other field, it would be unusual if not obscene for a medical doctor to rely on his own sex appeal to sell his patients on an expensive elective surgery. But in a field where the doctor-patient relationship still so often breaks down across gendered lines, it remains the case that plastic surgery trends are closely tied to male desire, male notions of beauty—and that the women who seek out cosmetic surgery often fully embrace this dynamic. The opinion of a straight male doctor becomes a proxy for the desires of men at large; the plastic surgeon's expertise is not just in medical technique, but in being able to tell his patients how they should look if they want to be wanted by men.

At the same time, the concept of beauty itself has undergone an extreme makeover, fueled by the rise of social media, the dawn of influencer culture, and the ubiquity of pornography, among other factors. In some cases, the new beauty standards are female-driven and arguably positive, corresponding with an increased diversity in the range of looks and body types that are considered desirable, as well as the increased accessibility and affordability of cosmetic procedures. We've come a long way from the days when doctors believed that looking too "ethnic" was a psychologically distressing deformity that required surgical correction.

But in many cases, the desires of men, their particular preferences, are still the elephant in the operating room. What breast implants were to the 1960s, the Brazilian butt lift is today—not only in terms of reshaping women's bodies into a caricature of sexual desirability but also in the unregulated, Wild West–like atmosphere surrounding the procedure. As the popularity and visibility of BBLs exploded, so did a cottage industry of "discount" surgical facilities offering deals on multiple procedures, and unlicensed recovery centers that sell post-op patients on packages with names like The Dream, The Peach, and The Vixen (the latter includes round-trip airport transfers as well as transportation to and from the surgery, which patients make lying facedown on a mattress in the back of an unmarked van). Eventually, the situation got dire enough that the ASPS put together a task force to address it, standardizing techniques to improve the safety of the BBL—but before that happened, the procedure boasted a horrifying death rate of one in every three thousand patients.

And yet, women continue not only to seek out these procedures but actively participate in marketing them to future patients, showing off their results in videos that are edited, set to music, and blasted across the internet by their plastic surgeon and his social media team. Where Drs. Gerow and Cronin had to sell Timmie Jean Lindsey on implants after encountering her at the hospital, doctors like Jimerson reach women on social media, racking up thousands of views with photos and videos of patient transformations. The shift from breasts to butts in beauty culture has also inverted an existing surgical pipeline: where surgeons once augmented women's breasts using fat grafts from their buttocks, the Brazilian butt lift reshapes the buttocks using excess fat from the upper body.

◆ ◆ ◆

And then there's labiaplasty, for which one of the most popular search terms is "Barbie vagina." Like the breast implants of old, labiaplasty is the surgical solution to something that has only lately been deemed a valid problem: women who find their genitals visually displeasing, usually owing to asymmetrical or undesirably long labia minora. Recent years have seen a 40 percent increase in women having labiaplasties; even ten years ago, it was practically unheard-of. And while there are functional reasons to have the procedure (labiaplasty is especially popular among female cyclists, for whom protruding labia can cause discomfort and sometimes injury while riding a bike), the vast majority of women cite aesthetic reasons for wanting the surgery—raising the question of whose aesthetics, exactly, should dictate the appearance of a body part that is rarely in a position to be seen by anyone, including the woman herself.

The social factors that lead women to seek this procedure are myriad, but the willingness of doctors to provide it is another matter, one with uncomfortable callbacks to the early practice of legitimizing surgery by describing healthy, functional body parts as medical deformities. How many of the women who show up at doctors' offices in search of labiaplasties would still choose to have the procedure if they knew that longer or asymmetrical labia are not outlying conditions, but something a majority of women have? How many doctors, knowing this, would still operate on patients requesting "Barbie vaginas"?

But while a medical education teaches doctors to recognize the diversity of "normal" shape and size when it comes to other body parts—including, notably, men's penises—there is no analogous recognition of the normal diversity of women's genitals, nor is that information available to anyone who might try to seek it out. The average medical student doesn't see many vulvas; his education might include one elderly female cadaver, one mass-produced plastic model of female genitals, one anatomy textbook that serves only to teach how women's genital structures functionally compare to men's (the labia are analogous to the scrotum, the clitoris to the glans of the penis, and so on), and one limited gynecology rotation. There is virtually no instruction on anatomical diversity—a dearth of knowledge only exacerbated by the taboo surrounding physicians observing (or making comparisons between) the shape, size, and aesthetic appearance of a patient's body parts. What may be good advice in some contexts—"don't gawk"—is nevertheless transformed in this one into a problematic knowledge gap.

All told, the average graduate of a medical school is entering an industry in which female genital cosmetic surgery is on an unprecedented upswing—but with no concept whatsoever of how normal anatomy might vary from woman to woman, no basis for being able to reassure a patient on the fence about having surgery that there's nothing medically wrong with her. What they have instead, based on some combination of personal experience and pornography consumption, is a highly personalized and probably misinformed notion of what labia are "supposed to" look like.

And indeed, we can't talk about labiaplasty, or about its predominance in the field of plastic surgery, without talking about porn. Here, once again, we see how surgical standards come to be influenced not by what is healthy but by what is considered attractive: the average labiaplasty has very little to do with medical necessity and a great deal to do with what men like to look at. Doctors have long struggled to comprehend that women's genitals might come in a normal diversity of shapes and sizes, in a history infused not just with misogyny but also no small amount of racism. Labiaplasty no doubt has its roots in culturally loaded notions of a "civilized" vulva versus a "savage" one, dating back to the eighteenth century, when the enlarged labia of some African women were christened the "Hottentot apron" and presumed to be a sign of race-specific sexual depravity.

One colonial traveler to South Africa in the late 1800s lamented that the women he encountered there were reluctant to indulge him in close examination of their genitals, seemingly surprised that a woman whose traditional garb left her legs and belly exposed would nevertheless not appreciate having her private parts ogled or groped by a stranger. Attempts to pay the women to be examined, he wrote, were "rejected with contempt by Hottentot maidens almost naked." The women who consented were treated as human novelties, and often cruelly exploited. One woman, Sarah Baartman, was brought to England by surgeon Alexander Dunlop and displayed naked in public—or, for select wealthy families, brought to their homes, where patrons could pay to touch her. The indignity inflicted on Baartman persisted even after her death: instead of being buried, her remains were displayed at the Musée de l'Homme in Paris, along with a wax mold of her labia.

Modern medicine hasn't done much better: in 1975, Professor Sir Norman Jeffcoate, a physician and former president of the Royal College of Obstetricians and Gynaecologists, compared elongated labia minora to a dog's ears and concluded, erroneously, that women were causing the condition by masturbating too much. Almost fifty years later, the notion persists that longer labia are a reflection of depravity or sexual promiscuity, particularly among religious conservatives still fighting the purity wars. It's not uncommon in 2024 to encounter a particular brand of viral post in which a picture of a ham sandwich with its meat spilling out is described as representing the vagina of a sexually experienced woman (usually any woman, although the meme is sometimes, bizarrely, specifically aimed at Taylor Swift).

Oddly enough, the cultural breakout moment for the concept of the "designer vagina"—which arguably heralded the popularity of labiaplasties—came in 2008, amid a sex scandal that resulted in the resignation of New York governor Eliot Spitzer. The escort with whom Spitzer had been involved, Ashley Dupré, was reportedly the possessor of "the most beautiful vagina in New York," leading to much speculation about just what a beautiful vagina might look like. And even now, in the golden age of labiaplasties, the place where a person is most likely to encounter one of these perfectly symmetrical, understated vulvas is on a porn star (an irony that appears to be lost on the participants in this particular culture war). At the end of the day, medicine still has no standard for delineating what a "normal" vulva looks like—but the culture has entirely changed its mind about which types of labia ought to be put on display.

There is still some paternalism present in plastic surgery. But there are also patients who look for that doctor-patient interaction. They may be having surgery to appear more attractive to men, and they value the perspective of a male surgeon saying, "This is what you're going to look like," and "This is going to look great."

—Aviva Preminger, MD, plastic surgeon, New York City, excerpt from interview 2022

The revision cosmetic breast surgeries Aviva Preminger performs—and she performs a lot of them—often stem from the same problem: they're too big. Big enough to cause tissue damage, sometimes, or just bigger than the patient wanted. In some cases, the problem is subjective, and aesthetic. The doctor believed bigger was better, more beautiful, and the patient who preferred a smaller implant either acquiesced or just didn't understand that she'd been overruled.

◆ ◆ ◆

Preminger understands better than almost anyone how important it is to strike a balance between what is beautiful and what is possible, and to know when a cosmetic procedure might veer too far into impairing function. The too-large implants are one form of this; overzealous labiaplasties are another.

"The labia minora have a function," she says—a fact that patients don't always seem to recognize. If too much tissue is removed, the patient can experience chronic vaginal discharge, irritation, chafing, and debilitating pain. And worst of all, this is a problem with no easy solution; one of plastic surgery's foundation principles is that it's relatively easy to remove tissue from a body but extremely hard to add it back in. For this reason, when Preminger performs

labiaplasties, she steers patients away from the "Barbie vagina" aesthetic that might create a medical issue where none previously existed.

In cases such as a botched labiaplasty or a too-big breast implant,
the question of whose idea it was is ultimately irrelevant. Whether
a woman was talked into an ill-advised procedure or requested one,
it's the job of Preminger and doctors like her to advise against it or
fix the problem that someone else created.

◆ ◆ ◆

On the other hand, there are still disturbing echoes of plastic surgeries past visible in the field today. It's TikTok influencers posting
advertorial videos about how Botox is a form of self-care; it's a breast
implant patient, with a surgical cap on her head and an IV already
in her arm, shimmying for her doctor's Insta followers before the
general anesthesia kicks in; it's the common understanding, little
discussed but broadly accepted, that breast implant surgeries trend
larger when performed by men.

One thinks again of Timmie Jean Lindsey, saying she would have
preferred having her ears pinned to having her breasts augmented.

One thinks of her doctor, waxing nostalgic: "She trusted us without any hesitation."

How do the doctors of Preminger's breast implant revision patients remember them? Do they believe they gave the patient what
they wanted? Do they think they knew better than she did what
that was?

One need only compare numbers—the number of plastic surgeries done per year, versus the number of patients who return
dissatisfied—to understand that cosmetic surgery now occupies a
permanent place in our social fabric. Many women are choosing to
have work done, and few ever come to regret it. The numbers have
only increased as the procedures get better, and cheaper; the cosmetic surgeons whose practices once piggybacked off the facial reconstruction of mutilated soldiers have given way to medspas where
licensed aestheticians dole out injectables to women on their lunch
breaks. A delicate euphemistic vocabulary has sprung up alongside
these new procedures: lifting, plumping, smoothing, filling. It all
sounds so gentle, less like medicine, more like self-care. And yet

we are still no closer to disentangling what women want for their faces and bodies from what doctors, or husbands, or social pressures might tell them they're supposed to want.

It is possible to deplore the pressures that women feel to conform to a stereotyped standard of beauty, while at the same time defending their right to make their own decisions.

—Marcia Angell, MD, editor in chief, *New England Journal of Medicine*, 1992

I meet Amrita on a normal day, but she's an unusual patient: after receiving a cancer diagnosis in her home state, she has traveled more than a thousand miles to New York for a second opinion. She's alone; her husband has stayed behind with their teenage children. Most striking is how put together she is, despite being clearly exhausted from her journey the previous day. Her hair and makeup are neatly done, including a matte plum lipstick that flatters her deep brown skin.

Despite the metastatic cancer that has spread to her bones, Amrita is doing remarkably well. The greatest challenge of her condition is the uncertainty of it: the availability of new and effective treatments for her cancer mean that she might live a normal, healthy life for years yet, but her cancer could also mutate, starting with one treatment-resistant cell that spreads like wildfire and kills within months. On that front, I can't offer her any more reassurance than her doctors back home, but Amrita handles our difficult conversation gracefully, asking incisive questions and remaining poised throughout. It's only when I turn to leave that she says she has one more question—and bursts into tears.

"I'm too embarrassed to ask my oncologist back home," she says, and for a while, I'm afraid that she won't be able to bring herself to ask me, either. It takes a lot of coaxing and several false starts before she finally tells me what's troubling her: she desperately wants to get Botox, but she doesn't know if that's something she can do while also undergoing chemotherapy.

Amrita begins to cry again: she says she knows she should be grateful just to be alive, that she's ashamed to admit how much her appearance matters. But of course it does. My patient is already living with the burden of knowing what will kill her. She has seen its shadow on her scans. Why should she also have to see it on her face, every time she looks in the mirror? Why shouldn't she take this one small step to look less old, less sick, less haunted by the knowledge she's already living with? The cancer had already taken so much: her health, her peace of mind, an unknowable number of years. By refusing to let it take her beauty, Amrita wasn't just giving herself the gift of a more youthful appearance; she was reclaiming a sense of control over her life.

Ultimately, the referral I gave her for a dermatologist—along with the assurance that getting Botox would not compromise her cancer treatment—was the most important piece of medical advice I dispensed that day.

Doctors can forget that our patients have lives beyond the confines of their appointment, lives in which how they look on the outside matters much more, day to day, than how healthy they are under the skin. Indeed, that complex interplay between beauty and health can make the difference between a patient who is living, versus merely surviving. Long before I became a practicing oncologist, as a pre-med college student working at the Dana-Farber Cancer Institute, I came to understand that cosmetic interventions were where we could get to know patients as people, not just a collection of malfunctioning body parts in need of fixing. The boutique at the institute, where patients were fitted for wigs and breast prostheses, did not do anything to treat the cancer itself—but these interventions, far more than radiation or chemotherapy, made women feel whole again. The single professional in her thirties who wondered how she would date again after a mastectomy, the mother who cried as she explained that her children were frightened by the way she looked without hair or eyelashes: these patients were experiencing a devastation to their sense of self that was just as debilitating as any other cancer symptom, only these symptoms, many doctors refused to take seriously. During my residency, I would recoil when fellow MDs scoffed, "It's just hair, it'll grow back," at a patient who had been so transformed by chemotherapy that her reflection in the mirror looked like a stranger's. As far as we may have come from the days when doctors referred to amputated breasts as "useless appendages," the legacy of those days rears its ugly head every time we dismiss a patient as vain for caring about how she looks. And where cosmetic surgeons have long held to the ethos that aesthetics matter, oncology and other fields of medicine have much catching up to do when it comes to how we weigh the impact of treatments on our patients' quality of life—in which psychological and cosmetic concerns are just as meaningful as adverse health effects or toxicities. Even now, the treatments we do have that can help prevent hair loss in some chemotherapy patients may be overlooked by physicians—or seen as valueless by insurance companies who refuse to cover them.

As much as I have sought to understand cancer itself at the most microscopic level, I remind myself every day: the insidiousness of this disease is not in how deadly it is, but how it destroys a woman's life, her sense of self—externally, internally, and everywhere in between. For some patients, the biggest milestone in their treatment is not a clean scan, a successful surgery; it's when they wake up to find that their hair, eyebrows, and eyelashes are finally growing back. It's when they finish getting nipple tattoos on their reconstructed breasts. It's when they look in the mirror and see themselves looking back.

You know, we're living in a society!

—George Costanza, *Seinfeld*, "The Chinese Restaurant," aired 1991 on NBC

Men's cliché midlife-crisis cars and affairs are seen as embarrassing, febrile grasps for youth, sure—but not as embarrassing as a woman who tries to get her face from 1985 back.

—Frances Dodds, Coveteur, 2018

Our fraught relationship with vanity and aesthetics in medicine reflects our fraught relationship with these things on a societal level: there are rules, and expectations, oftentimes in conflict with one

another. It's hard to know where to draw the lines between deformities that are "worthy" of correction to simply undesirable features
that aren't, and that's before we even consider the changes to a person's appearance wrought by illness, injury, or age. The fact that a
person can have cosmetic surgery to improve these things does nothing to solve the moral conundrum of whether she should, especially
as the social consensus is so often that she shouldn't—that there's
something gauche about buying beauty, or buying it back when it
begins to fade. Even as our society fetishizes youth, or the appearance of youthfulness, to acknowledge this too openly—to let it show
on your face in the form of having had obvious work done—is still,
somehow, a bridge too far.

Women, we are told, should age gracefully. And yet the notion
of aging gracefully requires grace, in the form of a sort of passivity
that is just as feminine-coded as full lips or perky breasts. The alternative to engaging with the medical establishment in this case is
resignation. A choice not to fight back against the vagaries of time,
of gravity, of too much laughing or smoking or sunlight. And why?
Because cosmetic surgery is too costly? Too painful?

Or is it that it's undeserved?

After all this time, we remain caught up in the same questions of
legitimacy that plagued aesthetic medicine in its infancy: When is
it right to intervene? The surface of the body doesn't just protect us
from the world; it's the intermediary through which we experience
it, and through which the world experiences us. Some people are
born beautiful and welcomed with open arms; some are less fortu-
nate, and are received with less forgiveness. If a doctor could turn
someone from the latter category into the former—if the patient
herself knocks on the cosmetic surgeon's door to request as much—
who are we to deny them?

If women's bodies are the battlefield, we're told, then the noble
thing, the graceful thing, is to wave a white flag and turn away—
riding off, wrinkles and all, into the sunset of our lives. But then by
that note, aesthetic surgeons could come to seem like brothers-in-
arms, the warriors fighting bravely at the sides of those who refuse
to go quietly, helping women take control of their facial features,
their body contours, the effects of time itself.

All of this is complicated by the fact that cosmetic surgeries are often empowering to the women who choose them, quite literally endowing them with greater influence than if they'd left their faces untouched, unattractive, or aged. A bad facelift might be embarrassing, but a good one buys you something immeasurable: a few more years of being seen, in a world where women of a certain age tend to become invisible.

And of course, these days, the women who show up in medical spas and surgeons' offices are more likely to be accompanied by their mothers than by men.

◆ ◆ ◆

Simran is twenty-six years old when she learns that death is coming for her.

There had always been cause for concern: her mother was diagnosed with breast cancer at the age of thirty-three. Other women in her family, the ones who still lived in India, had similar stories: breast cancer, ovarian cancer, a shared history of aggressive malignancies that suggested a genetic connection. When her mother tested positive for one of the BRCA mutations that causes breast cancer, it was no surprise.

When Simran tests positive for the same mutation, a countdown begins. As a palliative care physician, she understands better than most what's at stake. Cancer is all but a certainty unless she undergoes surgery, and soon; her mother's age at diagnosis is not just a tragedy but a benchmark, the date by which she needs to remove her breasts if she hopes to avoid the same fate. The doctors all give her the same advice: have children, then have a mastectomy—and then, they say, get breast implants.

But Simran doesn't want implants.

And she's not getting them, no matter what they say.

◆ ◆ ◆

"Oh, it was horrible. It was horrible," Simran says. It has been two years since her surgery, but the memory of this moment is still vivid, her anger and frustration still palpable.

The days of doctors shrugging off a mastectomy as the no-big-deal loss of "useless appendages" are long gone. That a patient undergo reconstruction, via either fat grafts or implants, is not just encouraged but assumed; when Simran began to plan for her mastectomy, the plastic surgeon she saw even suggested they incorporate the reconstruction into the same procedure, swapping out the removed breast tissue for an implant. "He basically was like, 'Yeah, direct to implant is best for you based on, you know, you're young, healthy, beautiful,' those were literally his words," she says.

Simran already knew that implants were not in her future. As a doctor, she had more insight than most into not just her own medical options but the likely outcomes of what she might choose, and she had all kinds of reasons for choosing not to replace her missing breasts with silicone. She'd always been small-breasted, especially after having children. She didn't like the idea of having a foreign body inside her. The women she knew who'd received implants all seemed dissatisfied; their new breasts were cold to the touch, or sat unevenly on their chests, or just didn't feel like theirs. Her own mother, who'd had a flap reconstruction using fat grafts from her abdomen, had been plagued by belly and back pain ever since— and not only that, her new breasts were too large. What Simran wanted was a different type of reconstruction, called aesthetic flat closure, which leaves the patient flat-chested but with little scarring and her nipples intact. But her surgeon's attitude, his fixation on giving her implants right there on the table while she was having her mastectomy, caught her off guard, and so she sought a second opinion—from a woman this time, who she assumed might be more open-minded about her various options. At the appointment, Simran carefully explained what she wanted, and why.

But far from being understanding, the female surgeon balked. She told Simran that being flat-chested would psychologically scar her.

"I was appalled," Simran says. "In that moment, I was of course sad for myself because I left that visit in tears, feeling like I was not heard at all."

◆ ◆ ◆

Simran's story has a happy ending: her breast surgeon ultimately gave her the flat aesthetic closure she wanted, and the result was so successful that she often gets calls from other patients who are considering forgoing implants in favor of flat reconstruction. But what makes this story remarkable is how it fits into the evolution of plastic surgery as not just a medical field but a form of female empowerment, culminating in a moment where the patient not only chooses exactly what she wants to look like but chooses to step outside conventional notions of beauty, of desirability, of where her value to society truly lies. What she loves about the result of her surgery is not that it makes her look sexy or beautiful, but that it makes her feel like herself.

If you talk to people about how plastic surgery and what their experiences are, how they're doing now, they don't really talk about how they look. They talk about how they feel.

—Charles Galanis, MD, plastic surgeon, excerpt from interview, 2022

All of this and more makes plastic surgery, and its history, uniquely complicated in context. Unlike our other bodily systems, which are plagued by diseases and disorders for which we must seek a cure if we want to live, cosmetic surgery and medicine are fields with which women engage by choice. The woman on the operating table is there because she wants to be, or thinks she does.

Maybe, like Timmie Jean Lindsey, she simply feels lucky to have the opportunity and the means to make herself more beautiful. And maybe the cosmetic surgeon who likes big breasts or small labia isn't some all-powerful inflicter of punishing beauty standards on his hapless patients, but a doctor helping patients to live the lives they desire. In any event, we continue to chase beauty, even as it eludes us, escapes us, fades away. The battle will continue. And there will be blood.

bones

SKELETAL
SKULLS AND WHALEBONES

We may congratulate ourselves as a Society on the possession of so fine and rare a Cesarean specimen.

—Maurice Fitzgibbon, MD, 1879

While Mary Ashberry is alive, people hardly look at her. To many, she's literally beneath notice: an achondroplasiac dwarf in her early twenties, she stands three and a half feet tall, the height of a five-year-old girl. The details of her short life will remain a mystery, alluded to only after her death by a doctor who examines her corpse and pronounces her "a helpless thing," the victim of unspecified misfortunes at the brothel in Norfolk, Virginia, where she makes her home. There will never be a record of how she found her way to the brothel, or the nature of her tenure there; nobody will ever know how she lived, happily or unhappily, or with whom.

When Mary falls pregnant, and her belly begins to swell, there will be no record of who the father was—or even who he might have been.

◆ ◆ ◆

It's the spring of 1856 when her labor begins, the sunlight hours growing longer. In another week, the magnolias will be in bloom, their branches heavy with waxy flowers in shades of pink and white.

By then, both Mary and her baby will be dead.

It's the labor that kills her—that, and a doctor's ignorance. Mary's pelvis is too small for the child to pass through; her only hope of survival is for the physicians attending her to abort and dismantle the skull of the fetus, an operation they take too long to attempt and then fail to complete. Later, a doctor named Fitzgibbon will examine what is left of Mary Ashberry and note, dispassionately, that "as the operation was commenced and carried so far as the destruction of the child's life, it is to be regretted that it was not carried further." Instead, the doctors cut into Mary's womb. She expires three days later, perhaps from the trauma, perhaps from infection.

In this moment, Mary dies as she lived: unnoticed, overlooked, unseen. Her corpse is piteously small—remarkably small.

Perhaps this is why they don't bury her.

Instead, what's left of Mary travels north. Her nameless baby travels with her. By the time she arrives at the Philadelphia museum that will be her final resting place, Mary is no longer a "she" but an "it": the only thing left of her is her skeleton, with its disproportionately large head, its shortened arms and legs, its unusually narrow pelvis. It is, as Fitzgibbon notes, a fine, rare specimen. The human woman it once belonged to has been forgotten entirely.

They bleach her bones until they gleam. They lift her upright, suspending her in a standing position with a line that runs through a hole in her skull to a pipe ten feet overhead.

In life, Mary died with no partner, no family. In death, she has both. Beside her, in the glass case that holds her bones, is the skeleton of a giant—a nameless man who stood at least seven and a half feet tall in life, whose remains were put up for sale in Kentucky in 1877. And in her hand, she holds something small and white and grinning: the skull of her baby.

For more than a century, Mary's skeleton has stood behind glass at the Mütter Museum in Philadelphia, where more than a hundred thousand people come to look at it each year. They approach. They stare. They observe the strangely curved line of her humeri, the way her femurs bow inward. They see the bones that gave her body its shape in life, now stripped of skin and muscle, the star attraction in a curious tableau. They are interested in what she was—but not *who* she was.

And so, like the people who surrounded her in life, they don't see her. Not really.

◆ ◆ ◆

I remember sawing her skull into two halves. My anatomy instructor placed his hand on my shoulder, gentle and reassuring: "This will be the hardest part."

I remember the scent of menthol balm clinging to my upper lip, sharp and overpowering, yet still not quite enough to mask the ubiquitous smell of formaldehyde.

I aligned the bone saw against the base of her skull and began to cut.

The dissection was nearly complete. For months, we had been peeling open the elderly woman's body layer by layer, revealing muscle and tendon, organs and bone. The skull we'd saved for last, because it was one of the most physically demanding tasks and because the instructor—a male physician overseeing the work of four female first-year medical students—believed it was the part we would find the most upsetting.

It was not. That part, which had come many weeks earlier, was the moment when we understood what had ended her life. The woman had several tattoos on the right side of her chest, not decorative but tiny pinpoints, a telltale sign of prior radiation treatment to her breast for cancer as well as a small scar on her breast indicative of a lumpectomy. In the months we spent dissecting her body, memorizing every vein, nerve, and muscle, we came across countless rubbery white nodules: tumors. Her body was riddled with them. The cancer had likely started in her right breast, and then spread to her lymph nodes, her bones, her brain, until it killed her.

Of course, there was no satisfaction in diagnosing her. And knowing how she had died still told us nothing about her life: who she had been, how she'd lived, who she'd loved. Our cadaver was not a patient, but a lesson. Inside of her lay the same systems that lie inside us all. After we concluded our work, my fellow students and I clasped hands over her body, thanking her for her selflessness and promising to honor the gift of knowledge she had given us. It was the first and last time I would dissect a cadaver, and my medical career would ultimately be dedicated to saving the lives of women with the same cancer that had killed this one.

Mary Ashberry, whose skeleton has been on display at the Mütter Museum in Philadelphia for the better part of two centuries, died in 1856. It would be twenty years before she caught the attention of the medical establishment, but unlike the elderly woman whose body I dissected as a first-year medical student, Mary's life—and the way it ended—were of little interest to the physicians who were entrusted with her remains. The doctor, Fitzgibbon, who was so delighted by the condition of her bones, spared only a passing thought for the path that led her from a young woman living and working in New Orleans to a medical artifact. "The little creature was nothing but a helpless thing," he wrote—not as an expression of sympathy, but by way of explaining why the doctors who attended her lacked the necessary tools to deliver her baby and save her life. Her body was simply too small for the usual instruments.

And when her skeleton was mounted for display, it was apparently done not in the name of medical knowledge, but of morbid curiosity. At the time of Mary's death, preserved bones were a valuable tool for doctors and medical students. Being able to engage with the human skeleton offered important insights into how the body was structured, how to set bones and repair joints. But the skeletons used as anatomical guides were held together with wire; it was important not just to see them but to touch them, to see how they moved. Mary Ashberry, on the other hand, is held together by the calcified remains of her own soft tissues. If someone attempts to move her, to turn her head, to lift her hand and hold it, she will break. Instead, she stands motionless, holding the skull of the baby she died giving birth to, in a macabre tableau that is as medically useless as it is shocking.

Mary's body was not a lesson; it was an object to be gawked at.

◆ ◆ ◆

But in the context of medical history, Mary Ashberry's bones not only contain knowledge but serve as an embodiment of all the tension and strangeness with which a woman's skeletal system was viewed by the establishment. The same forces that led doctors to regard Mary as a grotesque object also wrought their influence on depictions of the female skeleton more generally, fueling a widespread (or, perhaps, bone-deep) ignorance whose effects can still be observed today.

The skeletal system in itself holds a unique place in our understanding of both medicine and mortality. In life, it gives shape and structure to the body; in death, eventually, it is all that remains. As such, it is the anatomical system with which ordinary people, not just doctors, have the greatest familiarity; it's hard to think of any comparable system that is both as medically important and as culturally ubiquitous.

With rare regional exceptions (namely, Italy and the South of France), dissecting human bodies was largely illegal until the sixteenth century, which created both an air of mystery and a great deal of misinformation surrounding human skeletal structure; human dissections before this time were done rarely, and when they were, covertly, as obtaining specimens often involved robbing graves. Before then, anatomical knowledge of human beings was predicated largely on the work of Galen, a physician from the Roman Empire whose theories dominated Western medicine for more than a thousand years. But Galen's work was heavily reliant on assumption and extrapolation about human anatomy based on the dissection of animals, and many of those assumptions were incorrect.

A revolution in the field of anatomy began in the mid-1500s, when Dutch physician Andreas Vesalius became not only an open advocate for the dissection of human bodies but an illustrator of remarkable, vibrant, vivid depictions of the body's hidden layers. These illustrations betray a fascination with anatomy that goes beyond mere medical knowledge; Vesalius's work is as laden with cultural and religious symbolism as it is with anatomical detail. In one series, he illustrates a forlorn man pointing heavenward as he holds his own skin, dripping, in his other hand; in the background, a church can be seen. In another illustration, famously nicknamed "the Skeletal Hamlet," he details a human skeleton contemplating a decapitated skull that rests atop a tomb; the inscription on the tomb reads, in Latin, "Ingenuity will live, all the rest will die."

Unlike many anatomists, Vesalius did consider and appreciate the differences between male and female bodies; his work includes nude renderings of each. But his understanding of sexed anatomy didn't penetrate deep enough; it did not go down to the bone. Accompanying his anatomical nudes, Vesalius illustrated just one skeleton, and labeled it, *HUMAN*.

But of course, the skeleton wasn't only human.

It was male.

What fueled this omission? It's possible that Vesalius didn't know that the female skeletal system differs in certain crucial ways from the male's. But it is also equally possible that he knew but didn't consider it important enough to merit a separate, anatomically accurate illustration of those differences. In the latter case, he would not have been alone in his judgment: depictions of the female skeleton are few and far between in early anatomical texts, but perhaps more importantly, those that do exist tend to sacrifice accuracy for aesthetics. The study of anatomy seems to have been permeated early on with a double standard: the depiction of men's bones conveyed medical knowledge about the human body, while the depiction of women's bones conveyed aesthetic, cultural, and social concerns.

In these early texts, the adult female skeleton is often rendered as if it were a child's: underdeveloped, frail, breakable. It's worth noting that this view of women's bones was not the exclusive purview of men: when the French scientist Marie-Geneviève-Charlotte Darlus Thiroux d'Arconville published her drawings of the female skeleton in 1759, she exaggerated the sexed differences to the point of caricature. The skull was vastly smaller, the pelvis much wider. Embedded in the depiction was a message: women, with their smaller skulls and larger hips, were clearly intended by nature itself to be mothers, not thinkers.

It was a message that thoroughly permeated the medical thinking of the time. The French medical *encyclopédie* of 1765, rather than omitting the female skeleton, dwells heavily on the differences between the bones of men and women before drawing this final conclusion: "All of these factors prove that the destiny of women is to have children and to nourish them." In 1796, German anatomist Samuel Thomas von Sömmerring famously—and inaccurately—

illustrated the female skeleton with a disproportionately tiny head, an enormously broad pelvis, and an improbably narrow rib cage. The inaccuracies were so marked that some doctors did in fact step in to criticize Sömmerring's illustrations as misleading, but they were overruled by the remarkable defense that Sömmerring was an artist, not an anatomist. The fact that this was considered a compelling argument is revealing of how the medical establishment viewed skeletal knowledge vis-à-vis women: if the illustrated skeleton was beautiful and rich with symbolism, it simply didn't matter if it conveyed the anatomical truth. Sömmerring's female skeleton wasn't accurate. It was something better: an object to be admired, not a system to be understood.

This trend in the depiction of women's bones continued into the nineteenth century. When Scottish anatomist John Barclay tackled sexed illustrations of the skeleton in 1829, he not only engaged in the same exaggerations as his predecessors but adorned each illustration with the skeleton of a corresponding animal: a powerful horse for the man, an ostrich for the woman. At the same time, anatomy and artistry began to diverge, with women's bodies being relegated to the latter category and excluded from the former. Since the time of the ancient Greeks, medicine had been captive to the idea of the male default: men's bodies were the healthy standard. Women's bodies, in their differences, represented deviations from the ideal.

Now, this notion permeated not just the minds but the texts of medical knowledge-seekers. With the exception of reproductive organs, the bodies depicted in textbooks—including the gold standard *Gray's Anatomy*, and even within the past twenty years—were invariably male.

All psychologists who have studied the intelligence of women, as well as poets and novelists, recognize today that they represent the most inferior forms of human evolution and that they are closer to children and savages than to an adult, civilized man.

—Gustave Le Bon, MD, 1879

At the same time as women's bones were being overlooked as a source of medical knowledge, their skulls were coming in for special scrutiny thanks to the nineteenth-century twin obsessions with phrenology and craniology. These pseudoscientific fields, whose practice was inextricably entwined with the rise of anthropology, Darwinism, and eugenics, posited that the size and shape of a skull held telling details as to the character, capabilities, and intelligence of its owner.

Perhaps unsurprisingly, many of the same characters who were willing to sacrifice anatomical accuracy in order to make women's skeletons align with a feminine cultural ideal were also possessed of the notion that the topography of a person's skull revealed proof of genetic inferiority. Also unsurprisingly, many of these men were racists. Before Samuel Thomas von Sömmerring made his famous skeleton illustration, he was an early craniology enthusiast and strong proponent of the theory that the skulls of dark-skinned "moors" were smaller than those of whites, reflecting the former's inferior intellectual capacity. In this case, Sömmerring's defense was that he was not just an artist but a bold truth-teller, one who would not be deterred from his studies simply because they invariably led to wildly racist conclusions. (On this front, very little has changed since the eighteenth century: these same arguments are in use today by the modern race scientists who hope to uncover a connection between racial background and IQ.) A 1786 engraving depicts a beatific Sömmerring examining a human skull with a pair of calipers, ignoring a Medusa figure who slings snakes at him from above while holding a banner reading *DIE GUTE SACHE*—in English, "the good cause."

As is so often the case in medical history, where racism took root in the scientific community, misogyny was not far behind. Anthropologists led the charge here, scrutinizing skulls belonging to people of various races and concluding, predictably, that white men like them were the most intellectually evolved creatures on the planet. One of the fathers of physical anthropology, Samuel George Morton, collected hundreds of human skulls from all over the world in the early 1800s and eventually claimed to have found a link between interior cranial capacity and intelligence. The literature of the time is rife with commentary so wildly racist and sexist that it reads like caricature, the monologue of some mad scientist from a schlocky horror film. In one representative musing about the intersection of race, sex, and species, nineteenth-century anthropologist James Hunt wrote, "It cannot be doubted that the brain of the Negro bears a great resemblance to a European woman or child's brain, and thus approaches the ape far more than the European, while the Negress approaches still nearer to the ape."

A fixation on the skull began to overtake the anthropological and medical communities in the middle of the nineteenth century. At the same time, practitioners began to pay particular attention to women's skulls, scrutinizing them for signs of inferior intelligence. In 1868, Parisian anthropologist and surgeon Paul Broca determined that the study of women had become a specific and urgent necessity. The women's rights movement was beginning to pick up steam in Europe and North America, which was a sinister development in Broca's view: women reformers seemed set to interrupt the natural order of things, cause a "perturbance of the races," perhaps even divert evolution entirely. But if doctors and anthropologists could point to scientific evidence of women's natural inferiority— a destiny literally written into the curves of their skulls—surely these intemperate ladies would see reason, go home, and cease their silly agitating for things like voting rights, temperance, or an end to child labor.

Broca's disciples immediately took up this cause. Fast-forward to 1879, when a French anthropologist named Gustave Le Bon compiled the data and published what contemporary historian Stephen Jay Gould calls "the most vicious attack upon women in modern scientific literature." Women's lesser status, Le Bon wrote, "is so obvious that no one can contest it for a moment; only its degree is worth discussion." They were "the most inferior forms of human evolution"; they were "closer to children and savages than to an adult, civilized man."

"Without doubt," Le Bon concluded, "there exist some distinguished women, very superior to the average man, but they are as exceptional as the birth of any monstrosity, as, for example, of a gorilla with two heads; consequently, we may neglect them entirely."

This was obviously quite convenient for Le Bon, given that his mentor had all but demanded that women's inferiority be confirmed by science, as soon as possible, lest their delusional quest for equality lead society—and even humanity itself—to the brink of collapse. But the pressure to find a scientific basis for women's subservient social role wasn't only coming from Broca; it's not a coincidence that a vogue for phrenology took hold among physicians alongside the rise of Darwinism, which advanced the exciting but also frightening notion of biology inextricably linked with destiny.

The more the scientific community understood about evolution, the more vital it seemed to simultaneously prove that women were less evolved, even if one had to indulge in pseudoscientific quackery and human skull–collecting to do it. Darwin himself weighed in on this topic, noting that women's physiology appeared "characteristic of the lower races, and therefore of a past and lower state of civilization"; man, he wrote, was necessarily destined to achieve "a higher eminence, in whatever he takes up, than can women—whether requiring deep thought, reason, or imagination, or merely the use of the senses and hands."

At every turn, a study of the female skeletal system was essential to these conclusions. A central tenet of craniology held that brain size—and hence skull size—indicated mental ability. To the medical men of the moment, all those illustrations of female skeletons with their wide pelvises and tiny skulls looked not just like the embodiment of delicate femininity but like divine Darwinian truth. (The issue of skull size did present a problem, briefly, as scientists realized that women's skulls could sometimes be bigger in proportion to their bodies—but in these cases, they simply pivoted to argue that these large-skulled women resembled children, and hence were still clearly inferior. Heads I win, tails you lose.)

The only constant was a forgone conclusion: that women's bones revealed them to be primitive and frail, underdeveloped and inferior, and above all, in need of watchful protection by male stewards.

After all, they had to be. The alternative—that women might be equal, or, God forbid, more evolved—was too horrifying to entertain.

[If] a girl who is "not of the period" seeks to taste the delight of being laced too tightly to breathe, it may be as well for humanity if she carries out the experiment effectually . . . like an occasional accident to a railway director, her actual death by suffocation might even do more good than her theories will do harm.

Lancet, letter from the editors, 1869

While some doctors went all in on the phrenology fad, others became obsessed with a different sort of fashion: corsets, and all their attendant (and sometimes imagined) ills. Some of the most famous images from this era are still in circulation today, illustrating the alleged effect of corseting on the female skeleton. You've probably seen these pictures: there's the skeletal torso, its ribs compressed and drawn downward like wilting leaves, tapering to an improbably small waist. There's the simple line drawing of a female silhouette with ribs and viscera visible, her liver and intestines squeezed like toothpaste out of the protective enclosure of the rib cage and down into the place where her womb should be.

These images, provocative as they were, captured the imaginations of doctors and laypeople alike. It was an issue tailor-made to stoke a moral panic: Young women were permanently disfiguring their bodies, their bones, and for what? For fashion!

The physicians sounding the alarm on the dangers of skeleton-deforming fashion included John Lee Comstock, a surgeon who had operated on the battlefields in the War of 1812 before turning his attention to education. His book *Outlines of Physiology* was among the first anatomical textbooks to be widely used in American schools. In 1848, he published another anatomical tract that included the ominous heading: "DRESS, ANOTHER SOURCE OF DEFORMITY," in which he bemoaned "the recent fashion of dressing so wide across the neck as to leave one, or perhaps both the acromion processes, or shoulder tips, in a state of entire nudity." Comstock's concern wasn't modesty, however; it was that women would hunch and squirm in order to keep their dresses from slipping down, developing a habitual slump, "until [one shoulder] became permanently higher than the latter."

Perhaps needless to say, the wide-necked, shoulder-exposing dresses Comstock observed with such concern were hardly worn often enough, for long enough, to result in permanent disfigurement; even if women were doing strange things with their shoulders to prevent dress slippage, the dresses in question were evening gowns that would be worn only for dinners or parties, and only for a few hours at most. That Comstock did not bother to ask any women about this before opining on the scourge of shoulder-deforming fashion is a remarkable early entry into the annals of mansplaining, but it also reflects the general bent of male doctors at the time, and nowhere is this more evident than in the panic around corsets and tight-lacing.

While those alarming images of rib cages permanently altered by corsets were technically accurate, if doctors had actually asked women about this, they would have learned something vitally important: most women didn't, and couldn't, lace their corsets tightly enough to cause skeletal deformities. A tightly laced corset was an impediment to walking, cleaning, cooking, interacting with children, performing manual labor—in short, to any activity except the quiet, seated leisure pursuits of upper-class women. A tight-laced figure was a hallmark of a lifestyle few women could afford, and with it, an elite socioeconomic status.

For this reason, it's not surprising that the horrors of tight-lacing became a matter of mainstream concern; then, as now, the concerns of upper-class women received a disproportionate amount of attention, both medically and culturally. But when ordinary women observed that their own experiences with corsets bore little resemblance to the harms attributed to corseting by the medical profession, things got tense.

In late August 1869, the medical journal *Lancet* published a short, cranky piece in its "Medical Annotations" section, bemoaning that despite continued admonitions from the medical community, women continued to make bad decisions about how to wear their underwear—to the detriment of their looks, their health, even their very lives.

"If the evils of tight-lacing were confined to the distorted appearance which it never fails to produce we might regret indeed to see the female form divine so defaced, but it would scarcely be in our province to comment upon it," they wrote. "But, as medical practitioners we see its effects every day in the train of nervous and dyspeptic symptoms by which it is constantly indicated and in the still more grave internal mischief of permanent character which is often caused by it."

Of course, while the authors of the letter protested that the impact of corsets on women's physical appearance was the last thing on their minds, they couldn't seem to stop bringing it up. They lamented the ugliness of corseted women who moved "in a stooping position, unable to even hold [themselves] upright in consequence of the constraint upon the muscles of the back." They cursed women's foolishness and lack of education in their own physiology, without which "it is of little use to protest against the cruel injury to health which women thus inflict upon themselves."

"Worse than crime—it is folly," they concluded, "for beauty is destroyed by the process which is intended to increase it."

For those counting, that's about one and a half complaints as to the impact of corseting on women's health, and three complaints that it makes them hideous. But more importantly, this medical note contains zero testimony from women themselves, a fact that did not go unnoticed when it was reproduced in the *Times* of London. One woman, hoping to correct the record, wrote a fairly scathing letter in reply. The anti-corseting op-ed, she wrote, "has naturally excited some discussion among those affected by it, [and] I request to say a few words in our defense." Among her countercriticisms: that the stooped posture the *Lancet* writer found so offensive was not the result of tight-lacing—indeed, one of the few benefits of a tightly laced corset was that it made this literally impossible—but of wearing corsets "with weak steels in front."

The punch line: these corsets, which did not constrict the front ribs in the same way as a traditional corset, were the ones recommended by doctors.

The letter writer, who signed herself "Not a Girl of the Period"—which is to say, not a frivolous trend-chaser—pleaded that the author of the *Lancet* article familiarize himself with the history of corsets, by no means an undergarment worn only by women, and to "for once, consult instead of advising those who have had real experience of it."

Between the lines of this extremely nineteenth-century conflict lies a far more familiar, and timeless, frustration: one of women being lectured to by doctors who did not listen to them, even when the women possessed information, and firsthand experience, that the doctors did not. These young women could attest to effects of wearing corsets daily. They could have demonstrated to doctors that corsets with weaker front supports produced a certain type of posture. They could have, in partnership with the medical system, come to a mutual, beneficial understanding of both the impacts of corseting and how best to mitigate them, if needed.

But for that to happen, doctors would have had to be willing to see women as, if not equals, then at least possessors of valuable information about what it was like to be a woman. And, perhaps needless to say, this did not happen.

Instead, the *Lancet* editors published a response to "Not a Girl of the Period" in which they expressed the earnest hope that she be strangled to death by her corset.

Dear Beth: I have scoliosis, and my doctor wants me to wear a brace. My friend said she just did exercises and went to a chiropractor and now she's all better, but my parents say I have to do what the doctor says.

—"Ask Beth," *Los Angeles Times*, 1990

The photographer lifts his camera, then lowers it. He backs away three steps, then one more.

"Can she," he starts to say, then stops. Whatever he was about to say, the answer is obviously no. Can she turn this way? Twist that way? Bend over, sit down, take a bath?

Can she move?

Of course she can't.

She is fourteen years old. She'll be fifteen before she leaves the hospital, nearly a year after she first came. A year inside this plaster prison, a year confined to her bed. The cast she's wearing covers her from the crown of her head to her knees, with only a few strategic openings: one big one between her legs, for the bathroom. Two tunnel-like holes on either side of the head, so she can hear. And the most important one, a complete break that runs the circumference of her rib cage, where the cast has been sawed in half and then connected on one side by a metal lever, a turnbuckle, which gives the whole apparatus its name.

When they first put her in the cast, the opening with the lever was the length of her forearm. But now, it's down to just a few inches. In another few months, they'll cut the cast off, and then cut her open to fuse her vertebrae together.

Until then, there's not much to do but lie there. Sometimes she talks to the other girls, or tries to, but they're all in casts, too, and even with the earholes cut in the plaster, it's hard to hear beyond the next bed. There are ten of them on the ward, a neat line of girls encased in plaster, caterpillars in white cocoons. They're something to look at, which is why the photographer is here. In another week, there will be a story in the newspaper, and they'll all take turns looking at it. The headline says, "Spine welders," a reference to the surgery that comes after the cast. But it's the cast that everyone wants to see, that the photographer is stepping backward to capture because he wants to get the whole thing, and it doesn't quite fit in the frame.

He lifts the camera again.

"Okay," he says. "Smile!"

She does.

But when the newspaper comes the next week, she'll see that smiling didn't really matter. Between the angle of the photograph and the thickness of the cast that covers her head like a helmet, you can't see her mouth at all.

◆ ◆ ◆

It's remarkable, even within a system that often sidelined, ignored, infantilized, and silenced women, how little we know about the ones who suffered from scoliosis. We glimpse them here and there in the literature, usually from behind, as they stand facing away from the camera and naked from the hips up—the better to display a spine in need of correction, no doubt, but these images are invariably more erotic than clinical. In some, the patient's draping has slipped down to expose the cleft of her buttocks; in others, her head is just barely turned, as though she were on the verge of glancing coquettishly over her shoulder at the viewer. One striking triptych from the late 1800s shows the patient standing topless beside a bureau; her hair is in one thick braid, draped over her left shoulder, which sits lower than the right owing to the snakelike curvature of her spine. Then, the setting changes: the woman stands beneath an iron tripod with her arms drawn up and bound above her head. Her doctor, a man with a beaked nose, luxurious head of hair and massive sideburns, stands close beside her. Observing the progress of her treatment, perhaps, but between the angle of the photograph and the shadows that obscure his eyes, he could just as easily be staring at her bare breasts.

In the last photograph, apparently taken after the conclusion of treatment, the patient remains facing away from the camera. Her spine is straighter, but she's also no longer naked: in curing her, the doctor has restored her health and her dignity alike—but we never see her face.

Occasionally, in later images, the patient turns toward the camera. She peers out from beneath the turnbuckle cast that covers her head like an oversized nun's wimple; sometimes she's even smiling, if only out of habit or at a photographer's request. But even when they smile at us, these women are uniquely voiceless. Perhaps it's because in other fields, with other kinds of maladies, doctors were obligated to at least inquire as to their patients' symptoms and histories in order to make a diagnosis—even if they ultimately dismissed those symptoms as fabricated, psychosomatic, or a product of hysteria. But nobody needed to ask a woman if her spine was crooked; here was a diagnosis doctors could make not just without speaking to the patient but without ever even looking her in the face.

And perhaps this is why the history of medicine and the female skeletal system is not just particularly objectifying, but particularly paternalistic. Scoliosis, a condition that overwhelmingly afflicted women, seemed to prove the phrenologists right: women's skeletons were not just less evolved but so primitive that they could not walk upright like men without medical intervention. Structural garments, the cause of such consternation when women wore them of their own accord in the form of a corset, suddenly became in-dispensable when recast as medical devices which women must be forced to wear. The preferred treatments for scoliosis were often brutally disruptive to the lives of the young women who endured them—and who, even as recently as 1990, were told in response to their objections that they had to do what the doctor said.

One of the few medical professionals who was an early supporter of corsets, Dr. Henry Robert Heather Biggs, was the closest thing to an ally as envisioned by the "Not a Girl of the Period" letter writer; in 1905, he wrote that "women do not require to be told that corsets are unnecessary when they have accumulated experience of centuries to prove the reverse." Unfortunately, Biggs was also convinced that the structural indispensability of corsets was owed to women's inability to look normal without them, particularly after puberty and childbirth. Women were just too frail, too weak, to support the weight of their own bodies—and in the absence of proper corseting, he wrote, would inevitably devolve into "hideous objects of disfigurement."

But even the physicians who took all those semi-pornographic pictures of their faceless female patients were often quite progressive for their time. One such doctor was Louis Bauer, a German-born orthopaedic surgeon who emigrated to the United States after spending several months in prison in 1848 for his opposition to the Prussian monarchy. But his forward-thinking views did not extend to his scoliosis patients, whom he characterized as frail and evolutionarily deficient (or, if they were boys, effeminate), and who he believed were at least partly to blame for bringing on their spinal deformities. The risk factors for scoliosis identified by Bauer included a poor diet or sedentary lifestyle, but also "violent dancing and late hours," suggesting that the true causes of spinal curvature were basically anything Bauer himself found morally disagreeable. Scoliosis also continued what would ultimately be an irresolvable conflict over whether women's undergarments were a cure for disfigurement, or its cause; Bauer cited the work of another physician, Beuring, who blamed "improper dress, more especially the wearing of corsets" for scoliosis.

And then, of course, there's the Victorian doctor's favorite culprit for all ills: masturbation. Bauer claimed to have two patients whose condition stemmed from a penchant for self-abuse, while Dr. Robert Tuttle Morris (a surgeon and eventual president of the American College of Obstetricians and Gynecologists) hypothesized that women afflicted with "clitoral adhesions" would develop masturbatory habits, which led to laziness, which would in turn lead to curvature of the spine.

By the turn of the twentieth century, some doctors were starting to look more closely at the relationship between weight-bearing exercise and scoliosis. In his 1899 publication, "The Treatment of Lateral Curvature of the Spine," London physician Bernard Roth lamented that girls were not more encouraged to be physically active: "In addition to being much handicapped by their dress, [girls] do not have, as a rule, one-forth [sic] of the amount of physical exercise, such as cricket, football, hockey etc allowed to and enjoyed by boys and men." Roth examined a thousand scoliosis case studies and concluded that it was best to treat the condition purely through exercise, and exercising proper posture. He was joined in this belief by Lewis Albert Sayre, the physician with the huge sideburns who appears in photographs beside his topless patient as she hangs by the wrists from a large tripod: Sayre, who worked at Bellevue Hospital in New York City, recommended gymnastics to strengthen the muscles on whichever side of the body the spine curved toward.

But even among doctors who believed in exercise as a cure, the belief in female frailty as an obstacle to proper treatment persisted. An 1895 case study by Dr. Jacob Teschner displays the utter contempt with which women were often treated by their physicians. Teschner laments that his patient, a fifteen-year-old girl named Martha, is "awkward, indolent, lazy, slow of perception, and took no interest" in his prescribed exercises—before going on to casually mention that she had greatly improved her scoliosis through weight training and had recently lifted a fifty-pound bar above her head a total of ten times (for those not in the know, this is well above-average strength for a woman even by 2024 standards).

The fact that Teschner could observe a fifteen-year-old girl performing a fifty-pound standing overhead press for ten reps and still call her "awkward" and "indolent" suggests that some doctors were predisposed to see their scoliosis patients as weak, lazy, and unmotivated, even in the face of compelling evidence to the contrary.

And this may in part explain why debilitating measures like the turnbuckle cast ultimately eclipsed all others as the preferred solution to scoliosis and remained in vogue well into the twentieth century—including at the Hospital for Special Surgery, from which reporter Karl Kohrs filed his "Spine welders" dispatch in June 1950.

Kohrs dutifully reported the surgeons' claims that the teenage patients "do not seem to mind" spending the better part of a year immobilized in a cast, but one notes that he never bothered to ask the girls how they felt about it. What also seems increasingly likely is that the doctors didn't, either. Not because they didn't care, but because teenage girls were simply assumed to be content with a quieter, less active life. The landmark Title IX statute that would revolutionize girls' athletics was still two decades away; a young woman who enjoyed formal exercise or yearned to play sports would have been seen as odd, unfeminine, even a bit uncouth. Surely these plaster prisons weren't such a hardship, then, when their occupants didn't really care to move in the first place.

The adolescent girl is undergoing rapid development. For this reason her posture must be carefully watched.

—Morris Fishbein, MD, American physician, 1937

From the late 1800s through the 1950s and beyond, the social, cultural, and moral baggage associated with the female skeletal system coalesced into a preoccupation with posture. Standing up straight was not just a mark of good health, but of high class and strong moral character; slouching, conversely, suggested that something was wrong in body and soul.

As class consciousness began to creep into the already-complex interplay of Darwinism, racism, eugenics, and gender norms that informed the study of the skeletal system, doctors hurried to incorporate it into their practice. A piece on posture appeared in 1922 in the medical journal *Lancet*, which noted, "Some primitive races who have the squatting habit, and even many country people at home, keep the knees and back bent and have a carriage and gait not much better than that of the higher apes. As a general rule, the more highly civilised the people the better is the carriage, but a perfectly erect carriage cannot be attained without drill."

As per usual, a certain contingent of physicians took this opportunity to argue that education was therefore deleterious to women's health, in this case causing spinal curvature as a result of spending too much time hunched over schoolwork. The proper place for a book, per these men, was not in a woman's hands, but balanced on top of her head, the better to perfect her posture.

Here, too, it became impossible to separate notions of health from those of morality, and of beauty. Just as a healthy (read: slim) figure signaled a woman's ability to control her appetites, excellent posture revealed a certain level of bodily discipline. Of course, that wasn't all it revealed, as the male physicians of the era were quick to note. The 1937 edition of the *Modern Home Medical Adviser* included the following note on posture from editor Morris Fishbein:

"The chin and abdomen should be kept in and the chest forward. Many young girls worry about the development of breasts and, not understanding the changes that occur, attempt to hide them. Poor posture may result from holding the shoulders in such a manner as to draw in the chest."

Despite the limitations of his writings on female posture, Fishbein was a shrewd and insightful physician, particularly when it came to the cutting edge of women's reproductive care: in 1937, thirteen years before the introduction of the birth control pill, he declared the prevention of pregnancy to be a matter of medical and scientific interest as well as social, and predicted that the time would come when women could receive an "injection of some substance into the bloodstream" that would prevent pregnancy long term, maybe two or three years. Yet for all his ability to comprehend the importance of birth control to women, he nevertheless assumed that a young woman who slumped to shield her chest from view must be suffering from an inability to comprehend what was happening to her body—rather than experiencing the entirely rational desire not to be leered at.

Granted, the objectification of women's bodies has always been beyond the reach of doctors to solve. If there's a cure for this, it's cultural and social, not medical, and when Fishbein and others instructed women in proper posture, they were not making a normative judgment; they were only describing what was, not what ought to be. And yet, women of the time surely noticed that a "healthy" posture was also one that put their bodies on display.

A girl throws a stone awkwardly, less from want of practice than from a natural peculiarity of physical structure.

—John Harvey Kellogg, MD, *Plain Facts for Old and Young*, 1881

John Harvey Kellogg, an early twentieth-century celebrity doctor who we'll get to know intimately in the chapter on the GI system, famously believed that constipation caused brain poisoning—so it should surprise no one to learn that he also had some peculiar notions about how women's skeletons worked. In addition to theorizing that the female body was constructed so as to make throwing a stone impossible (see above), he suggested that skeletal differences rendered women "generally less graceful and naturally less skillful in the use of the extremities than man, and hence less fitted for athletic sports and feats requiring great dexterity." (This section of his book also ends with a nod to phrenology, making it a veritable buffet of sexist skeletal nonsense.)

At the time, Kellogg's comments fell perfectly in line with the long-standing medical consensus that women were less evolved, more delicate, and possessed of a bodily structure that was designed for the exclusive purposes of looking pretty and bearing children—all of which would cause a riot if said in a medical classroom today. Osteology has long since evolved past the notion of women as inherently skeletally primitive.

So why, then, do we still refer to poor athletic form as "throwing like a girl"?

As always, the beliefs that shaped the study of bones back in the 1800s are still embedded in the specialty today. The notion that women are not built to move has long since given way to the related one that women don't *like* to move, that physical activity isn't important or essential to their lives in the way it is to a man's. In the 1950s, we saw this manifest in the conviction among spinal surgeons that a girl with scoliosis wouldn't mind being immobilized in a cast for months on end—but it's with us today, too, in the way the medical profession approaches many of the most common orthopedic issues in women.

One of these issues is "frozen shoulder," a capsulitis of the shoulder joint that is most common in women over the age of forty. The condition not only causes greatly reduced mobility, but is so painful that it keeps patients awake at night—and yet, until recently, the most common treatment for this painful and disruptive disorder was to not treat it at all.

"They called it 'benign neglect,'" says Beth Shubin Stein, codirector of the women's sports medicine center at the Hospital for Special Surgery in New York. "Because it got better, eventually, on its own. They had done some research that showed that it was a time limited problem—meaning it would usually resolve within two years. But the truth is, in that era, 98 percent of the orthopedic surgeons and shoulder surgeons were men. They weren't afflicted by it."

This approach was originally proposed in the 1940s, but it had two major flaws. For one, the very notion of benign neglect was predicated on doctors' assumption that it was "benign" for a woman to have her mobility restricted for months, if not years, on end.

But more importantly, they were wrong: the problem didn't actually go away.

In 2017—that is, nearly sixty years after doctors first decided that middle-aged women need not be treated for frozen shoulder since they didn't really need to be able to move their arms—a paper published in the journal *Physiotherapy* found no supporting evidence that frozen shoulder would resolve on its own. Indeed, far from the promise of benign neglect—an easy, painless resolution accomplished by doing nothing—patients were suffering from "persistent limitations lasting for years."

. . . Oops?

In addition to the idea that being immobilized was no big thing for women, patients suffering from frozen shoulder also appear to have been up against another form of prejudice that is by now familiar to any student of medical history: the notion that any problem mainly afflicting women must have a psychosomatic component. In 2006, Jo Hannafin, an orthopedic surgeon who had long been pressuring the medical community to take a closer look at the causes of frozen shoulder, published a paper that referenced, among other things, an evaluation of the mental health of patients treated for the condition. It included the following remarkable line, which seems to answer a question one can't imagine really needed to be asked: "The investigators suggested that female patients who overcome adhesive capsulitis do not have an intrinsic emotional, psychologic, or personality disorder."

Today, frozen shoulder in women is beginning to be taken more seriously, and to be treated more like similar injuries in men: with a steroid injection. But as Shubin Stein says, "That was a long time coming."

Meanwhile, the science is still struggling to catch up when it comes to skeletal problems that genuinely afflict women differently. One of the best examples of this is the torn ACL, an injury that not only afflicts young women versus young men by a ratio of ten to one, but which I suffered myself at the age of fourteen. Even though I was under the care of an excellent and thoughtful doctor, a gendered double standard reared its head in the examining room: rather than fix the tear, the doctor thought we should wait a few years until I was certain that I really needed my knee. He patted my hand.

"Let's see how active you end up being," he said.

Fortunately, even within the past twenty years, things have gotten better on this front; an active fourteen-year-old girl presenting with the same injury today would have it reconstructed immediately. Unfortunately, the gender parity in treating ACL tears still remains lacking—particularly in cases where equality requires paying attention to what makes women's skeletal structure unique. Women tear their ACLs for different reasons, in different ways, than men. They need different forms of physical therapy to heal, and they need different lines of research to determine how to not just treat ACL tears but prevent them. And even then, the scientific community still gets bogged down in the question of what constitutes useful information about the female body. At one point, Beth Shubin Stein tells me, researchers became fixated on the notion of the menstrual cycle as a contributing risk factor for ACL tears, and began investing enormous amounts of money into investigating this.

Is this as bad as the bad old days in which scientists analyzed the topography of women's skulls to prove that they were too intellectually inferior to be treated as equals? Of course not—and the researchers investigating a possible link between the menstrual cycle and ACL injuries would almost certainly be horrified and indignant at the suggestion. And yet, focusing on menstruation nevertheless holds echoes of that archaic idea: that women are anatomically unsuited to certain activities, certain roles.

"At the end of the day, that's a non-modifiable risk factor," Shubin Stein says, meaning that there's no changing it. On the other hand, one of the most common contributing factors to ACL injuries in women is how they position their feet and legs when they're doing something that stresses the knee joint—in other words, an extremely modifiable risk factor. But when it comes to investigating how women might modify their exercise routines or foot placement to mitigate damage to their knees, says Shubin Stein, "the money behind it just doesn't happen."

◆ ◆ ◆

They're playing *Swan Lake* in the waiting room at the endocrinologist's office. She recognizes it from the first note, the plaintive moan of the oboe that always sounded to her like a woman crying. Soon the music will rise and Odette, dressed all in white, will step out of the wings and into the forest. She'll come across a man, a stranger, who bows to her, and reaches for her as the music swells. Odette doesn't know it, but her fate is sealed. She shouldn't have gone to the woods; she shouldn't have danced with the stranger. Within minutes, he casts a spell that transforms her into a swan.

The urge to rise, to dance, is overwhelming. It's been decades since she danced the part of Odette, but she remembers every step. Some people call this muscle memory, but to her it feels like something deeper, the music vibrating down in her bones.

But her bones are why she doesn't rise. Why she won't dance, and hasn't in years. Her feet in their orthopedic sneakers will never know the grip of a pointe shoe again.

And so she sits, listening to the music soar, until they call her name.

Like Odette, the patient's fate was sealed long before she knew it, from the moment she stepped out of the wings; the damage to her body was done many years ago, when she was a young woman at the height of her career. It had been a point of pride when she stopped getting her period. A level of bodily control that was something beyond the grace of her carriage, the precision of her footwork. This was mastery over nature itself. Nobody told her there would be a price.

At twenty, she could defy gravity, leaping and twirling under the stage lights like a creature made of air. At fifty, gravity is a punishment: she walks in a careful shuffle, her spine bowed, her shoulders hunched. At her first scan, her bone density was that of an eighty-five-year-old woman who'd been confined to her bed for years. A strong handshake will fracture her fingers. An ordinary stumble could shatter her hip.

If someone had told her that this was her future, would she have listened? Maybe. Maybe not. She was only doing what was expected; she was hardly the first dancer to lose her period as she honed her craft. But they didn't tell her.

Instead, they praised her. They admired the body she'd built, its strength and grace, its jutting clavicles and scapula so pronounced they looked like wings.

"You were born to dance," they said.

"I can count your ribs," they said.

And when they said it, they smiled, and so did she.

◆ ◆ ◆

The notion of the female skeleton as a frail and beautiful object is less overt now than it was in the literature of the eighteenth century, but it's still with us—as is the cultural baggage it carries. Being so slender that your clavicles pop remains a mark not just of beauty but status; you can never be too thin or too rich, but if you're one, you're probably the other.

The sanctified status of a bone-thin body has its own medical repercussions, in the form of osteoporosis, a condition that dispro-portionately afflicts women. This is partly due to natural changes in the body that occur during menopause—the loss of estrogen causes women's bones to weaken—but also due to cultural factors. The elite ballerina who trains so fiercely and eats so little that she loses her menstrual cycle is doing untold damage to her bones even as she's held up by society as a paragon of female strength; so is the woman who avoids weight-bearing exercises all her life because she's afraid of getting "bulky." Additionally, osteoporosis is a risk factor for women of all ages undergoing estrogen deprivation therapy as part of their breast cancer treatment, a looming threat that waits in the wings for my patients even as they fight for their lives.

The medical landscape surrounding osteoporosis is so muddled, and so entangled with the original conflation of a feminine skeleton with a frail one, that diagnosing and treating this disease continues to be a challenge. Many of my patients who are aware of the risks of accelerated bone loss are also aware, and deeply fearful, of some of the devastating side effects of osteoporosis treatment, including a rare but ghastly condition called osteonecrosis of the jaw. And knowing the proper course of action remains difficult for doctors; the science surrounding which treatments are safest and most ef-fective is still playing catch-up. Some women will avoid treatment of osteoporosis even after a diagnosis. Others, active women who "look" so healthy that it never occurs to anyone to investigate the condition of their bones, might not receive a diagnosis at all until an accidental fall results in a catastrophic injury.

The gap between outward appearance and internal anatomy is also a particular plague on the type of women who excel in female-dominated pursuits like gymnastics, figure skating, and dance, where what looks like the pinnacle of athletic achievement can mask the presence of debilitating connective tissue disorders like Ehlers-Danlos syndrome (EDS). Ehlers-Danlos patients, 70 percent of whom are female, suffer from such extreme hypermobility that they can eventually dislocate their joints while asleep—but they also often wait more than a decade to be diagnosed, owing to the tendency of people, including physicians, to assume that their flexi-bility is not just a natural feminine trait but a desirable gift. One of my classmates from medical school, a former dancer who had suffered from joint pain for years and had dislocated her kneecap half a dozen times, wasn't diagnosed until she was a faculty member at Hopkins—when she recognized her own symptoms during a grand rounds lecture on connective tissue disorders.

That said, awareness of these disorders that disproportionately affect women is growing, and women's skeletal health is treated with more curiosity and concern today than it ever has been. Of course, some progress is visible purely in the absence of open contempt for women that once defined this field—no doctor today would hope (as the *Lancet* editors did in 1869) that a woman be suffocated by her underwear as punishment for flouting his recommendations, or diagnose teenage girls as having caused their spines to curve by masturbating too much—but the greater difference comes in the form of active pushback, from within and often by female physicians, against the twin forces of objectification and paternalism that have dominated for too long in orthopedic medicine.

Doctors like Beth Shubin Stein are working to dispel the lingering sense that orthopedic medicine is something of a boys' club. Women are discouraged by pervasive myths about the field—"You have to be a bodybuilder to be an orthopedic surgeon. You have to like working with power tools," she says, citing some common misconceptions that discourage female doctors from specializing in orthopedics. The source of these misconceptions isn't hard to trace; in years past, orthopedic surgical instruments were standardized for the size and grip strength of male hands, and other equipment, like the radiation shields employed in most orthopedic labs, didn't adequately protect the breasts of female doctors because they were designed for male torsos. But the increased presence of women in medicine means that these problems no longer fly under the radar—nor do some of the more unsubtle manifestations of the archaic idea that women's bones and bodies are best understood in terms of aesthetic value rather than as a source of medical knowledge. As recently as 2014, the *Examination Techniques in Orthopaedics* textbook published by Cambridge University Press included images of buxom female patients being examined (except in some cases, it's more like groped) by the hands of an unseen man; the women in the photos were wearing nothing but underwear and vaguely come-hither expressions. Clearly, the authors of this textbook failed to consider that some of the aspiring surgeons consulting these texts might be women; after the lampooning they received by female doctors and in the international press, it's a mistake they certainly won't make again.

And when it comes to their needs as patients, women are finding their voices—and finding that the world is, at last, beginning to listen to them. Women with connective tissue disorders like EDS are using social media to connect and mobilize in search of better diagnostics and treatment for diseases that have long been overlooked by the medical establishment. Influencers like Paralympian Jessica Long are raising awareness every day of the challenges that female amputees face when it comes to finding prosthetics that are properly designed for women's bodies and women's lives. And Omri Ayalon, a hand surgeon and co-director of the Center for Amputation Reconstruction at NYU, tells me that doctors are learning to challenge their own biases when it comes to outfitting prosthetics for female patients, simply by allowing those women a greater share in the decision-making process surrounding their own care. The field of prosthetics has advanced by leaps and bounds in recent decades, and doctors are often understandably excited by the prospect of outfitting patients with cutting-edge bionic body parts that restore unprecedented levels of function.

"It's like science fiction, where we are able to give these people working hands," Ayalon tells me. It was a woman who had lost all four fingers to a workplace accident who opened his eyes to the fact that function has its own limitations: not everyone wants a hand that looks like it once belonged to the Terminator.

"It turned out that she didn't care at all about the function, but did care significantly about the appearance, the cosmetic," he says. "But it's not like they're going to make one silicone restorative nicer for a woman than they would for a man. They make what we tell them to make."

In this case, because that patient was insistent that she wanted a beautiful hand more than a functional one—and because her doctor trusted her to know her own priorities when it came to restoring her lost fingers—what Ayalon told the lab to make was an astonishingly lifelike prosthesis that allowed his patient to move through society without her disability drawing attention. The result was a revelation, not just to the patient but to her physician. Today, Ayalon describes these cosmetically focused prosthetics with the same awe as he does the "science fiction"–grade bionic limbs with articulating joints.

"I'm telling you, these silicone hands—you cannot tell that they had an amputation," he says. "They're amazing!"

Once upon a time, doctors and anthropologists alike posited that women were so frail and primitive at a skeletal level as to be not fully evolved. They scrutinized the interior volume of women's skulls for evidence of their intellectual inferiority. And as a result, they developed a field of specialization founded on the belief that women were simply not built for the world. Today's challenge—one that orthopedic physicians and patients must face together—is to abandon those biased foundations in favor of a new paradigm: one in which the world, and the medical system, is built for women, too.

CHAPTER 3

muscle

MUSCULAR

WHO'S THE WEAKEST OF THEM ALL?

In all of medical history, there is perhaps no more tragic case than the woman whose mind, body, and overall health have been destroyed by bicycling. Physically broken, mentally deranged, as grotesque as she is pathetic. Her bloodless lips are set in a permanent grimace; her eyes bulge from their sockets; her face is pale and splotchy, with dark purple circles under the eyes and scowl lines deeply etched on her forehead. Beneath her chin, the unsightly bullfrog-like swell of a goiter may be observed, a telltale sign of overexertion. Her body is overmuscled, stout, and shapeless, and she walks with an ungainly shuffle, owing to the deformation of her pelvis caused by too much time in the saddle.

The worst of the damage, however, is hidden: the patient's labia have hardened as a result of repeated bruising by the bicycle seat, her reproductive organs are in disarray, her appendix is beginning to rupture. And then there's the matter of her mind, dangerously unhinged, veering ever closer to lunacy.

The prognosis is grim. The patient's health will continue to decline. Her mental instability, now made manifest in her bizarre predilection for wearing unflattering and unfeminine cycling fashions, will eventually take on more and more sinister forms. Compulsive masturbation. Homicidal mania. If she survives, she will never marry, never have children, never know the fulfilment of a good and righteous life.

The medical literature from the turn of the nineteenth century is rife with warnings about the dangers posed by cycling to women's physical and mental health. This patient—wrecked by too much exercise, with her bulging eyes, broken mind, and disfigured genitals—occupies page after page in medical journals, in newspapers, in urgent letters from physicians hoping to steer vulnerable women out of harm's way. She is what you don't want to become; she is what you must do everything in your power to avoid.

There's just one thing the doctors never mention amid all their urgent warnings: this patient doesn't actually exist.

◆ ◆ ◆

Where in other chapters we've met and will meet real patients, real women, whose cases became the blank page onto which so much early medical bias was projected, the consensus that exercise in general (and bicycling in particular) was deleterious and dangerous to the health of women was a complete fabrication. The teenage girl sexually corrupted by cycling; the woman suffering from a terrifying condition known as "bicycle face": these patients never walked through the door of any doctor's office. They were phantoms, boogeymen, conjured by a medical establishment and a society that were deeply alarmed by the mere possibility of a woman developing physical strength, stamina, or, God forbid, muscles.

Curiously, the neglect of women's muscular health has a more complex legacy than many comparable indignities in medical history, as ancient societies appear to have been torn on the question of whether physical fitness in women was a help or a hindrance. On one hand, there were the teachings of Hippocrates, which advanced the notion that the human body contained a finite amount of energy and hence that an athletic woman was diverting valuable resources from her reproductive organs—and, of course, risking a dangerous imbalance of her bodily humors if she perspired too much. On the other, the existence of female gladiators in ancient Roman society suggests that the taboo against female athleticism nevertheless allowed for exceptions, and some of the literature of

the time indicates positive associations between a woman's reproductive prowess and her competency in physical combat: a woman
strong enough to fight was, presumably, also more likely to survive
childbirth.

Even then, however, the spectacle of women wielding swords
and shields spurred fears of disruption to the social order should
they begin to take athletics, and sports, more seriously. In 200 CE,
Emperor Septimius Severus officially outlawed women's participation in the arena, citing concerns that a populace who had grown
too used to hooting and hollering at the spectacle of female gladiators would soon broaden their horizons to widespread disrespect
for women in general. Yet his other, perhaps more urgent, aim was
keeping the athletic ambitions of women themselves in check. The
arena was one thing, more performance than sport (much like the
contemporary farce of the WWE bears little resemblance to actual
competitive wrestling). But if women were permitted to train for
the former, they might eventually want to partake in the latter, up
to and including participation in the Olympic Games. And while
the sight of women beating one another up in a game of theatrical
swordplay was one thing, the prospect of them actually competing
was quite another, the kind of disruption that would shake society
at its very foundations.

Some sixteen hundred years later, these same anxieties manifested around a new threat: the bicycle. The horrifying notion of a
woman with visible muscles (not to mention a penchant for wearing pants) was only the beginning. The bicycle was a vehicle upon
which a woman might exercise not just her body but her autonomy.
It represented freedom, competition, and the possibility of a woman
straying far from home under her own steam—and hence, also
represented a host of burgeoning fears about the alarming effects
of liberation on women's role as wives, mothers, and guardians of
the domestic realm. And while doctors might have come around to
appreciate the positive effects of cycling on women's health if left to
their own devices, the culture of the moment demanded the opposite response: then, as now, controlling women's bodies was much
easier (and seemed much less sinister) if it was seen to be supported
by science.

Don't be a fright. Don't faint on the road. Don't wear a man's cap. Don't wear tight garters.

Don't boast of your long rides. Don't criticize people's "legs." Don't wear loud hued leggings. Don't cultivate a "bicycle face."

Don't refuse assistance up a hill.

Don't use bicycle slang. Leave that to the boys. Don't go out after dark without a male escort. Don't scratch a match on the seat of your bloomers. Don't discuss bloomers with every man you know.

Don't appear in public until you have learned to ride well. Don't overdo things. Let cycling be a recreation, not a labor. Don't ignore the laws of the road because you are a woman.

Don't imagine everybody is looking at you.

—excerpted from guide for women on bikes, published in multiple newspapers in 1895

While bicycles had been around in various forms for the better part of the nineteenth century, the sudden ubiquity of cycling as a leisure activity beginning in the 1890s—and its particular popularity among women and young people—spawned a widespread moral panic. In addition to etiquette guides like the one excerpted above, newspapers published graphic accounts of bloody cycling accidents and editorials lamenting the threats posed by bicycles to civilized society. In this hothouse of anti-cycling sentiment, the medical establishment was under enormous pressure to condemn bicycling, especially by those members of society seen as most frail, most vulnerable to corruption, and most in need of protection. It wasn't long before a vast body of literature sprang up to condemn women's cycling as both physically dangerous and morally depraved.

In 1896, one year after the *newspapers around the country* identified "bicycle face" as a fashion don't, British physician Arthur Shadwell gave it the additional imprimatur of a medical condition with a *National Review* article titled, ominously, "The Hidden Dangers of Cycling."

"Some time ago I drew attention to the peculiar strained, set look so often associated with this pastime and called it the 'bicycle face,'" Shadwell wrote. "The general adoption of the phrase since then indicates a general recognition of its justice. Some wear the 'face' more and some less marked, but nearly all have it, except the small boys."

Per Shadwell, bicycling carried the risk of physical and mental derangement for anyone, but it was women for whom he reserved the most chilling cautions. The article included many accounts of purported case studies that read more like urban legends, like that of a hapless young woman who was "healthy, rather stronger than average" until the fateful day she took up cycling: "To all appearances she can do as much as anybody in short flights. One day they go farther, nothing much, perhaps ten miles: the result, utter collapse, with bed for several days."

Utter collapse was just one of the risks posed by bicycles to young women; Shadwell also warned that cyclists risked exhaustion, nervousness, anxiety, goiters, internal inflammation, chronic dysentery, and infertility, to name a few. Notably, these cases were often associated not with the mechanics of cycling, but with doing it for longer distances. Shadwell and the like might grudgingly acknowledge that a woman could ride a bike, but it was impossible to miss the subtext: on a bicycle or otherwise, great dangers awaited the woman who colored too far outside the lines, who strayed too far from home.

Meanwhile, despite the exhortations of the *New York World* not to "imagine everybody is looking at you," women cyclists would have been forgiven for concluding that a lot of people, including physicians, were, in fact, looking at them, and levying extraordinarily harsh judgments based on what they saw. Much was made by both the media and medical classes alike of women's cycling outfits, which were seen as representative of the wearer's apparent insanity: "If the commissioners in lunacy have classed every woman whom they have seen in bicycle costume as a person of unsound mind, they have clearly done what it was their duty to do," declared an 1896

New York Times article. That same year, the *Journal of the American Medical Association* was host to a debate on bicycle riding, with former US surgeon general John Hamilton bemoaning "a costume and posture which make ninety women in a hundred absurd spectacles."

As for posture, many physicians became especially fixated on bicycle seats, and what effects they might have on the female body, with particular attention paid to the impact of cycling on pregnancy, childbirth, and parenting. The aforementioned article in the *Journal of the American Medical Association* made sweeping pronouncements about the physiological impact of cycling, declaring that "a woman, especially an adolescent girl, can not be suspended on the summit of a wedge without injury to the structures above, and deformation of the pelvis," but even doctors who disagreed with Hamilton as to the injurious effects of bicycle seats struggled to frame their argument in anything but reproductive terms. Like the defenders of female gladiators more than a thousand years before, those who argued that women could safely cycle did so from the position that it would strengthen the pelvis, and thus make them more effective at bearing and birthing children. And even then, critics scoffed. In 1898, the *Journal of the American Medical Association* again featured an editorial, this one by Dr. A. C. Simonton, grumbling that all this discussion of pelvises was entirely beside the point. While cycling "may deform the pelvis," he insisted, "it will have little to no effect as regards the ease of childbirth"—because the siren song of the bicycle would render women far too busy riding bikes to ever get pregnant anyway: "Will the female rider throw aside her wheel long enough to have a baby, let alone to rear a respectable sized family?" he asked rhetorically, going on to complain that a woman cyclist having children was so preposterous that he'd never even heard of such a thing.

But because this was the Victorian era, the anatomical impact of bicycles was ultimately far less interesting to doctors than the behavioral one. And on this front, they were in agreement: the worst thing about bicycles was that women could, and would, use them to masturbate.

It was not only bicycles, of course. Physicians of this era were obsessed with the specter of female masturbation as either a symptom, a cause, or sometimes both, tied to an astonishing array of maladies (a phenomenon that is explored at length in multiple sections of this book). But here, the sexually exciting nature of bicycle seats makes for a remarkable example of the medical establishment reaching a conclusion before doing the research—and writing off the women who contradicted their assumptions as untrustworthy liars.

Among the doctors convinced of a link between bicycles and self-abuse was Dr. Robert Latou Dickinson, a gynecologist who we'll meet at greater length in the Reproductive chapter. In 1895, Dickinson authored a journal article titled "Bicycling for Women from the Standpoint of the Gynecologist," with specific attention to the impact of cycling on women's sexual health. Ironically, his was one of the first and few arguments broadly in favor of allowing women to use bicycles, yet his defense of cycling was in many ways more absurd and offensive than the diatribes against it. Dickinson readily admitted he could find no cases in which riding a bike turned a woman into a chronic masturbator, but this didn't sway him from his belief that all possible steps should be taken to prevent it from happening: "It is perfectly conceivable that under certain conditions the bicycle saddle could both engender and propagate this horrible habit," he wrote.

Of course, those certain conditions existed primarily in Dickinson's imagination, which was vivid indeed. (He also believed he could identify a masturbator from the size and shape of her genitals, a theory he attempted to prove by making detailed sketches—and eventually, clay sculptures—of his patients' private parts.) But he did believe, assuming the risk of women deriving sexual satisfaction from bicycling could be mitigated, that it was otherwise a beneficial activity in moderation, and even a cure for everything from a nervous disposition to menstrual cramps. Here he was joined by Dr. George S. Brown, who in 1896 penned a rebuttal to the former surgeon general's anti-bike diatribe in the *Journal of the American Medical Association*: Brown believed that little girls, confined to nurseries where they spent their time playing quietly with dolls and other "inane amusements," were becoming "pale faced, dull eyed and constipated" as a result of too little physical activity. And however bad cycling might be, he argued, surely leaving young women to twiddle their thumbs at home would beget far worse consequences—given that "idleness and erotic thoughts always go together." In other words, far from bicycling serving as a gateway drug to masturbation, Brown believed it might be a useful preventive.

The confused and conflicting discourse around the medical hazards of the bicycle was, of course, founded not in science but in the ordinary societal nervousness that coalesces around the new; the same fear that fueled horror stories about "bicycle face" can be found throughout history, animating panics over everything from trains to telephones to televisions to 1980s hair metal bands. And, crucially, the participants in this panic were not exclusively male; groups like the Women's Rescue League also came out against the scourge of bicycle-riding women, with founder Charlotte Smith writing an impassioned letter which appeared in newspapers all over the US in 1896, the same year as the debate over bicycles raged in medical journals.

"Bicycling by young women has helped to swell the ranks of reckless girls who finally drift into the standing army of outcast women of the United States," Smith wrote. "The bicycle is the devil's advance agent morally and physically in thousands of instances."

In the end, both the medical community and the moral authoritarians of the moment conspired to agree that bicycling was an activity that a woman should participate in only with her doctor's permission, an admonishment that swiftly made its way out of medical journals and into the mainstream press. "No woman should ride a bicycle without first consulting her medical man," announced *Harper's Weekly* in 1896.

But in between the lines of the claims that a woman who exercised unsupervised risked her health by doing so, it's clear that what was truly being perceived was not a bodily threat, but one to the status quo. When in 1897 male undergraduates at Cambridge University staged a protest against the admission of female students to the college, they hung an effigy of the "New Woman," that terrifying avatar of social progress, from a window in Market Square.

The effigy was riding a bicycle.

1. ALWAYS appear in feminine attire when not actively engaged in practice or playing ball. This regulation continues through the playoffs for all, even though your team is not participating. AT NO TIME MAY A PLAYER APPEAR IN THE STANDS IN HER UNIFORM, OR WEAR SLACKS OR SHORTS IN PUBLIC.

2. Boyish bobs are not permissible and in general your hair should be well groomed at all times with longer hair preferable to short hair cuts. Lipstick should always be on.

—All-American Girls Professional Baseball League, Rules of Conduct for
Players, 1943

Although the specific panic surrounding the medical dangers of the bicycle faded into the background in the early twentieth century, the anxiety surrounding women exercising persisted. It's a testament to the mindset of the time that doctors spoke as urgently about the risks of women being masculinized by exercise as they did about its purported threats to their health—even the ones who believed that physical activity could be beneficial to women. One doctor, Dudley A. Sargent, was refreshingly skeptical of the notion that women were too frail to exercise, challenging both the Victorian stereotype of women as fragile and prone to fainting and the Victorian conventions of dress, including corsets, that made it difficult for them to move.

But even Sargent, who was an outlier in recommending vigorous exercise for both sexes, was careful to make a distinction between exercise and athletics, fueling a general sense that women were unsuited for the latter. In 1912, he penned a massive article for the *Ladies' Home Journal* titled "Are Athletics Making Girls Masculine? A Practical Answer to a Question Every Girl Asks," in which he emphasized that women should exercise only in very particular ways, lest they overtax their bodies or, worse, begin looking like men.

As tempting as it is to see Sargent as a rank chauvinist—he described the "danger" of sporty women taking on "marked masculine characteristics" and recommended that athletics be modified, and competition de-emphasized, to accommodate for the female propensity toward "great emotional disturbances"—it's worth noting that he was not personally troubled by the prospect of women becoming more muscular, so much as aware that this was a major concern for other people, including women themselves. In fact, Sargent's opinions about women's physical capabilities were not just contrary to the conventions of the time but extremely controversial:

in the 1910s, he caused a series of uproars by declaring that the supposed physical frailty of women was a myth, an affectation designed to cultivate male attention, and one in which women themselves were complicit. His remarks included the declaration that "women's timidity and her traditional inferiority in physique and courage are, consciously or not, a pose. It is her method of inviting pursuit."

In fact, Sargent insisted, a woman was less evolved than a man— "Nearer to nature and more of a savage"—and hence more capable of withstanding physical discomfort, perhaps even better suited for military service. When the St. Louis Post-Dispatch ran Sargent's comments, it was under the provocative headline: "The Weaker Sex? No, Not Woman, But Man!"

And people were provoked, indeed; every time Sargent advanced the notion that women were more than capable of becoming athletes, laborers, or soldiers, it was received with condemnation and mockery. "Manly men should oppose such pernicious doctrines," declared one letter to the editor, while another columnist quipped: "The assertion of Dr. Dudley Sargent of Harvard that women are stronger than men and can endure more encounters widespread contradiction, but perhaps he is right. Look how women endure their husbands!"

Compared to his comments just a few years later, Sargent's writings on women's athletics in 1912 are far less confrontational, and evidently designed to address not his own fears but that of his audience:

"I have no hesitation in saying that there is no athletic sport or game in which some women cannot enter, not only without fear of injury but also with great prospects of success. In nearly every instance, however, it will be found that the women who are able to excel in the rougher and more masculine sports have either inherited or acquired masculine characteristics," he wrote.

Yet even despite the pervasive worry that sports would make women look mannish—one still in evidence today among those who avoid lifting weights lest they get too "bulky"—the first half of the twentieth century was marked by the steady normalization of exercise thanks in no small part to the efforts of women themselves, who began to form informal athletic clubs on US college campuses beginning in the late 1800s. By 1920, 22 percent of universities in the US had women's athletic programs. At the same time, the ideal female figure had evolved from the buxom, wasp-waisted vision of the Victorian era to the more svelte, boyish flapper, while the confining garments of the former were replaced by shorter, drop-waisted dresses that left plenty of room to move.

All told, muscular fitness for women remained a fraught and tension-filled topic for the first third of the twentieth century, a tension complicated but not eradicated by the onset of World War II, and the mass exodus of the nation's able-bodied young men out of athletics and into military service. Out of necessity, the 1940s saw female strength recast as an asset rather than an embarrassment, with women stepping into the various roles vacated by enlisted men. The best-known mascot for this moment was Rosie the Riveter, her jaw set, her jumpsuit sleeve rolled up to reveal a muscular forearm and bicep.

And yet, that embrace did not quite extend to dismantling the taboo surrounding competition and sport. Before the country went to war, a cultural backlash against women's athletic programs in the 1930s contained shades of the ancient Roman edicts against women fighting as gladiators: exercise for the sake of leisure or theater was one thing, but actual competition was quite another. Many college sports programs for women were dismantled and replaced with game days or fitness classes, the latter being considered more feminine and hence more socially acceptable.

If Rosie the Riveter was the visual embodiment of America's relaxed attitude toward women as manual laborers, the All-American Girls Professional Baseball League serves the same purpose when it comes to showing its comparative nervousness about women athletes. The country's first women's professional sports league, the AAGPBL walked a tightrope when it came to the image of its players, who were subject to the strictest standards of both dress and behavior. The first two rules of the league—which forbid players from wearing pants and required the wearing of lipstick at all times—sent a clear message: to make up for her athleticism on the field, a woman had to be seen as a caricature of femininity off of it.

It was in many ways a radical reimagining: of competitive sports, of social mores, of how femininity and physical fitness could permissibly intersect, and of the role of physicians in drawing these new parameters for women's lives. On the surface, it seemed women were freer—and stronger—than ever. But while the boundaries had shifted, they were no less narrow, no less punishing, and no less preoccupied by the notion that there was something unseemly, and unnatural, about a woman with muscles.

◆ ◆ ◆

The runner knows she's being watched. She can feel people's eyes on her, an insistent gaze that grazes the length of her body and follows her out of every room, that assesses the width of her hips, the breadth of her shoulders, the athletic flatness of her chest. Whispers trail her, even into the locker room; the other women, her competitors, talk about her as much as if not more than the officials do.

The stares and whispers go on for days, until it's clear that the question is not if they'll summon her, but when.

The examination room is cold and sterile. There are three doctors there to perform the assessment, or at least, she hopes they're doctors; all men, all wearing the same stone-faced expression, all scribbling notes on identical pads. They don't introduce themselves, and they don't ask her name; they just tell her to undress.

She does.

They stare.

If she's lucky, staring is all they'll do. If not, the staring is only the beginning; if she's not lucky, they'll put their hands on her, or inside her. They'll take notes on the size of her breasts and the shape of her genitals, and if she shows any signs of discomfort, they'll take notes on that, too. When the examination is done—after they've poked and prodded and groped her naked body without asking her a single question or even looking her in the eye—they'll confer and render their verdict.

A long time ago, the runner sat in front of a doctor who listened to her lungs, took her pulse, and told her, shruggingly, that she was certainly healthy enough to train competitively if she wanted to. It was the first barrier she had to break, but since then, she has broken many. She's earned her place over and over, race by race, proving that she's strong and fast and good enough to hold her own, proving that she belongs here. She has won at the regional level, the state level, the national level. But in this room, her lean and powerful body is no longer an asset. It is a liability. In this room, her strength and speed and stamina will not benefit her, because what these doctors intend to determine is not whether she's strong enough to run against the world's fastest women.

What they intend to determine is whether she's a woman at all.

And when they render their verdict, it will be a loss like none other. Not just of opportunity, but identity—stripping the runner of her womanhood as easily as they stripped her of her clothes.

◆ ◆ ◆

Over the course of two centuries, the medical debate over the nature, the limits, and the acceptability of women's strength remained in constant and often self-contradictory flux, as the early conviction that women couldn't work out gave way to fears that their bodies and brains would be perverted by exercise (except for those who were convinced that a lack of exercise would make the perversion even worse). But when it came to the existence of elite female athletes, the scientific community was generally in agreement: nature did not intend for women to excel at competitive sports—and if a woman did excel, it was because she was, herself, a perversion.

In 1896, Baron Pierre de Coubertin, the founder of the modern Olympics, insisted that "no matter how toughened a sportswoman may be, her organism is not cut out to sustain certain shocks." A few years later, de Coubertin doubled down: "In our view, this feminine semi-Olympiad is impractical, uninteresting, ungainly, and, I do not hesitate to add, improper." Fortunately, he didn't get the final word—the 1900 Olympic games welcomed women in five events: tennis, sailing, croquet, equestrianism, and golf—but his opinion was nevertheless representative of a consensus view that women didn't belong in high-level sporting competition.

As always, the cultural arguments against female athletes—that they were uninteresting, unladylike, and unattractive—were bolstered by dubious medical justifications. Even the most forward-thinking scientists could end up circling this particular intellectual drain when presented with the question of women competing in traditionally male-dominated sports. In 1926, as female athletes agitated for inclusion in a greater range of events including winter sports, a group of German physicians issued a categorical edict against women's ski jumping: "At this time," they wrote, "there is no need or reason to organize jumping competitions for ladies. Because of the unanswered medical question as to whether ski jumping agrees with the female organism, this would be a very daring experiment and should be strongly advised against."

In short, whether women could safely jump was deemed an unanswered question, but also a question too "daring" to explore via the usual course of medical study. The result was a self-reinforcing state of ignorance that persisted among doctors for decades, even as the existence of uninjured female ski jumpers suggested that this theory didn't exactly hold water.

But when doctors weren't worrying that the physical strain of competing would overtax a woman's reproductive system—or, in the case of ski jumping, cause her uterus to fall out—they were tasked with enforcing the boundaries of womanhood itself. At the center of the debate surrounding female athletes was an impossible, and preposterous, question: How athletic could a woman be before she didn't count as a woman anymore?

It is a testament to both the complexity and the intractability of this issue that Olympic officials and physicians have spent a century wrestling with it, and have yet to reach a satisfactory conclusion. In 1968, the International Olympic Committee instituted mandatory testing to verify the sex of female athletes—but long before that, women who didn't look feminine enough were subject to humiliating examinations calling their sex into question. In the 1920s and 1930s, officials would visually inspect any female competitor whose appearance aroused suspicions; in 1948, the IOC began to require that women prove their sex via a doctor's note.

Meanwhile, the normalization of sex testing by the IOC led to its widespread implementation by other sporting organizations, including the 1967 Pan-American Games in Winnipeg. American shot-putter Maren Sidler was present for the Winnipeg incident, and gave a disturbing account of the "science" behind women's elimination from competition:

"They lined us up outside a room where there were three doctors sitting in a row behind desks. You had to go in and pull up your shirt and push down your pants. Then they just looked while you waited for them to confer and decide if you were OK. While I was in line I remember one of the sprinters, a tiny, skinny girl, came out shaking her head back and forth saying. 'Well, I failed, I didn't have enough up top. They say I can't run and I have to go home because I'm not 'big' enough."

And complicit in this humiliation of female athletes were doctors, who advised that a woman's eligibility for competition be determined via roughly the same methods that farmers use for sexing livestock. A 1968 *Journal of the American Medical Association* article titled "A Medical History of the Olympic Games" devotes only a few brief lines to women, but they are telling: "There has been concern for a number of years that among the more successful female competitors many would be found who exhibited male characteristics, and who might be pseudohermaphrodites," it reads, citing the need to confirm the sex of women athletes via genital examination.

◆ ◆ ◆

Then, as now, there was a genuine conversation to be had about how best to ensure a level playing field. It is a question complicated by the existence of intersex athletes who defy conventional categorization along a strict male/female binary—and in more recent years, transgender athletes who wish to compete in the category that aligns with their identity—as well as ongoing concerns about doping by aspiring Olympians. But in too many cases, this conversation devolved into crude stereotyping rooted not in science but in sexism. And doctors, tasked not with diagnosing disease but rather enforcing the boundaries of femininity, too often erred on the side of stigmatizing strength.

We want to prepare girls for their role of being the mothers of strong, healthy men.

—Tenley Albright, MD, 1964

By the 1960s, the question of whether exercise itself was medically recommended was no longer in dispute; doctors agreed that physical activity was beneficial to everyone, regardless of sex. But for women, this advice had acquired an aesthetic, and decidedly unscientific, gloss: the exercises recommended for women were meant to make the body not stronger, and not healthier, but smaller.

America's flirtation with female strength as represented by Rosie the Riveter had fallen out of style after the war, giving way to something at once much sillier and much more insidious. In one newsreel from the 1940s, a group of women wearing swimsuits and heels demonstrate the newest fitness technology: a "workout" that involves standing still while your body is contoured and kneaded by hydraulic machinery. A male announcer cheerfully quips that having helped win the war effort at home, women must now wage war on their own bodies: "The battle of the bulges is still on!"

Although the body-pummeling machines seen in this newsreel were a short-lived and ridiculous fad, they reflected a deeply entrenched set of beliefs about what women's workouts were for. Vigorous, sweaty exertion was considered unnecessary and unladylike; the ideal form of exercise for women was non-strenuous (or even, as with this "gym," entirely passive), and the desired outcome was thinness, full stop. It's not hard to see how this type of workout eventually gave way to the vogue for things like jogging and aerobics—or, later, barre and Pilates and spinning—all of which promised to make women thin ("like a sea nymph," the newsreel announcer simpers) rather than muscular.

At the same time, the conventional wisdom about women and exercise was that they lacked all motivation to do it, being possessed of weak motivation to go with their weak bodies. The way doctors approached women's physical fitness was of a piece with a broader medical paternalism, and a tendency among physicians to assume that if a woman was unhealthy, it was her own fault. In 1968, a physician and former air force lieutenant colonel named Kenneth Cooper wrote a book called *Aerobics*, which single-handedly introduced millions of Americans to the benefits of cardiovascular exercise—but while Cooper did write a section of his book tailored specifically to women, it ultimately revealed far more about the author's condescension than it did about the best path to cardiovascular health.

The entire section is short on practical information, instead taking the form of an extended lament.

"One of the greatest disappointments of my career is the general indifference of American women toward exercise," Cooper wrote. "American men are indifferent to it, obviously—four out of five of them are out of shape—but at least they sit home and worry about it once in a while. Women don't."

And even when Cooper managed to stop bewailing that women would rather spend four hours in a beauty parlor than ten minutes running around a track, his advice was framed in such a way as to leave no question as to his dim view of his audience: "If running is not your cup of tea, swimming is second best and definitely lady-like."

To Cooper's credit, his next book was titled *Aerobics for Women* and opened with an apology to all the female readers he alienated with his ill-considered remarks—but he's just one guy. The culture that produced those remarks, on the other hand, did not correct for its errors, and continued to shape the medical consensus around women's fitness, even among the pioneering female physicians who might have known better.

In 1971, nearly sixty years after Dudley A. Sargent first attempted to persuade fearful *Ladies' Home Journal* readers that they could exercise without turning into men, a doctor named Tenley Albright revisited the same topic—this time in a report commissioned by the US Department of Health. But where Sargent assured his readers that "I have no hesitation in saying that there is no athletic sport or game in which some women cannot enter," Albright brought the hammer down:

"The muscle-building type of exercise, such as weight lifting, does not suggest itself to any of us as suitable for girls, partly because a woman would not look attractive performing and partly because she would have to look unattractive to us if she had the muscles she'd need to perform well," she wrote. "While this kind of exercise would not cripple a woman or decrease her ability to keep house well, it certainly would not add to her feminine image."

For Albright to come out so strongly against strength training for women—and to do so while promoting the antiquated view that a strong female body must necessarily be ugly to others—was especially outrageous considering her credentials: not only was Albright a Harvard-trained surgeon, she was a former Olympic athlete, having won gold in figure skating at the 1956 Winter games in Italy. Yet despite being both an elite athlete and no stranger to shattering convention in a male-dominated field, Albright took the most outdated notions of what constituted "suitable" exercise for women and gave them not only a medical stamp of approval, but the imprimatur of a government recommendation. Of course, she could hardly be accused of sexism; she was a woman herself.

At the time, Albright's view was shared by everyone—from politicians to governing bodies in sports, and from women's physicians to women themselves. In addition to stigmatizing weight lifting as unattractive and hence undesirable, a bias persisted within the medical profession when it came to women athletes as a category. Where doctors had once been coaxed by panicked culture warriors to issue warnings about the medical inadvisability of bicycles, now they were the ones stuck in the past, even as the rest of the world began to accept that they'd been wrong, that women could compete. Female distance runners were finally granted access to the Olympic Games in 1960; the medical profession, meanwhile, held fast to the belief that a woman was physically unfit to run long distances, lest she damage her uterus, well into the 1970s.

In 1967, runner Kathrine Switzer became the first woman to complete the Boston Marathon. It almost didn't happen: a few miles into the race, she was physically assaulted by a race manager named Jock Semple who tried to forcibly remove her from the competition.

"I heard the scraping noise of leather shoes coming up fast behind me, an alien and alarming sound amid the muted thump thumping of rubber-soled running shoes," Switzer wrote of the experience. "When a runner hears that kind of noise, it's usually danger—like hearing a dog's paws on the pavement. Instinctively I jerked my head around quickly and looked square into the most vicious face I'd ever seen. A big man, a huge man, with bared teeth was set to pounce, and before I could react he grabbed my shoulder and flung me back, screaming, 'Get the hell out of my race and give me those numbers!' Then he swiped down my front, trying to rip off my bib number, just as I leapt backward from him."

This story is famous for its account of the biases faced by female runners at a time when the phrase "like a girl" was still in wide-spread use to describe a lack of athleticism. But it's remarkable for another reason, too: Jock Semple wasn't just a race manager, but a longtime professional in the fitness industry. He had worked as a masseur and physical therapist for the Boston Bruins and the Boston Celtics, and as a trainer for Olympic athletes. Surely he had come into contact with gifted female runners before; surely he knew there were women who not only wanted to run marathons but were entirely capable of doing so. Why, then, did he attempt to brutal-ize Kathrine Switzer? What made the rules barring women from racing so important that they needed to be enforced by any means necessary, even violence?

Semple told *Sports Illustrated* the following year, "The amateur rules here say a woman can't run more than a mile and a half. I'm in favor of making their races longer, but they don't belong with men."

Where might Semple have gotten this idea? It's not hard to guess: at the time, it was just what the doctors ordered.

◆ ◆ ◆

I meet Susan at the first follow-up appointment after her mastec-tomy. She's a youthful fifty, very blonde, and slender; she's traveled to see me from Connecticut, where she works in fashion retail at a high-end boutique where both customers and employees alike all look a bit like Gwyneth Paltrow.

By the time Susan's cancer was diagnosed, it had already begun to spread: her mastectomy included the removal of the lymph nodes from her underarm, putting her at risk of a condition called lymph-edema. Lymphedema isn't a threat in the way that cancer is, but it can be debilitating and makes her case more complicated. I'm glad to see, as I join Susan in the exam room, that she has her husband with her—and surprised when, as I ask her to step on the scale so that I can determine her proper medication dosage, she tells him to leave. Even now, she's embarrassed at the idea of him seeing how much she weighs.

As it turns out, Susan fits the profile exactly of the patient whose muscular risk factors go overlooked: she's thin by appearances, and her BMI is normal. It's only because she's participating in a clinical study including non-routine body composition scans that we learn the truth: a hidden cache of visceral fat puts her actual fat-to–lean mass ratio in dangerous territory. Her bone density scan reveals osteoporosis.

Because Susan learned early on to equate good health with a smaller body, a lower number on the scale, she has never exercised outside of occasional walking; when it's cold outside, she sometimes does cardio on the elliptical machine. She has never lifted weights. She has always worried about being thinner. She avoids most physical activity, including cycling, because she's afraid it will make her thighs big. When I tell her she needs weight training to improve her bone density, she panics: she doesn't know how. She's afraid she'll bulk up. She read somewhere that lifting weights would increase her risk of lymphedema.

Susan is the living embodiment of all the ways in which the medical system fails to address women's muscular health. All of the information she should have known, information that is even more essential to her healing now, after a life-altering surgery, is information no doctor ever told her. And the result of having been deprived of this information is something worse than simply not knowing: everything she believes about exercise is either needlessly terrifying, woefully inaccurate, or both.

As challenging as it is to treat Susan's cancer, undoing this damage—caused not by disease but by a two-hundred-year history of incuriosity, ignorance, misinformation, and shame—will be more difficult by far. I know this because I have fought this battle not only as a doctor treating women, but as a patient myself.

During my first pregnancy in 2010, my doctor gave me a series of stern and frightening warnings about the dangers of physical activity. I was told never to elevate my heart rate above one hundred and forty beats per minute, the equivalent of a brisk walk. Lifting weights was completely out of the question. Raising my body temperature too high—in other words, working out hard enough to sweat—was also forbidden. All of this was in spite of the fact that I had always exercised vigorously, and always found it beneficial not only to my physical health but my mental well-being. My body, it was understood, was no longer mine; the energy I spent on exercising was energy I wasn't giving to the baby growing inside me. (Meanwhile, after I had given birth, I was praised for returning to my pre-pregnancy weight as fast as humanly possible, without a word from my doctor about preserving muscle mass or the injuries I sustained as a result of neglecting it.)

How different is this, really, from the Victorian edict that riding a bicycle would render a woman unmarriageable, infertile, insane? How different are the contemporary anxieties surrounding women exercising in pregnancy from those that gripped Dr. A. C. Simonton when he asked fearfully, "Will the female rider throw aside her wheel long enough to have a baby?"

In some senses, we have come a long way from the bad old days when doctors believed that women would deform their pelvises or detach their uteruses by doing the wrong kind of exercise. In others, we are still beholden to all the same foolish fears: That a woman with a strong and capable body cannot also be a good mother. That the time and energy a woman spends exercising is time and energy wasted. That a woman's strength is unsightly, unseemly, and unfeminine. That the most important thing a woman's body can be is small.

[Women] can move in dignity, in grace, in airy lightness, or conscious strength, bodies erect and firm, energetic and active—bodies that are truly sovereign in their presence, the expressions of a sovereign nature . . .

—Elizabeth Blackwell, MD, first female US recipient of a medical degree,
   1859

Today, many of these misguided ideas—the Victorian plague of bicycle face, the disembodied uterus left behind on a ski slope— have long since been corrected in both medical and mainstream understanding. What lingers on is the myth that women and muscular development don't mix, which can manifest in everything from school athletics to medical research to the BMI chart hanging in your doctor's office. But in recent years, doctors have at last begun to rethink using thinness as a stand-in for health, and to reexamine the diagnostic tools they use to determine whether or not a patient has a healthy body composition. The body mass index (BMI) chart that compares height and weight to determine whether a patient is underweight, normal, overweight, or obese has been around for a long time, but its use in medical settings often overlooks as much as it reveals, particularly for women.

Dr. Neil Iyengar, a medical oncologist at Memorial Sloan Kettering Cancer Center, tells me that the BMI chart, which was developed in the 1830s, was never intended as a substitute for a more in-depth assessment of an individual patient's health: "BMI was originally developed as an epidemiologic tool," he says. "So at a population level, it is useful for understanding disease patterns—but we also have to remember the bias through which research has been conducted, which is essentially focused on men and male diseases."

Women, on the other hand, carry more fat but also carry it differently than men do, which makes the BMI chart a markedly ineffective measure of what's happening inside their bodies. Consider two hypothetical patients: on one hand, a woman with healthy body fat levels and above-average muscle mass; on the other, a woman with elevated body fat levels but so little muscle that she can barely lift a ten-pound bag of groceries. It's the latter patient who is actually at elevated risk of multiple medical problems, but it's the former who will register on the BMI scale as overweight—and who will be wrongly instructed by physicians that she needs to be thinner.

Iyengar says, "To this day, almost every single weight loss intervention in women is geared towards body weight loss and achieving that skinny ideal. And we're learning that that is not always the best approach, especially with some of the new fad diets like fasting, for example. You lose fat, but you'll lose muscle as well."

For many reasons, this is a damaging paradigm, and one that is fundamentally disempowering to women who have been systematically misled as to what a healthy body should look like. Doctors like Iyengar are working to help patients understand that maintaining a certain amount of muscle mass, even if it means sitting at a higher weight, is far more important to overall health than keeping the number on the scale low. That resistance training that builds muscle will make the body far more resilient than the calorie-burning cardio exercise to which most women gravitate. That this is especially true after menopause, when weight-bearing exercises become increasingly important for helping to maintain bone density, and when maintaining a healthy body composition is essential to lowering the risk of certain diseases. In 2018, a study found that women with a normal BMI but elevated levels of body fat—women like the latter patient in the hypothetical above—were at nearly double the risk of developing breast cancer. These are also the patients who would most benefit from increasing their level of exercise, as the dangerous combination of a thin physique but high body fat percentage is almost invariably associated with a lack of physical activity. This is where the medical establishment still needs to catch up: these women are the least likely to be advised to exercise, and most likely to have their risk overlooked, simply because they don't "look" unhealthy.

Indeed, the guidance most women receive from their doctor when it comes to physical activity is a blanket recommendation to exercise for thirty minutes, five times a week, which has been standard advice for decades. The average medical education still includes little formal training on this front: in 2015, a survey of medical schools found that only 21.2 percent offered courses centered on exercise, and in only about half of these cases was the course required. Additionally, most of the available courses were centered on exercise physiology or sports medicine; information on how to exercise for better health was vanishingly rare. Instead, what information doctors know about exercise tends to be self-taught as a result of personal interest, and for many, that interest is virtually nonexistent. The famously demanding standards of a medical career leave little time to hit the gym, and the average doctor is often out of shape himself; the desire not to appear hypocritical on this front leads many to avoid straightforwardly advising their patients to exercise.

In this way, the medical ethos surrounding how and how much to exercise still contains echoes of what it was a hundred years ago. Not because nothing has changed—today's doctors aren't consumed by the fear that you might be deriving erotic enjoyment from your Peloton—but because even once the taboos surrounding exercise faded away, the ignorance created by those taboos persisted.

A world in which women's athletics are valued and celebrated is a world in which we can begin making long-overdue inquiries into how sport interacts with women's health, from brain function and memory to bone density, joint stability, hormone levels, and more. Does a woman who plays sports in her younger years age differently than one who doesn't? Do female soccer players risk the same cumulative effects of repetitive head trauma as men who played football or hockey?

Until recently, we had no way of knowing: virtually all of the science in this area was based on studies of men. When the *Women in Sport and Physical Activity Journal* examined the gender composition of more than 5,200 publications between 2014 and 2020, it found that only 6 percent of the studies were solely focused on women—compared with 31 percent that included only men. And sports medicine as a field remains admittedly dominated by men, even when the athletes are women. As of this writing, every team physician in the National Football League (NFL), National Basketball League (NBA), and Major League Baseball (MLB) is male—as are 82 percent of Women's National Basketball Association (WNBA) team physicians.

But as the medical stigma surrounding women as elite athletes has faded, the medical interest in caring for those athletes has finally begun to catch up. This is a positive and necessary development, since as women began to exercise more, and to excel at physical pursuits, they began to present at doctor's offices with a condition known as the Female Triad: disordered eating, irregular menstruation, and loss of bone density. The condition is common among dancers, gymnasts, elite runners—any sport where an exceptionally lean physique is considered an asset—and left untreated, it can lead to serious long-term consequences including infertility, stress fractures, a compromised immune system, a slowed metabolism, cardiovascular damage, and mental health issues.

Kathryn Ackerman, an associate professor of sports medicine at Harvard Medical School, tells me, "I have athletes who think they should have a certain BMI, but they don't get their period when they're at that size. The big focus [for] everybody has been to be as lean as possible. And have your weight be nice and low. They're like, but your BMI is normal, so I guess you're fine. There's just this disconnect about what's actually important."

The emphasis on having a small body rather than a strong one has been heightened by the increasing ubiquity of technology like DEXA scans, which used to be a diagnostic tool available only to medical professionals but have since made their way into the world of college sports, where coaches use them to keep tabs on the body composition of female athletes. In 2022, the *New York Times* reported that the pressure on young women to be as thin as possible is so strong, and the "leaner is better" mindset so entrenched, that athletes would be congratulated for dropping body fat even when it made no difference to their actual performance—and even when they got so thin that they stopped menstruating and started losing their hair.

Only recently has awareness begun growing that these symptoms are a sign of a body in distress—and that the desire to be lean above all else is nothing more or less than the insidious legacy of the persistent notion that women should exercise not to be strong, but to be thin. Ackerman says, "Everybody's focused on the leanness rather than strength. They're asking, do I have thigh gap? And do I look as thin as everybody else on the team? Rather than focusing on actual training, on performance improvements."

For too long, a woman could be in the best shape of her life, but this wouldn't be seen as a positive thing—even by her physician—unless that shape was also exceptionally small. The physicians working to transform the relationship of the medical establishment with women's bodies suggest a new paradigm: one that measures improvement not by how much weight a woman loses but by what she gains in strength, in speed, in power. Here, Ackerman leads the charge: her recently launched Female Athlete Program at Boston Children's Hospital is a groundbreaking venture that brings together doctors from multiple specialties to address the needs of female athletes at every stage of life. A sign of how far things have come: many of the physicians involved in the project are former competitive athletes themselves.

Meanwhile, research scientists have begun to turn their attention to the gender gap in sports injuries, with downstream effects in areas ranging from medical education to sporting equipment centered on the goal of addressing the unique needs of female bodies. The "shrink it and pink it" approach to creating gear for female athletes is increasingly out of style, in favor of designs that not only consider but center women's anatomical differences. Even the cultural standards that once spooked women away from the weight room out of fear that lifting would make them "bulky" have given way to a world in which female fitness influencers publicly celebrate how much they can squat. And that bug-eyed, clench-jawed, be-goitered bicycling grotesque of the Victorian era? She's finally gone from the medical consciousness and the public imagination alike. What we need now in her place is not a new boogeyman, but an icon: one who is strong, fast, fearless, and ready to take up space.

blood

CIRCULATORY
MATTERS OF THE HEART

If a young girl on the brink of womanhood stops eating, her blood will thicken and move sluggishly. If she eats too much, or eats juicy foods, she will cause an excess of blood. If she eats perverse foods, she will block her veins.

—Hippocrates, as paraphrased by Helen King, 2002

The circulatory system comprises all the organs that move blood through the body—the heart that pumps it, the veins and arteries that transport it. It also includes, crucially, the blood itself, and for this reason it's one of few systems of which humans have always had some awareness, long before the advent of modern medicine, and even long before ancient societies first began to explore the interior of the body and investigate how best to heal it. No medical training was necessary to observe the way that blood would bead from a perforation in the skin, to lay your ear against someone's chest and hear the echoing thud of their heart, to feel a pulse jumping beneath your fingertips, or to observe the arterial spurting where a limb (or a head) had been severed.

In the teaching of Hippocrates, blood was one of the four humors (along with phlegm, black bile, and yellow bile) that the body was known to contain, the balance of which was considered necessary to maintaining good health. To be sure, this represented only the most fractional understanding of the circulatory system, one that overlooked or misunderstood far more than it intuited—but as with the anatomical knowledge that doctors once gained by dissecting animals and applying what they found to humans, what they knew was still enough to prove useful, even to save lives. Cauterization, for example, used to stanch hemorrhaging and close amputations, was developed in antiquity based on the accurate understanding that burning a wound with a hot iron or blade would stop the loss of blood. References to the procedure appear in ancient texts from Hippocrates to Leonides of Alexandria to the Chinese *Su wen*.

But when it comes to women's medicine, the limitations of the time stand out more starkly—and the propensity of doctors to fill in their knowledge gaps with guesswork fueled as much by bias as by science proved far more problematic, in keeping with that famous line from Alexander Pope about a little knowledge being more dangerous than none.

The "humorism" that dominated medicine for more than two thousand years was particularly rife with sexist nonsense that stood in the way of science, to the point where the humors themselves were assigned a gendered valence. The common medical wisdom was that female bodies were "phlegmatic" (which is to say, full of and/ or ruled by the humor phlegm) while male bodies were "sanguine" or "choleric," ruled by blood and bile. Even as doctors understood that every human body contained all four substances, blood itself was seen, medically speaking, as more of a guy thing. A man with a preponderance of blood was virile, healthy, a magnificent specimen. A woman, on the other hand, needed her blood kept in check, or even drained on purpose, lest it render her dangerously unbalanced.

Advancements in medical knowledge and the advent of germ theory in the nineteenth century eventually relegated humorism to the dustbin of medical history, but its attendant prejudices proved far more entrenched. There are multiple medical specializations in which humorism continued to manifest in subtle ways; in urinary medicine, for instance, the notion that women's phlegmatic constitution made them naturally leaky contributed to centuries of apathy surrounding female incontinence, and to generations of women suffering needlessly from treatable conditions. (For more on how women are still peeing on themselves today thanks to the dismissive attitudes of various male doctors circa 2050 BCE, see the Urinary chapter.) But for ailments of the circulatory system—blood disorders, cardiac issues, and the like—the influence was far more overt, fueled by the conviction that a woman's blood, much like a woman's body, was something at once different from and inferior to the healthy male default.

Some diseases continued to be coded as explicitly female, owing to women's assumed, inherent frailty, while others (like heart disease) were believed not to affect them at all. Most importantly, women afflicted with these maladies—like the hypothetical girl described by Hippocrates, whose predilection for juicy foods causes her body to become engorged with an excess of blood—were generally assumed to have somehow caused them, or at the very least allowed them to happen, through weakness of either constitution or will. And once it had been established that women were simply too fragile, whether anatomically or morally, to care for their health, the cure was obvious: they needed to cede control of their blood, their bodies, and their lives to men.

I do not know, but we have some physicians who say that chlorosis in girls is the result of that pleasure indulged in to excess.

—Giacomo Girolamo Casanova, 1792

The disease commonly known as chlorosis is one of the original enigmas of the female circulatory system, a consummate example of a socially constructed disease. Medically speaking, chlorosis is best understood to describe the symptoms of iron deficiency anemia and assorted similar ailments. The associated symptoms were both widely variable and wildly nonspecific: weakness and pallor were the most common, along with shortness of breath, palpitations, and fainting, but all of these could be caused by any number of conditions. What really made chlorosis recognizable was less how it manifested than in whom: adolescent girls and young women.

In Hippocrates, the condition is included in a text titled "On the diseases of virgins," while Casanova (yes, *that* Casanova) mentions it in his autobiography as being caused by "pleasure indulged in to excess"—if not quite a sexually transmitted disease, then certainly on the same spectrum in its connection to carnal appetites.

It also wasn't always called chlorosis; before the seventeenth century, the condition was known as "green sickness," with the word "chlorosis" first appearing in a 1615 tract by Jean Varandal. Varandal, a professor of medicine at France's University of Montpellier, one of the oldest medical schools in the world, named the ailment after the Greek *chlôros*. It's a clever double entendre: the word means green, as in the color, but also as in new, fresh, and sexually inexperienced.

Varandal noted that the disease could be found first and foremost "among the noblest and most beautiful young girls," in keeping with the existing wisdom that chlorosis was primarily a pretty girl's problem. It was also around the same time, in the final years of the sixteenth century, that William Shakespeare entered chlorosis into the literary canon, where it's recognizable by description if not by name. In *Romeo and Juliet*, Shakespeare conjures the image of a wan, sick, and female-coded moon who envies the radiance of the beautiful Juliet:

> *Be not her maid, since she is envious;*
> *Her vestal livery is but sick and green*
> *And none but fools do wear it; cast it off.*

That sick, green vestal livery? A cheeky reference to Juliet's virginity, reimagining it as a garment as foolish as it is unflattering. Cast it off, indeed!

Chlorosis is hardly the only condition in women's medical history with a strong social and cultural element, in which what made a woman healthy was treated as more or less synonymous with what made her beautiful. It is, however, one of the few conditions for which sex as cure was not only fodder for a bawdy Shakespearean jape but quite literally what the doctor ordered.

In 1554, a German royal physician named Johannes Lange wrote to a friend on the topic of the friend's firstborn daughter, a young woman named Anna. The girl was of an age to be married, but her father had been turning suitors away on account of Anna's ill health: she was easily winded, nauseated by food, and above all, noticeably pale. The family's doctors could not agree on a diagnosis, but Lange recognized the condition immediately: clearly, Anna was suffering from what Hippocrates called the "disease of virgins."

Lange's theory of what was happening inside Anna's body made up in imagination what it lacked in medical accuracy: because Anna was on the verge of womanhood, he wrote, "at this time, by nature, the menstrual blood flows from the liver to the small spaces & veins of the womb: which when from the narrow mouths, which are not yet distended, also obstructed by thick & crude humors, & finally from the thickness of the blood, cannot escape."

In Lange's view, Anna's symptoms traced back to "the filthy blood of the menses," which was slowly flooding her body and bathing her liver, her bowels, and her heart in toxic sludge. The idea of a woman being slowly poisoned by her own unexpelled menstrual blood is remarkable, and darkly absurd, yet also unsurprising in context: not only does it echo the ongoing influence of humorism (as a woman, Anna was obviously full of phlegm, a "thick and crude" substance that plugged up her body's egresses so that the blood had nowhere to go), it also foreshadowed the later (and equally misinformed) medical vogue for autointoxication, which posited that a constipated woman would develop brain poisoning from her own unexcreted feces.

But while the physicians of the Victorian age battled autointoxication with bran flakes and yogurt enemas, the sixteenth-century solution for chlorosis was far more rudimentary. As Lange communicates, Hippocrates' "trusty advice" was that women suffering from the disease of virgins be cured via bloodletting.

Of course, there's more than one way to make a virgin bleed . . . if you know what I mean.

"I instruct," wrote Lange, that "virgins afflicted with this disease, that as soon as possible they live with men & copulate."

Granted, Lange's advice makes a certain, twisted sort of sense in line with the scientific mores of the time: if you believe that the "narrow mouths" of a woman's body are too blocked up by phlegm to allow her "filthy" menstrual blood to escape, then inserting something to clear the blockage—like, say, her husband's penis—would indeed seem a logical course of action. But while Lange undoubtedly meant no harm, to prescribe sex and marriage as a cure imbued the entire field of circulatory medicine with a paternalism that would not be easily dispelled.

Over the course of the next few centuries, chlorosis would continue to afflict young women, and to confound physicians who found the condition at once mystifying and titillating, synonymous as it was with virginity, desirability, and sex. And while the idea of marital intercourse as a chlorosis panacea would eventually go out of style, the idea that chlorosis was a lifestyle disease that required the patient to surrender her autonomy to a male authority did not.

As for Lange, he signed off on his letter to Anna's father in full confidence that marriage would cure her: "In the treatment of this disease of virgins I have never been deceived or my hopes frustrated," he wrote. And then, perhaps feeling it was only fair, he took the liberty of inviting himself to the wedding.

◆ ◆ ◆

In the late nineteenth century, nearly three hundred years after the word "chlorosis" emerged into the medical lexicon, a young woman afflicted with the condition sits in conversation with her physician. She has recently returned from the seaside, a trip that was supposed to restore her but instead seems to have had the opposite effect: she returned even paler, even thinner, in such a weakened state that even her fiancé couldn't hide his alarm when he caught sight of her.

Her doctor is a man named Simon, a specialist in gastrointestinal diseases who has recently returned from a voyage himself: an extended period of study in Germany. He's an unusual-looking man, fair-complected and blond in a way that one usually only sees on children, his thinning hair matched by eyebrows that virtually disappear against his skin. His lower lip looks like a little boy's, too—very full, almost pouty—and his eyes behind his wire-rimmed glasses are a pale, unsettling shade of blue. The young woman is relieved that he mostly looks at his notes instead of at her, and so she never notices that the doctor is avoiding her gaze, too, that he seems almost nervous in her presence.

For now, he takes a history of her condition: digestive upset followed by an overall listlessness, then weight loss and diarrhea, then the pallor and weakness that several weeks by the sea failed to cure. He asks after her diet, her menses, and her sexual proclivities, seeming most keenly interested in the latter. When she finally admits that something did happen one evening before she left for the shore—something she never thought she'd tell anyone—he nods knowingly as he writes it down.

In 1897, this young woman will appear as a pseudonymous patient in *The American Journal of the Medical Sciences*, in an article titled "A Study of Thirty-One Cases of Chlorosis, with Special Reference to the Etiology and the Dietetic Treatment of the Disease." Perhaps owing to the particulars of her case, Dr. Simon will be painstakingly opaque in describing not just the onset of the condition but her identity; where other patients are identified by their initials, this one he refers to only as "Miss X." But despite his discretion, Simon is no more enlightened in his diagnosis than the medieval doctors who referred to this same condition as a "disease of virgins." Indeed, he believes the patient's condition to be self-induced; masturbation, in his opinion, is a prime and "frequently overlooked" cause of chlorosis.

"In this case," he writes, "an attack of profound chlorosis developed from ungratified sexual desire."

◆ ◆ ◆

Despite subscribing to the peculiar conviction, so common to doctors of the era, that female masturbation was the secret root cause of virtually every health issue under the sun, Charles E. Simon may have been one of the more insightful and less judgmental physicians to explore the condition known as chlorosis. Even Miss X, who ostensibly developed the disease as a result of being pathologically horny, was accurately understood by Simon to be ultimately suffering not from lack of sex but from anemia, for which a high-protein diet was his recommended (and effective) cure. Indeed, her case in Simon's 1897 article is followed by the forceful conclusion that irrespective of the particulars of this or any case, "chlorosis is in the great majority of cases the result of malnutrition."

As for what led Miss X to become so malnourished that she developed anemia, Simon was so discreet as to render himself incomprehensible, writing that the attacks of chlorosis occurred after several occasions on which "she had become highly excited sexually, and . . . an orgasm had occurred without intercourse." Whether this happened in her sleep, while masturbating, or even as a result of fooling around with her fiancé, is a mystery—but then, so is Simon's rationale for describing a woman having multiple spontaneous orgasms as "ungratified." (Some people, needless to say, would consider this the definition of gratification.)

But if Simon put too much stock in sex (or rather, lack thereof) as a root cause of chlorosis, he was hardly alone in this. Even as humorism was widely discarded by nineteenth-century doctors in favor of more sophisticated medical theories, chlorosis retained its reputation if not its name as a virgin's disease, and remained synonymous in the medical community with youth, beauty, and sexual desirability. In 1852, physician Frederick Hollick described chlorosis patients as "delicate and interesting," noting that the disease not only did not detract from their beauty, but "even heightens its attractions." In 1899, Sir Byrom Bramwell, who was among the first wave of British physicians to teach clinical medicine to women, described the "beautiful rosy-red tint" in the faces of chlorosis patients who blushed when being examined.

Unsurprisingly, at this time, chlorosis proliferated as a diagnosis not just for scientific reasons but via social contagion, thanks to its cultural cachet. If you were going to be ill, then surely it was preferable to have this disease, which even the medical literature referred to as "the anaemia of good-looking girls." In some cases, chlorosis functioned as a symbol not only of one's desirability but of elite status and membership in the upper class. In the Victorian era, particularly, adolescent girls were all but expected to develop chlorosis—and doctors, having been primed to look for it, were happy to oblige with a diagnosis.

As with Simon, Bramwell's lasciviously tinged views of chlorosis patients did not preclude genuine medical insight. He, too, understood that these women suffered from anemia; he, too, effectively treated patients by increasing the iron content of their diet (although Bramwell relied on iron pills where Simon recommended eating meat). Also like Simon, Bramwell acknowledged the common wisdom surrounding chlorosis as a young woman's problem—"It used to be thought that the disease was due to disappointment in love," he wrote—while expressing skepticism that this was a cause rather than a contributing factor. Both men observed that the link between heartbreak (or in the case of Miss X, horniness) and chlorosis had more to do with the impact of melancholia on a woman's appetite; an emotionally traumatized or grieving woman would develop the condition not because of her sadness, but because in her sadness, she'd stopped eating properly.

As for the bizarre-by-modern-standards observations about the beauty of chlorosis patients, the Victorian conflation of femininity with both physical frailty and impeccable self-restraint likely played a role. These attitudes were most impactful (and are explored at greatest length in this book) when it came to gastrointestinal medicine, in which the notions of medically advisable and morally righteous were often indistinguishable from each other, tangled as they were in the era's fear of sensual excess. These physicians, who expressed such tenderness and admiration for their anemic (and often anorexic) chlorosis patients, inhabited a world in which etiology and etiquette were given nearly equal scientific weight, such that a robust appetite in a woman was considered a signpost for poor health. To the Victorians, a predilection for eating was an entrée to depravity, the resulting dyspepsia reflecting a degradation of the soul and body alike. Meanwhile, the women who were afflicted with chlorosis—so pale, so delicate, so beautiful not just in their sickness but as a result of it—were almost invariably characterized by the nonexistence of their appetites. In the majority of Simon's thirty-one case studies, the chlorosis patient didn't just avoid meat; she explicitly did not like it.

Unfortunately, this conflation of good health with good etiquette—and of feminine propriety with an absence of appetite—created a catch-22 for chlorosis patients: what would have helped them medically (that is, eating red meat to improve their iron levels) was contraindicated morally (that is, eating meat was seen as a hallmark of a depraved and entirely unladylike craving for flesh). And unfortunately for Charles E. Simon, his insights into the plight of these women ended with Miss X; around the time of his publication on the etiology of chlorosis, his nervous disposition developed into a full-blown case of agoraphobia, leading him to abandon his medical practice and spend the rest of his days in relative isolation, working out of a small laboratory in the stable behind his home.

Meanwhile, even as some doctors accurately concluded that chlorosis was caused by malnutrition generally, and iron deficiency specifically, many others continued to treat the condition as a lifestyle disease that could only be cured by better behavior—which is to say, "better" as envisioned by men who believed they knew better than women how to live a healthy, virtuous life. As a result, the prescribed treatments for chlorosis in the hundred years or so leading up to 1920 were not just morally charged but often hilariously self-contradictory.

The "meat or no meat" issue was only the tip of the iceberg: women diagnosed with chlorosis were told to take a cold bath, and also a hot bath, and also to bathe less altogether. They were to go outside for fresh air, but also not to leave their beds under any circumstances. Exercise was recommended, except when it was proscribed. Dancing was forbidden—unless you danced during the daytime, in which case it was a possible cure. One patient was given iron pills; the next, emetics to make her vomit; the next, laxatives to purge toxins from the other end. Horseback riding was considered a palliative except when it was identified as a cause, but then again, the list of "causes" by now had grown to include virtually anything from which a woman might derive sensual pleasure, from drinking coffee to sleeping on a featherbed to reading novels. As was typical for the era, the medical understanding of chlorosis was haunted by the specter of uncontrolled female sexuality; the fact that iron deficiency was often accompanied by odd dietary cravings—for chalk, dirt, charcoal—only contributed to the idea that poor health in young women was fundamentally linked to a perverse and insatiable appetite.

Meanwhile, some of the original Hippocratic cures for the condition still remained in use, albeit with updated justifications: since many chlorosis patients suffered from irregular periods, doctors once again began to speculate that this was not just a symptom but a cause of the condition, that women were being poisoned by the toxic by-products of their own interrupted menstrual cycles. Unfortunately, this theory was not just misinformed but led doctors to treat chlorosis patients once again with bloodletting—which, like the medical stricture against eating meat, was more likely to exacerbate anemia than to cure it. The ubiquity of bloodletting as treatment was noted at length in 1853 by physician Edward John Tilt in his "On diseases of women and ovarian inflammation: in relation to morbid menstruation, sterility, pelvic tumours, and affections of the womb," where he described himself and his colleagues treating chlorosis through the application of leeches, sometimes on a woman's lower abdomen, sometimes on her vaginal labia.

Tilt, an original fellow and eventual president of the Obstetrical Society of London, was himself no stranger to bizarre and sometimes barbaric forms of treatment when it came to women; among other things, he was an early and avid proponent of medical clitorectomies. But even he seems to have picked up on the paradox of intentionally bleeding anemic patients, leading to one of the more fascinating instances in medical literature of a doctor taking one step forward and then, immediately, two extraordinarily sexist steps back:

"Nonwithstanding the anaemic state of this young lady," he wrote of one such patient, her irregular periods were causing "fits" that could only be relieved through the release of blood: "As soon as the menstrual discharge appears, the hysterical symptoms abate or disappear."

In other words, a little anemia was nothing when there was a case of hysteria to treat—and so, bring on the labia leeches.

By the turn of the twentieth century, the medical understanding of chlorosis had come full circle: what began in ancient Greece as a special derangement of beautiful young women caused by a buildup of blood was now, some two thousand years later, seen as . . . a special derangement of beautiful young women caused by a buildup of blood. Of course, doctors in the early 1900s would have been at pains to explain why menstrual autointoxication was a valid scientific phenomenon in a way that an imbalance of humors was not, and perhaps would have been eventually pressed to do so, had chlorosis remained a matter of concern for the medical community.

But it didn't. As a new century dawned, the world was changing: scientifically, socially, culturally. Many of the attitudes and practices that once made chlorosis such a ubiquitous diagnosis—the fashionable association between beauty and fragility, the strictures against eating meat that left so many young women iron-deficient, the practice of bloodletting pregnant women leading to their babies being born with anemia, and the restrictive corsets that exacerbated many chlorosis symptoms—were increasingly out of style, as were the Victorian mores that kept women so tightly confined. Hemlines rose, conventions fell, and young women, finally endowed with the freedom to move more independently in society, no longer coveted a diagnosis that was synonymous with frailty and fainting fits, nor did they want this for their daughters. A chlorosis diagnosis, which once functioned as something of a status symbol and rite of passage for young women, now conjured a very different image of a pale, sickly, listless creature whose poor health was not only a social liability but a negative reflection on her mother, who was assumed to have caused her condition through either neglect, incompetence, or both.

At the same time, advancements in medical technology made it easier to identify and treat the anemia that was the real root cause of so many chlorosis symptoms, until the term itself began to fade out of popular use. And the chlorotic girl, an archetype of femininity whose pale skin, bright eyes, and fragile body had excited the sympathies of medical professionals, documentarians, and poets alike for more than two thousand years, also began to fade from the annals of medicine, and from public consciousness, until she was nothing but a memory.

Now her bosom rose and fell tumultuously. She was beginning to recognize this thing that was approaching to possess her, and she was striving to beat it back with her will—as powerless as her two white slender hands would have been. When she abandoned herself a little whispered word escaped her slightly parted lips. She said it over and over under her breath: "free, free, free!" The vacant stare and the look of terror that had followed it went from her eyes. They stayed keen and bright. Her pulses beat fast, and the coursing blood warmed and relaxed every inch of her body.

—Kate Chopin, "The Story of an Hour," 1894

Although the chlorotic girl began to disappear from the medical landscape in the early twentieth century, she left her mark on the culture when it came to lingering associations between femininity and frailty in matters of the blood and heart. The stereotype of women as constitutionally weak is a particularly central theme in Kate Chopin's "The Story of an Hour," which was first published in *Vogue* magazine in 1894.

"Knowing that Mrs. Mallard was afflicted with a heart trouble, great care was taken to break to her as gently as possible the news of her husband's death," the story begins, painting a picture of a young woman with an unspecified circulatory condition, one that has rendered her so fragile that upsetting news could pose a genuine medical threat. The truth, unbeknownst to Mrs. Mallard's family but soon revealed to the reader, is that the paternalism with which she's been treated by society in general and her husband in particular has made her life a misery, to the point where learning that he's been killed in a railroad accident is a welcome relief. Indeed, in the hour during which Mrs. Mallard believes her husband dead, she seems to shed not only the shackles of married womanhood but the limitations of her illness. Her heart, not so weak after all, beats hard, fast, and firm; blood runs warm and strong in her veins; her eyes grow bright. She is, for a brief moment, the picture of perfect circulatory health.

Then her husband—whose death was reported mistakenly—comes home, and she drops dead at the sight of him. Only the reader understands why; the physicians on the scene, who are themselves cogs in the patriarchal system that crushed Mrs. Mallard's spirit and took her life, do not. The final line of the story condemns the poor woman to be as misunderstood in death as she was in life: "When the doctors came they said she had died of heart disease—of joy that kills."

Insofar as heart problems in women were a subject of public awareness, this was more or less how they were imagined: as a congenital weakness that rendered a woman so fragile that an emotional shock could kill her. (While Chopin leveraged this trope to make a subversive point about how women suffer under a system that limits their freedoms "for their own good," it eventually made its way into horror stories, including the 1955 film *Les Diaboliques*, in which a man conspires with his mistress to scare his wife, who suffers from a heart condition, to death.)

But unlike the chlorotic girl, the weak-hearted women of fiction did not have a medical doppelgänger, nor a host of doctors eager to diagnose them. Indeed, the most influential scientists of the time believed that true heart disease in women was a fantasy, perhaps even one concocted by the women themselves. In 1897, the same year that Charles E. Simon published his comparatively insightful collection of chlorosis case studies, a renowned doctor named William Osler published his own classic text on cardiac ailments, *Lectures on Angina Pectoris and Allied States*. His argument, articulated explicitly and at length, was that women's hearts were nothing to worry about.

Curiously, Simon and Osler were contemporaries and friends; when Simon's phobias rendered him incapable of maintaining a normal medical practice, it was Osler who suggested that he convert the stable behind his home into a lab in order to continue his research. It's a touching story, and also a telling one: even as severe as his colleague's neuroses were, Osler saw no reason why they should interfere with Simon's ability to practice medicine, why he shouldn't be able to continue to contribute to the field despite his limitations. In light of this, it's not hard to see how Osler's compassionate temperament would have made him not just an excellent doctor, but an obvious champion of other medical professionals who were a little bit different, who faced challenges—including the enterprising young women who hoped to break into the boys' club of medicine.

Unfortunately, this, too, is a fantasy. Not that Osler wasn't a gifted physician—he was, described by biographers as the father of modern medicine, "one of the greatest diagnosticians ever to wield a stethoscope." But when it comes to his treatment of women, the truth is less flattering. Osler was no great champion of female doctors, and no savior to female patients. And when it comes to women's hearts, Osler is a chief architect of one of the most dangerous myths ever to pervade the medical system, which still remains present, and poisonous, as ever.

◆ ◆ ◆

It is September 1891 when the twenty-two-year-old "Miss C" makes her way from her hometown in the Finger Lakes region of upstate New York to the historic city of Baltimore, Maryland. It's a long journey, one that takes her farther from home than she's ever been before, but the novelty of watching the countryside flash by outside the windows of the train car is eclipsed by the urgency of the trip's purpose. The young woman is desperate for answers by now, even as she's also afraid of what those answers might be, what a diagnosis might reveal.

For years now, Miss C has been experiencing pain and numbness in her chest and left arm, sometimes more intense and sometimes less, but never entirely gone. Every few months, her heart itself seems to spasm, leaving her immobilized and gasping for breath. One doctor told her it was a tumor; the others couldn't even begin to guess. It was her family doctor who finally suggested she make this journey south, to a specialist whose brilliance in the field of cardiac medicine is second to none.

If anyone can tell what is the matter with her heart, he said, it's Dr. William Osler.

Osler, forty years old with a sharp widow's peak in his receding hair and a walrus-style mustache, is barely on the cusp at this moment of what will one day be a history-making career. But just two years into his role as the physician in chief of the newly created Johns Hopkins Hospital, he already has a reputation as a brilliant diagnostician owing to his careful taking of patient medical histories. His most famous quote, one that will eventually be part of the education of virtually every aspiring doctor to pass through the doors of a North American medical school, preaches the gospel of patient-centered medicine: "Listen to your patient, he is telling you the diagnosis." And when he meets Miss C, true to his reputation, Osler performs a thorough examination and makes careful, detailed notes.

A century later, we know quite a lot about Miss C: the precise date on which she was seen by Osler (it was September twenty-ninth, a Monday), her age at the first onset of symptoms (she was twelve when the pain first began), the way she jumped when he touched the skin on her left wrist to take her pulse. We know she was a diligent student and a recreational tennis player. We know that the symptoms she experienced were not just befuddling to her doctors but worrying to her friends.

But this is not Miss C's voice speaking; it is Osler's. Everything we know about this young woman is not everything she told him; it's just what he decided was important enough to write down. And in sketching this medical portrait, what Osler truly reveals is not who Miss C was, or even what she suffered from, but how she looked through her doctor's eyes—a doctor whose valuable belief in listening to patients coexisted alongside a second, far less enlightened set of beliefs about women's hearts, women's health, and women's trustworthiness as interpreters of what was happening in their bodies.

And as for the diagnosis Miss C has come so far to find, she will be sent home empty-handed. Insofar as Osler has answers, they are not to any question she asked, nor does he appear to have shared them with her.

"The patient was evidently very neurotic. She had no heart disease, no increased tension, and no sclerosis of the vessels," he writes, noting that her heart spasms, rather than the result of a physiological condition, were caused by "excitement and emotion." And when he sends her on her way, it's with a "favorable prognosis," the medical equivalent of a pat on the head and a *Don't you worry, sweetheart.* But then, how could it be otherwise, when he'd already decided that Miss C's problem wasn't her heart, but a nervous disposition exacerbated by studying too much? How could any doctor diagnose what he had already convinced himself didn't exist?

Are you entering the medical school? . . . Don't. Go home.

—Sir William Osler, MD, to female medical student Dorothy Mendenhall, 1900

The curious case of Miss C appears in William Osler's aforementioned text, *Lectures on Angina Pectoris and Allied States.* It was one of the most important teaching texts of Osler's career, but its publication was bracketed on either side by two other noteworthy incidents—incidents which were doubtless insignificant to Osler, yet offer vital context to his place in shaping women's relationship with the medical system.

The first of these came in 1894, three years before his lectures on diseases of the heart were published, when Osler stood before a crowd at the Harvard Medical Alumni Association annual dinner and declared the medical education of women to have been a fool's errand: "When I tell you that 33.3 per cent of the ladies, students, admitted to Johns Hopkins Hospital at the end of our short session are to be married, then I tell you that coeducation is a failure," he said. (The concept of "having it all" having not been invented yet, the possibility that women might get married and be doctors appears not to have occurred to him.)

The second incident came in the spring of 1900, when Osler encountered aspiring first-year medical student Dorothy Mendenhall as she traveled to tour the medical school at Johns Hopkins. Osler stared furiously at Mendenhall until she got off the trolley at the hospital stop, then followed her, interrogated her, and commanded her to go home.

Of course, Osler was hardly alone among men of his era in believing that women were unsuited to becoming doctors, and to his credit, he did teach women at the Hopkins school of which he was one of the founding fathers and first professor of medicine. (The then-twenty-five-year-old Dorothy Mendenhall was embarrassed when Osler accosted her, writing in her diary that "he literally stared me out of countenance, seeming to go over me from head to foot as if he were cataloging every detail for future reference," but not dissuaded: not only did she continue on to become one of the first woman graduates of Johns Hopkins School of Medicine, she was awarded a prestigious internship which she served under Osler's supervision. She would also go on to discover a key blood cell indicative of Hodgkin's disease, a type of lymphoma.)

Nor is Osler the only doctor to be leery of women as cardiac patients: in France in the 1860s, the proximity of the female heart to the female bosom made a physician named René Laennec so uncomfortable that he invented an early prototype for the stethoscope, just so he could avoid putting his ear to his female patients' chests.

But Osler's legacy, his outsized influence, means that he holds unique sway over women's lives—as doctors and as patients, in his time and in ours. More than virtually any other physician in history, Osler is responsible for having shaped the system that trains and educates doctors, for having decided not just what medical students learn but how. This includes some genuinely remarkable and innovative achievements: it was Osler who created the residency model that is still used today, with aspiring physicians rotating through each area of specialization before choosing their focus. He was also the first to insist on a bedside component to medical education, taking students out of lecture halls and into hospitals to learn.

But it is also thanks to Osler that cardiac medicine was designed with a male patient in mind, while women presenting with heart complaints were understood to be suffering from neurosis, anxiety, or hysteria. Heart attacks in particular were meant to be understood as linked not just to maleness but to masculinity, particularly tragic in their tendency to cruelly strike down a particular breed of virile, hardworking man in the prime of his adult life: "It is not the delicate neurotic person who is prone to angina," Osler declared, "but the robust, the vigorous in mind and body, the keen and ambitious man, the indicator of whose engines is always at full speed ahead."

Nearly all the case studies in Osler's 1897 text on heart disease are male, with the classic angina patient described specifically as "a well 'set' man from 45–55 years of age, with a military bearing, iron-gray hair, and a florid complexion." Women, meanwhile, were said to be afflicted with what Osler termed "pseudo angina"—literally, false angina—which described a collection of neurosis-induced symptoms masquerading as genuine disease. (Ironically, anxiety or emotional stress were still described as serious risk factors for a heart attack—but only in men.)

It's hard to overstate how dismissive Osler was of these women. Not only did he describe their symptoms as the cardiac equivalent of fake news, he also insisted that they were never fatal. This section of his lectures opens with a sweeping categorical declaration about any young woman who presents with heart complaints, one that gave any reader license to dismiss them out of hand: "The patients do not die."

"The extreme rarity of true angina in women must always be borne in mind," Osler wrote. On one hand, this comment can be seen as a variation on the classic medical maxim about considering the likely, common diagnosis before the rare one: when you hear hoofbeats, think horses, not zebras.

On the other hand, admonishing medical students to bear rarity in mind is often just another way of telling them not to think about zebras—or women's heart disease—at all.

And indeed, not only did physicians come to believe that heart attack in women was so vanishingly rare that it hardly needed consideration as a diagnosis, the study of cardiac medicine came to systematically exclude women as patients. In keeping with Osler's assertions, conditions ranging from heart attack to rhythm abnormalities were broadly dismissed in female patients as a symptom of emotional unbalance, rather than organic circulatory disease. In 1895, Sir Henry Thompson's *The Family Physician; A Manual of Domestic Medicine*—a key medical guide for practicing doctors at the time—instructed readers that cardiac arrhythmia (then called "palpitation") stemmed from a nervous disposition, occurring in patients who were "emotional or susceptible." Of course, we all know what that means:

"Thus the nervous constitution of the female sex renders women more liable than men," Thompson wrote, going on to note that women were especially prone to emotional instability—and hence symptoms of arrhythmia—when they were about to menstruate. As for the presence of arrhythmia in male patients, Thompson cagily explained that it was found primarily in a certain type of man: "The more the nervous system in men approached the feminine type, the more likely they are to suffer from palpitation."

In other words: heart attacks were for warriors; arrhythmia was for sissies. And as for women, they were simply left out of the discussion altogether. As far as the medical community was concerned, cardiac issues were the purview of men—and if a woman presented with complaints, the problem wasn't with her heart but all in her head.

The wife needs all the tact of a psychiatrist and all the self-control she can muster to induce her husband to shed pounds without nagging him into stubborn resistance.

—Paul Dudley White, MD, "On Hearts and Husbands," 1966

William Osler passed away in 1917 and left behind quite a mixed legacy: a model of medical training that still remains in use in 2022, and a latent incuriosity about heart disease in women that persisted for nearly as long. So convinced was the medical community that cardiac issues were almost universally the purview of men that the first American Heart Association conference for women wasn't held until 1964—and even then, this conference was for women but about men. Titled "On Hearts and Husbands," it instructed women in how to attend to (or manipulate) the men in their lives to live a heart-healthy lifestyle. (It was also, perhaps needless to say, a veritable buffet of classic midcentury sexism, replete with tips such as: "Your own daily housekeeping chores like sweeping, dusting, making beds and chasing toddlers, already place you way ahead of your husband in the exercise department; help him catch up.")

But as absurd as the Hearts and Husbands conference was, the entrenched attitudes it betrayed about women as cardiac patients were not just serious but deadly. In matters of the heart, women were routinely and systematically excluded: from diagnosis, from treatment, from research, and from the medical consciousness at large. When doctors conducted the first medical trial to establish a link between cholesterol and heart disease in 1982, their data set included 12,866 men—and no women. In 1995, the seminal study establishing that aspirin could reduce the risk of heart attack included 22,000 men—and, again, zero women.

Meanwhile, the "horses, not zebras" ethos surrounding the rarity of heart disease in female patients remained the consensus view in medicine for more than one hundred years, leaving women not just underdiagnosed but utterly in the dark about one of the greatest dangers to their health. The first governmental initiative to research heart disease in women specifically wasn't established until 1994. Go Red for Women, the American Heart Association's signature awareness-raising campaign for women's heart health, was finally established in 2004—at which point only 30 percent of women were even aware that heart disease was something they need be concerned about.

Since then, the scientific community has been frantically playing catch-up when it comes to treating women's hearts, trying to make up for a century of treating female cardiac patients like they didn't exist. In some areas, there has been genuine progress: today, 38 percent of cardiovascular research participants are women (which, while not quite achieving parity, is a massive improvement over the 0 percent it used to be). But on other fronts, doctors still haven't quite caught up to reality or escaped the lingering influence of Osler and his "pseudo angina." The woman suffering from heart disease will still receive far less aggressive treatment than a man. She is less likely to undergo diagnostic and therapeutic procedures like cardiac catheterization, balloon angioplasty, and coronary bypass. She is less likely to be prescribed medication to prevent heart disease (and more likely to be told to change her lifestyle, lose weight, or exercise). Her heart attack symptoms are considered "atypical," and are less likely to be taken seriously when she describes them to doctors. The machines used to diagnose her are still calibrated to the body of a standard (read: male) cardiac patient—and the doctor reading those results is also, in all likelihood, a man. Only 13 percent of all practicing cardiologists are women, and even fewer than that are electrophysiologists, who specialize in the arrhythmia that disproportionately afflicts women.

Today, fully one-third of women will develop heart disease at some point in their lives; for one woman in five, it will be the thing that kills her. That's not just more than breast cancer; it's more than all cancers, of every type, combined. A hundred years after William Osler declared that women's heart failure is all in their heads, it is their leading cause of death: all too real, and all too often overlooked until it's too late.

Heart disease is also a woman's disease, not just a man's disease in disguise.

—Bernadine Healy, MD, 1991

The year is 2004, late January, during one of the worst flu seasons on record. The ER at Elmhurst Hospital is overflowing with people coughing, moaning, sniffling, an extra layer of suffering on top of the usual late-night shuffle of accident victims, psychiatric patients, diabetics who've been trying to ration their insulin only to crash from skipping one too many doses. It's noisy and chaotic, the floor gritty with that dank mix of salt, mud, and melted snow that slicks the streets of New York in the winter. Patients can sit for hours on nights like this, while midnight becomes one o'clock, two o'clock, and the admitting staff struggles to triage, sorting the acute cases from the ones who can wait.

Most of the time, they get it right.

But not tonight.

Her name is Paula. She's thirty-eight years old, wearing a winter coat and hat over the pajamas she didn't have time to change out of before she left for the hospital. Like many patients, she's here alone; her husband, who she was sleeping next to when she woke up feeling shaky and short of breath, is still at home with their children. Her youngest, a daughter, is just three months old, which she explains in between apologies for taking up space in the ER. She's a nurse's aide, she says, and knows how busy it gets, especially at this time of year, especially at this time of night. There's fear in her eyes: she wouldn't have come, she says, if something weren't really wrong.

Something is really wrong.

The staff member who checked her in didn't realize, maybe because of the chaos in the waiting room, maybe just because her condition didn't raise the necessary alarms. She wasn't bleeding, feverish, or complaining of chest pains. Her symptoms—clammy skin, swollen legs, difficulty breathing that got worse when she lay down—seemed at a glance like nothing in particular, certainly nothing life-threatening. On a night like this, in a crowd like this, she was just one of dozens of patients who were left waiting, who seemed like they could wait.

It's not until hours later, when the supervising resident begins to ask more questions and Paula mentions her newborn baby, that the truth begins to dawn. Her pregnancy was plagued by these same symptoms, which doctors dismissed first as bronchitis, then as her own fault for being "out of shape." She had told her obstetrician repeatedly that she was exhausted, that her legs were swollen, that she was struggling to breathe. She has a family history: her grandmother died of an unspecified heart issue shortly after giving birth to her mother.

It has a name, this form of heart failure that afflicts women who are pregnant or have recently given birth, which often runs in families. It's even easy to spot if you know the symptoms: swollen lower legs, shortness of breath, fatigue, all classic signs of a heart that has stopped working effectively. When the supervising resident orders an echocardiogram, it will show that Paula's heart is pumping at 20 percent of normal capacity.

But Paula will not be diagnosed tonight. Not by the supervising resident, not by the cardiologist, not by the team of doctors who frantically work to revive her as she lies lifeless on the table, the words, "She has three small children at home," echoing back and forth between the clatter of medications being yanked from metal drawer, the frantic beeping of the heart monitors, the rhythmic hiss of the bag valve mask that covers her face. By the time anyone says the words aloud—peripartum cardiomyopathy—it will be to write them down on her autopsy form, a contributing factor to the massive pulmonary embolism that took her life.

◆ ◆ ◆

I was a twenty-six-year-old intern when I met Paula in the ER at Elmhurst. I watched the supervising resident's face darken with worry as he realized the urgency of the situation; I saw the anguish of the cardiology team as they arrived too late to save her from a death that could have, should have, been prevented. If only the triage nurse had realized that she had recently given birth; if only her obstetrician had recognized her symptoms during her pregnancy as the onset of cardiomyopathy; if only the medical community hadn't spent the better part of two centuries ignoring and dismissing female cardiac patients such that even in the year 2004 the manifestations of heart disease in women remained underresearched and misunderstood.

Paula's illness had advanced past the point of no return by the time she went to the hospital that night—but it wasn't just her heart that failed her. It was the system.

Ironically, the doctors who believed that women didn't suffer from cardiac issues in the same way as men do were half right: heart disease is different in women, with different symptoms, different risk factors, and different underlying causes. But that just makes it all the worse that women's hearts were ignored for so long; not only did women need to be included in cardiac research, they needed to be studied specifically, with an eye to understanding the difference between the sexes.

Dr. Hafiza Khan, one of the few female electrophysiologists in clinical practice today, describes the limitations of trying to diagnose women's heart disease using tools and standards that were designed with men in mind. Much of this comes down to the prime diagnostic tool in cardiology, the EKG, which is meant to measure electroconductivity of the heart and identify abnormalities. But the EKG's definition of "normal" is calibrated to a middle-aged, medium-weight male body—and when women are hooked up to it, things get complicated.

"A woman's arrhythmic risk varies according to her menstrual cycle," Khan explains. "When your estrogen peaks during ovulation, it's not only body temperature that goes up; the heart rate goes up, too, by about two to four beats. Meanwhile, we're at the lowest level of estrogen and progesterone right before the period starts, and that's the time that women are more likely to have arrhythmias."

Oddly enough, Sir Henry Thompson, who in 1895 declared that premenstrual women were prone to arrhythmia due to the emotional turmoil brought on by an impending period, almost got this one right—except that it's hormones, not hysteria, that affect a woman's heart rate. A woman's menstrual cycle is inextricably linked with her risk of fatal arrhythmia: patients with long QT syndrome, a disorder that can cause fast, chaotic heartbeats, are at greatest risk of death during pregnancy or just before menstruation. Another disorder, takotsubo cardiomyopathy—also known as "Broken Heart Syndrome," which can be triggered by extreme emotional distress— occurs predominantly in women who are postmenopausal. Still another, "Grinch Syndrome" (also called postural orthostatic tachycardia syndrome), which is allegedly characterized by an undersized heart, goes overlooked in the women it disproportionately affects because their hearts tend to be smaller to begin with.

The EKG doesn't accommodate for any of this, however. And the doctors who are most likely to be administering one, either during a primary care checkup or at the emergency room, often don't know it's a factor.

Meanwhile, even as the medical community has finally begun

to develop a broader awareness of women's heart disease, visibility is still a problem, in multiple senses of the word. Where men tend to suffer blockages in one of the heart's main arteries, women's coronary disease is often centered in smaller vessels, and less likely to show up via traditional imaging tools like an angiogram: it's quite literally harder to see. But it's also less visible culturally, which means that a woman having a heart attack often doesn't know she's having one, or even that she's at risk. Too many women remain unaware that pregnancy or hormone supplements can put their hearts in danger. Too many don't know that the systemic inflammatory and autoimmune disorders that disproportionately affect female patients also predispose them to heart conditions. Too many still fail to associate fatigue, nausea, and shortness of breath with heart attack symptoms, even though these are the ways such an attack most commonly presents in women. Today, a woman is still more likely to call an ambulance in response to her husband's heart attack than she is to call one for her own.

And like Paula, too many still die of preventable disease—because they don't know, and because nobody thought to ask.

Ygritte: What's fainting?

Jon Snow: When a girl sees blood and collapses.

Ygritte: Why would a girl see blood and collapse? . . . Girls see more blood than boys.

—*Game of Thrones*, "The Bear and the Maiden Fair," aired 2013 on HBO

The immense ignorance surrounding heart disease in women is one of the better-known scandals to come out of medical history, an egregious example of entrenched bias within not just circulatory medicine but science altogether, and one whose influence remains plainly visible today. By contrast, the days in which doctors attempted to relieve women of a toxic buildup of menstrual blood by opening their veins—or applying leeches to their genitals—seem very, very far behind us.

And yet, the legacy of humorism and its adherents, of the notion that women and blood don't mix, still makes for a subtle but confounding factor when it comes to diagnosing blood disorders in women, especially given their continued and somewhat taboo association with menstruation. There's iron deficiency anemia, which can cause a range of symptoms, including brain fog and fatigue, and which remains so underdiagnosed that it still afflicts nearly one in four adolescent girls.

◆ ◆ ◆

Consider the condition known as Von Willebrand disease, a clotting disorder that occurs in both sexes equally but is disproportionately severe in women. Some of the young women whose pallor and fatigue were diagnosed by Victorian doctors as chlorosis may in fact have been suffering from Von Willebrand or another clotting disorder, which went overlooked at the time owing to the common misconception that these conditions occurred predominantly in men—and because then, as now, the symptoms of the disease included heavy menstrual bleeding.

Dr. Rekha Parameswaran, a hematologist at Memorial Sloan Kettering Cancer Center, explains how bleeding disorders in women flew under the radar then and now, saying, "Women still do not talk about bleeding with their doctors. Either they're ashamed or embarrassed, or they think that what they're experiencing is normal."

One of Parameswaran's patients, a woman in her late forties, had spent her whole life with such heavy periods that she was soaking through five pads per day. But because this was the case for every woman in her family, she simply assumed it was normal—and none of her doctors ever asked the questions that might have let her realize otherwise. It wasn't until she nearly bled to death on the operating table during a hysterectomy and developed a wound that wouldn't close or heal that someone finally thought to evaluate her for a bleeding disorder. Dr. Ariela Marshall, a hematologist who specializes in treating women with bleeding disorders, tells me that the medical establishment is finally beginning to make progress on this front, at least when it comes to presurgical protocols: women are now routinely tested for Von Willebrand disease before undergoing hysterectomies, averting near tragedies like the one described above. It's a start, although gender parity in diagnosing clotting disorders is still a ways off.

Men with Von Willebrand disease are generally diagnosed by age ten; for women, it takes at least two years longer, and the average woman waits sixteen years from first onset of symptoms to find out what's wrong with her.

Even as doctors no longer speculate that women are being poisoned by an excess of "filthy" menstrual blood, this incuriosity about unhealthy bleeding and what it might mean remains embedded in the medical establishment. And women, meanwhile, continue to suffer—not for lack of treatments, but because they think they have to; because they don't know, and nobody tells them, that what's happening to them is not normal; and because the scientific community still shies away from the taboos that need to be shattered before we can empower women to live healthier lives.

◆ ◆ ◆

If William Osler is the father of modern medicine, Nanette Wenger might be described as its daughter and heir—including the part where it became her responsibility to clean up all the messes made by the men who came before her. In 1954, Wenger became one of the first female graduates of Harvard Medical School, having begun her medical education just five years after the school first opened its doors to women. As of this writing, she is in her nineties and a legend in her field as well as a keeper of its memories: pleased to see how far women's circulatory medicine has come since the days of Osler, but keenly aware of how much work remains to be done.

Wenger dedicated her career to women's cardiac health, beginning with her tenure as the first female chief resident in cardiology at New York's Mount Sinai hospital. It was there, in the late 1950s, that she first noticed the pervasive, systemic exclusion of women, not just from the research but from the medical consciousness altogether. When people talked about women's health, she says, they talked about breasts and reproduction.

"The rest of it was assumed to be the same as the men," she recalls. "As I started taking care of patients, I saw women in the hospital with coronary disease with myocardial infarction, not doing well. But when I went to the books, to the literature, there was nothing there."

The trajectory of Wenger's career serves as a poignant illustration of both how far we've come in unraveling the tangle of medical bias when it comes to women's circulatory diseases, and how far we've yet to go. After discovering that women had been left out of the literature on coronary disease, she set out to raise awareness of the issue among doctors and patients alike. It proved to be an uphill battle. In 1977 when Wenger put together a series of television presentations on heart disease in women along with another physician, Dr. Harriet Dustan, the only time producers would air them was at eleven o'clock p.m., when vanishingly few people were awake to see them. When she published a 1992 landmark paper in the *New England Journal of Medicine* that summarized how much cardiac disease in women remained underresearched and unexplored, coronary heart disease was not only the number one killer of women but an underdiagnosed, undertreated condition whose dangers the general public remained grossly unaware of. It wasn't until 2001, and the publication of a report from the Institute of Medicine titled *Exploring the Biological Contributions to Human Health: Does Sex Matter?*, that female mortality due to cardiovascular issues began to decline—and then it did so sharply.

Finally, doctors were asking the right questions.

In 1583, one of the earliest gendered illustrations of the circulatory system appeared in a text by the anatomist Felix Platter. The drawing is a curious artifact, anatomically inaccurate yet metaphorically astute: it depicts a heart-shaped hole at the base of the sternum, through which Platter believed that a pregnant woman's unexpelled menstrual blood was conducted from the uterus to the breasts, where it was turned into the milk that would eventually nourish her child.

If this alchemical theory of where breast milk comes from sounds preposterous and profoundly unscientific, that's because it is—but for all its medical uselessness, Platter's illustration is nevertheless laden with important meaning vis-à-vis which parts of a woman's anatomy were considered worthy of scientific study. Any physiological apparatus that spoke to a woman's role as mother and nurturer was deemed interesting; the inner workings of her heart, on the other hand, were insignificant and beneath notice. And while Platter's misguided notions about the workings of the female circulatory system were eventually (and rightly) discarded, it would still take nearly five hundred years before science finally developed the imaging technology to peer inside women's hearts, to see that they are indeed unique and distinct, but also no less susceptible to disease, no less in need of protection.

"I think we've just scratched the surface," Nanette Wenger tells me. "Cardiovascular disease, hypertension, coronary disease, heart failure: you name it, and there's a difference. And we're just beginning to look."

CHAPTER 5

breath

RESPIRATORY

PERHAPS WOMEN BREATHE DIFFERENT AIR

Consumption, I am aware, is a flattering malady.

—Charlotte Brontë, 1849

She has never looked lovelier. So pale, so frail, as precious and breakable as a china doll. There are shadowed hollows beneath the gracile curve of her protruding collarbones, and burning roses in her cheeks. Her eyes are bright, her lips a blushing red, only occasionally obscured by the lace handkerchief she holds in the tapered fingers of one delicate hand.

Poems will be written about how beautiful she was, here at the end of her short and tragic life. There will be odes, and sonnets, and songs. There is something otherworldly about her loveliness: like a flower so exotic, so fragile, you wouldn't dare touch it for fear of the petals falling away, but watch in tender and respectful awe as it blooms fiercely—briefly—and then dies.

On her last day, she lies back against the pillows. The rise and fall of her chest is so shallow as to be almost imperceptible; her skin is so white it seems almost translucent, as if some part of her has already slipped beyond the veil. She lifts the white handkerchief to her lips.

She coughs.

It won't be long now.

The blood that stains the linen, where it touched her lips, is the most beautiful shade of red.

◆ ◆ ◆

Despite its reputation for enhancing the beauty of the women it afflicted, and its continued, ubiquitous presence in fictional dramas about gorgeous Edwardian invalids, the reality of tuberculosis—or, as it was known colloquially in the eighteenth century, "consumption"—was decidedly unlovely. The disease, a bacterial infection that starts in the lungs, was lethal but agonizingly slow, destroying the body from the inside out over the course of months or even years. Patients, weak and emaciated, would ultimately cough themselves to death on bedsheets soaked with sweat, phlegm, blood, and sometimes feces (uncontrollable diarrhea, though it is never mentioned alongside the more romantic symptoms of tuberculosis, afflicts nearly 30 percent of sufferers). At its peak from the late 1700s through mid-1800s, tuberculosis is estimated to have killed off a quarter of the entire population of Europe, and proved particularly and tragically deadly for young adults.

And yet, due to the complex interplay of the era's cultural, medical, and social mores, tuberculosis—particularly in women—nevertheless developed a certain cachet that eventually rendered it almost aspirational, founded in the then-fashionable idea that there was something wonderfully feminine about being frail. The same forces that manifested in circulatory medicine as an obsession with chlorosis, and in orthopedics as a preoccupation with the smallness of women's skulls, reveal themselves here in a fascination with the consumptive girl, a pale and ethereal creature whose allure only increased as she drew nearer to her inevitable death.

With obvious exceptions (again, the diarrhea), the look of tuberculosis did tend to align with the beauty standards of the time: skin so pale it became transparent, emaciation brought on by lack of appetite, a natural blush in the cheeks and lips. Carolyn A. Day, in her book *Consumptive Chic*, writes, "Instead of the afflicted becoming unrecognizable as she deteriorated, the wasting associated with the disease was twinned with ideas of beauty." The imagined connection between tuberculosis and beauty was also a two-way street: the disease was not only said to make plain women more beautiful, but to be a particular threat to pretty girls, who were deemed more susceptible to it.

Between the purported sex appeal of tuberculosis and its special deadliness in young people, being afflicted with the disease—or at least, looking like you were—became associated with a certain status. This was a moment at which a woman's value was strongly tied to femininity, fragility, and purity alike. The consumptive girl lived at the tantalizing nexus of all three: being made at once sexually desirable by sickness yet also too sick to consummate that desire. And her death, heartbreaking as it was, only cemented her status as a sort of archetype of female purity, unsullied by the usual forces that conspired to slowly rob a woman of her value. It was possible, in this moment, to imagine that tuberculosis patients were destined for something greater, something more meaningful, than the ordinary vagaries of a mortal life: when the consumptive girl passed, it would be in a state of unpolluted grace—without having ever known the ravages of time, or lust.

The culture of the early nineteenth century was suffused with visions of these terminally ill beauties, languishing on their sickbeds while those around them swooned with pity and desire. Alexandre Dumas's *La Dame aux Camélias* and Victor Hugo's *Les Misérables* both feature tragic, heroic deaths for women with consumption, as do Verdi's *La traviata* and Puccini's *La bohème*. Emily Brontë's *Wuthering Heights* lingers on its description of the tuberculous Frances, who is "rather thin, but young and fresh complexioned and her eyes sparkled like diamonds." And when Henry James's beloved cousin, Minny Temple, died of tuberculosis in 1870, he channeled his grief into an homage: his 1902 novel *The Wings of the Dove* features a beautiful invalid heiress, Milly Theale, who is diabolically seduced by a man named Merton Densher in the hopes of inheriting her money when she dies, thus allowing him to marry the woman he really wants. But the joke is on Merton: Milly is so lovely, so good, so beautiful and pure, that her death is not only not a boon, it irretrievably destroys both him and the woman he meant to marry.

Even in the late stages of the disease, and even in real life, a woman with tuberculosis could still be the object of unmitigated adoration. In 1842, a passage frequently attributed to Edgar Allan Poe waxed poetic about how the disease had made his wife into a "delicately, morbidly angelic" creature, recounting how she'd suffered a hemorrhagic coughing fit at dinner: "Suddenly she stopped, clutched her throat and a wave of crimson blood ran down her breast . . . It rendered her even more ethereal."

Surrounded as they were by such rapturous depictions of tuberculous women, perhaps it's no surprise that doctors romanticized the disease, too. An 1833 article in *The London Medical and Surgical Journal* actually praises tuberculosis for being so wonderfully photogenic:

"Some diseases are borne in silence and concealment, because their phenomena are calculated to excite disgust; to others, the result of vicious courses, the stigma of disgrace is attached; unsightly ravages of the human frame, or the wreck of the mental faculties, inspire us with horror rather than with sympathy; but consumption, neither effacing the lines of personal beauty, nor damaging the intellectual functions, tends to exalt the moral habits, and develop the amiable qualities of the patient."

Of course, in comparison to diseases like cholera, tuberculosis was a more attractive ailment to suffer from—and given that it confined afflicted women to their homes and beds, if it didn't actually exalt their morality, it certainly kept them from getting into certain types of trouble. But more to the point, as long as its origins remained mysterious, it was possible to imagine that tuberculosis conveyed special status where other illnesses didn't. The prolonged timeline on which the disease progressed put tuberculosis sufferers in the peculiar position of knowing both how and (roughly) when they were going to die, even as they continued to live, work, and socialize in much the same way they always had—at least as long as they had the benefit of being a member of the upper class. As such, tuberculosis was not an uncommon presence in rarefied social circles, where the associations between being sick and being beautiful led many otherwise healthy women to cultivate the pale skin, feverish complexion, and slumped posture of tuberculosis sufferers.

By the dawn of the twentieth century, however, the mystery of tuberculosis was on the wane, and the romance associated with the disease along with it. The advent of germ theory led to the revelation that tuberculosis, far from being a mark of sophistication or sensitivity, was just another bacterial infection—a fact that swiftly took all the cachet out of consumptive chic. That young women with tuberculosis were ethereal, angelic creatures possessed of an otherworldly beauty and purity was a difficult notion to sustain once it was broadly understood that they were sickened by germs. In short order, both the cultural and medical consensus surrounding tuberculosis shifted: now, it was seen as a biological scourge to be battled against through sanitary reforms and public hygiene initiatives, just like any other illness.

And yet, in the decades during which tuberculosis was seen as the tragic, romantic affliction of the world's most beautiful girls, a crucial groundwork was laid. Together, medicine and culture had spawned an idea as potent as it was poisonous, one that the scientific breakthroughs of the day could mitigate but never entirely dispel. The idea was just this: that there is something beautiful, and wonderfully feminine, and powerful and empowering at once, about a woman who can't breathe.

Some women regard cigarettes as symbols of freedom. Smoking is a sublimation of oral eroticism; holding a cigarette in the mouth excites the oral zone. It is perfectly normal for women to want to smoke cigarettes.

—Abraham Arden Brill, MD, circa 1929

An Ancient Prejudice Has Been Removed. Today, legally, politically and socially, womanhood stands in her true light. AMERICAN INTELLIGENCE has cast aside the ancient prejudice that held her to be inferior . . . Gone is that ancient prejudice against cigarettes— Progress has been made.

—Lucky Strike advertisement, 1929

It's a brilliant, sunny morning in late March, and the avenue is thronged. Women in fashionable drop-waisted midi-length dresses, pearls, and cloche hats stroll slowly down the sidewalk, arm in arm with men wearing top hats and overcoats, their shoes freshly shined. They're here for the Easter Sunday parade, the year's best chance to see and be seen, as members of New York society exit their Fifth Avenue churches and make their way down the crowded street toward home, or the homes or friends, or a leisurely dinner at a nearby hotel. There is always gossip after the parade, usually about who was wearing the most exceptional—or exceptionally ridiculous—hat. But today, in 1929, the members of high society will have something far more scandalous to talk about.

Nobody notices at first, when Bertha Hunt reaches under her dress, hitching up her hemline until she can grasp the packet hidden there, strapped beneath her garter. No heads turn as she strikes a match and brings one hand to her mouth. She inhales, and exhales, releasing a delicate stream of smoke from between her pursed lips.

But then a murmur goes up. Beside Bertha, another woman is lighting a cigarette—and another. And another. Soon there are ten of them in all, strolling defiantly down the avenue, smoking and laughing and paying no attention as people mutter and stare. There'd been rumors of a protest, of course; everyone had heard them. But it's one thing to hear about a group of suffragettes protesting for equality with a public display of taboo flouting, and quite another to actually see it. Soon, the women are surrounded by reporters, peppering them with questions:

Why are they here?
What are their aims?
What is their preferred brand of cigarette?

Another murmur goes up: It's more than just these ten women. Something is happening. Something has been sparked. Everywhere, up and down the avenue, women are pulling cigarettes from beneath their hemlines. The writer Nancy Hale Hardin casually gestures with a cigarette as she walks with her husband, who is also smoking. Edith Lee, who is dressed to the nines in a fur-trimmed coat and matching cloche, holds the leash of her purebred sheepdog in one hand and a cigarette in the other. And everywhere, as journalists snap pictures and shout out questions, one word can be heard repeated over and over: freedom.

This is about freedom.

As she lights another cigarette, Bertha—the first to strike a match, the one who started it all—declares to a group of rapt reporters, "I hope that we have started something and that these torches of freedom, with no particular brand favored, will smash the discriminatory taboo on cigarettes for women and that our sex will go on breaking down all discriminations."

Tomorrow, those three words will be in all the papers: "torches of freedom."

Within the year, cigarette sales will skyrocket as women, inspired by the idea of freedom, equality, and fighting sexist taboos, start buying packs of "torches" themselves.

And Dr. Abraham Arden Brill, the psychoanalyst hired by Lucky Strike cigarettes—the one who coined the phrase "torches of freedom," and who told Bertha Hunt exactly how to smoke, and what to say, and how to say it—will be congratulated on a job well done.

◆ ◆ ◆

Long before he became the progenitor of one of the earliest known marketing campaigns founded on principles of psychology, Abraham Arden Brill was a striking example of the classic American success story: a scrappy immigrant who clawed his way up from nothing to become one of the most respected psychoanalysts of his time. Born to Jewish parents in what is now the Polish city of Kańczuga, Brill immigrated alone to the United States in 1890, at the age of fifteen. Even as a young man, he was renowned for his tenacity—Ernest Jones, a neurologist and longtime friend of Sigmund Freud, once admiringly referred to him as a "rough diamond"—and his hunger to learn. By the time he was thirty, he had worked his way through both college and medical school, and found a position at the Central Islip State Hospital on Long Island. In the early 1900s, he traveled to Zurich and became a disciple of Freud, whose works he was the first to translate into English. Photos of Brill from this time show a diminutive and mostly bald man with pointy features, wire-rimmed glasses, and a discreet puff of facial hair just below his lower lip (the style now colloquially known as a "flavor saver"). In one group shot, featuring Brill posed alongside several of the fathers of modern psychology, he's beaming over the shoulder of a cigar-smoking Freud, looking positively delighted to be there. (Side note: in addition to working as Freud's translator, Brill also trained early in his career with Dr. Adolf Meyer, who you'll recognize in the Nervous System chapter—using his influence to quash early reports of a medical scandal at the New Jersey State Hospital at Trenton.)

Brill was a giant in the field of psychoanalysis—not quite at the level of Freud or Jung, but influential nevertheless. Back in New York City, he lectured at Columbia, became clinical professor of psychiatry at New York University, and founded the New York Psychoanalytic Society & Institute, whose library is still named for him. He also married a fellow doctor, K. Rose Owen, and had two children.

But Brill has another legacy, too, not in psychiatry but in respiratory medicine: he is the doctor who first made smoking into a feminist cause.

In 1929, the year that Bertha Hunt sparked a mini revolution by lighting up at the Easter Day Parade, the notion that cigarettes represented liberation from the sexist days of yore was not entirely unfounded. Smoking was still considered an unseemly activity for women to engage in, a form of spiritual and moral corruption. In some places, including New York City, local governing bodies passed bills and ordinances that made it illegal for a woman to smoke in public—or even in the privacy of her own home if she had children.

If this was bad news for women's autonomy in the eyes of the law, it was also bad news for cigarette companies, who had an obvious, powerful financial incentive to smash the female smoking taboo. Enter Lucky Strike cigarettes and their main marketing strategist, a public relations pioneer named Edward Louis Bernays.

"The president of the largest tobacco company called me in and told me they were losing half of their market, because men did not permit women to smoke either in public or even at home," an elderly

Bernays recalled, in an interview conducted shortly before his death in 1995. "'What can we do about breaking down that taboo?' he asked."

Bernays, who was Sigmund Freud's nephew (small world!), naturally turned for advice to the nearest, respected disciple of his uncle, Abraham Arden Brill. What Brill said proved revelatory: shattering the cultural stigma around women smoking wasn't just about getting women to enjoy cigarettes. It was about getting them to identify as smokers, which is to say, as rule-breaking, taboo-flouting, feminist crusaders for freedom.

It is worth noting that Brill himself did not believe at all in this vision of taboo-shattering femininity. In his view, liberation was a booby prize for women whose true and natural ambitions—that is, to have as many children as possible—were being thwarted by modernity.

"Hence comes 'women's freedom,' 'women's rights,' women's entrance into politics 'business and the professions,'" he once wrote. "But no normal woman was ever satisfied without marriage and children."

She might, however, be satisfied by cigarettes, Brill suggested to Bernays—not just because they represented freedom, but because they "titillated the erogenous zones of the lips." (In other words, despite the insistence of his mentor Sigmund Freud that sometimes a cigar is just a cigar, Brill wasn't so sure that in a woman's mouth, a cigarette was always just a cigarette.)

As for Bernays, he immediately understood precisely how to translate Brill's insights into a marketing plan: "It occurred to me that any young debutante who was aware of the times and of herself as a woman being discriminated against would be delighted to walk in the Easter parade while smoking," he said, "to dramatize the idea that cigarettes were indeed 'torches of freedom,' and to validate that, and to invalidate the taboo against women smoking."

The ad campaign resulting from Bernays's conversation with Brill is an early, notable example of how doctors would lend their expertise—and sometimes even a medical stamp of approval—to marketing products that were the opposite of healthy. It also might be the first documented instance of the phenomenon known as "woke capitalism," in which corporations sold products to women under the guise of helping to liberate them. The so-called protest, in which women smoked openly at the Easter parade, was actually a stunt staged by Bernays, based on the ideas articulated by Brill. Before the parade, Bernays strategically spread rumors that a group of suffragettes planned to demonstrate there by openly smoking cigarettes. He carefully selected the group of ten women who would light up alongside Bertha Hunt—herself an employee of Lucky Strike—noting that "while they should be good looking, they should not look too model-y," lest ordinary women find the whole enterprise unrelatable. And before the parade, he enlisted the help of a committed feminist, Ruth Hale, whose invitation to her fellow activists to smoke at the parade could have doubled as ad copy:

WOMEN!

LIGHT ANOTHER TORCH OF FREEDOM!
FIGHT ANOTHER SEX TABOO.

While it's impossible to know precisely how much credit Brill and Bernays can claim for what happened next, it's safe to say that the parade stunt made an impact. The New York Times coverage in particular positioned the smoking women as part of something significant, a larger, exciting march toward progress: "Modern, prosperous New York was celebrating Easter. The models of the machines were 1929. The fashions on display were those of the future. A group of young women, who said they were smashing a tradition and not favoring any particular brand, strolled along the lane between the tiered skyscrapers and puffed cigarettes."

And within the year, rates of smoking among women had more than doubled, from 5 to 12 percent.

We make Virginia Slims especially for women because they are biologically superior to men.

—Virginia Slims advertisement, 1972

The connection between the 1929 "Torches of Freedom" campaign and the vogue, a century earlier, for consumptive chic, is a subtle one. Unlike the women of the early 1900s who adopted the stooped posture of the tuberculous patient, or used makeup to whiten their faces and redden their lips and cheeks, those who took up smoking in the name of equality were not trying to look sick. (It would be decades before the scientific community established a link between smoking and lung disease.) And yet they were trying to look like something; smoking represented a marker of status for the modern woman as surely as looking frail and feverish did for her Victorian counterpart. The only difference was that in 1929, fragility was out of style. Instead, a woman compromising her respiratory health through smoking became a symbol of liberation—and, crucially, continued to be treated as one by advertisers even after the link between smoking and respiratory disease was well-known.

As for Dr. Brill, if he had any misgivings about his legacy as the progenitor of the "Torches of Freedom" campaign, he never expressed them. Certainly, he would have balked at the idea that he was being insulting to women, or doing them harm; "I do not wish to imply that woman is inferior to man," he once wrote. "She is his superior in her own sphere. She does not rise as high as man in intelligence and creative power nor does she fall so low. She always pursues the middle course always."

And yet, his notion of cigarettes as tools of liberation became a standard element of the marketing for cigarette makers, who realized that they could flatter women into consuming their highly addictive product just as long as they positioned it as empowering—and particularly if the encouragement came with a doctor's seal of approval. When Lucky Strike launched a new campaign in the 1930s, this one centered on the use of cigarettes as a weight control device, they did so in collaboration with physicians who were all too happy to cite the evidence-based benefits of smoking when it came to staying slim.

The message was clear: smoking put women in control—of their lives, their futures, even their appetites. Lady Grace Drummond-Hay, a renowned journalist and adventurer, appeared in that new Lucky Strike campaign under a speech balloon: "I smoke a Lucky instead of eating sweets." Forty years later, Virginia Slims advertised its cigarettes for the "biologically superior" woman using a model dressed as Wonder Woman. Twenty years after that, the same company updated its ads for the 1990s feminist: "Equality comes with no apron strings attached," reads an ad depicting a smirking, short-haired woman smoking a cigarette while a man in an apron stands at the stove, preparing food.

Of course, by now, doctors had long since stopped encouraging their patients to smoke. (The 1995 "apron strings" ad is conspicuously emblazoned with the surgeon general's warning that smoking may cause fetal injury in pregnant women.) But the new medical conscientiousness around cigarettes was not accompanied by an equally robust commitment to taking women's respiratory health seriously.

Indeed, it still isn't.

As women, we wear various hats in our lives. Oftentimes, we forget to stop and take a deep breath to center ourselves.

—promotional copy for *The Mindful Woman: Gentle Practices for Restoring Calm, Finding Hope, and Opening Your Heart*, published 2008

The first time Sierra tells a doctor she can't breathe, it's at the urgent care center near her daughter's preschool. She's walked here straight from drop-off, and while it's a beautiful spring day and the distance is only a few blocks, she's already winded. She's always winded, she says, and it's getting worse. She used to run for exercise, even trained for a half marathon; now she has to stop, bent double and gasping for air, before she's even gone a mile. At home, her children run circles around her. She can't keep up.

The doctor gestures toward the window, and the budding trees beyond it.

"Allergies," he says. "I'm struggling with them myself."

He sends her home with an antihistamine.

The second time comes weeks later. Same clinic, different doctor. Again, she lists her symptoms—shortness of breath, decreased stamina, and now a steady ache in her shoulder that gets worse whenever she coughs. The doctor squeezes her shoulder and diagnoses her with a strained muscle. He points to her chart, the notes from her last visit.

"You have seasonal allergies, yes?" he says. "Try not to cough so hard."

The third time, the doctor is the same one who diagnosed her with allergies. It's been months now, and Sierra's cough is worse. She hasn't exercised in ages, and can barely walk a block or lift up her daughter without gasping for air. She's lost fifteen pounds anyway. The doctor frowns and says it looks like acid reflux. He sends her home with a prescription antacid. He says she'll be better soon.

The fourth time, Sierra doesn't go to that clinic. It's winter now, the blooms on the trees long since fallen, the antacid she was given six months ago long since finished. If it helped at all, it was only for a moment; now, a single breath of cold air causes her to cough uncontrollably. When she drives to the emergency room, it's partly because it's easier, but also partly because she wants to see a doctor she hasn't seen before. One who won't wave her away, telling her it's allergies, or muscle strain, or heartburn, when all she wants—all she's ever wanted—was for them to actually look at her lungs.

The X-ray takes just a few minutes.

The doctor's face is grim.

"I'm afraid it's not good news," he says. "It's a shame you didn't seek care sooner."

◆ ◆ ◆

From the rah-rah feminist smoking ads of yesteryear to the rise of contemporary wellness culture, attending to the respiratory system has increasingly become coded as a matter of self-care for women, rather than healthcare. Women are inundated with pseudoscientific suggestions to meditate, to download a breath-counting app, to get more exercise. There's even a magazine called *Breathe* (subtitle: "and make time for yourself.") Granted, this began as more a cultural problem than a medical one, but as in eras past, the medical community now ends up taking its cues from the culture—in this case, one that says respiratory health is a woman's problem to solve, rather than a doctor's to diagnose. The same medical establishment that told women in 1929 that smoking was a path to freedom, now responds skeptically when women say they can't breathe, despite their disproportionate exposure to environmental factors that can cause pulmonary disease.

As a result, women's respiratory ailments frequently go undiagnosed, sometimes with the worst kind of results. Rates of lung cancer, for which the imagined "standard" patient is a male smoker in late middle age, have risen 84 percent in women since the late 1980s, even as they drop in men. Women are more likely to suffer from lung cancer despite never having smoked, as well as remain at greater risk even after quitting smoking.

Every year, more women die from lung cancer than from breast, uterine, and ovarian cancers combined, and some of them surely don't have to. Sierra, the patient you met in the vignette above, was sent away by doctors three separate times, with three inaccurate diagnoses, all while the cancer in her lungs continued to spread. By the time I met her, as a first-year fellow at Memorial Sloan Kettering Cancer Center, the disease had metastasized to her bones, her liver, and her brain. Sierra was dead within a year. If someone had taken her early symptoms seriously, she may not be.

Respiratory medicine is plagued by the same tendency as other fields to write off a woman's symptoms as anxiety without searching more deeply for an organic cause. Lindsay Lief, an ICU/critical care/pulmonary specialist at NewYork-Presbyterian/Weill Cornell Medical Center, tells me she's trying to change this, saying, "I'm constantly drilling into my residents: anxiety is a diagnosis of exclusion in the hospital. You must first prove that you have explored everything else. I don't want to hear, 'I think she's just anxious,' when a patient presents with shortness of breath."

Lief's insistence on this front is born of harrowing experiences, close calls in which pulmonary doctors were summoned only at the last possible moment—or, tragically, too late. Many respiratory ailments, including asthma, can look a lot like panic disorder to a doctor who hasn't opened his mind for the former, with symptoms including dizziness, chest tightness, choking, or the sensation of being smothered. Some can cause mental confusion and heart palpitations. One patient, who seemed agitated and kept complaining that she couldn't breathe, spent nearly eight hours being incorrectly dosed with anti-anxiety drugs while she slowly went into shock and pulmonary failure. When she lost consciousness, they chalked it up to the sedatives—until a scan revealed massive fluid buildup in her lungs. Another patient, whose asthma attack was misdiagnosed as a panic attack, was still being scolded by medical staff to just calm down until she went into respiratory distress from lack of oxygen.

This is even more troubling given that more than one in ten women suffer from asthma, as compared with just over 6 percent of men, and their symptoms are usually more severe. Asthma-related death rates in women, particularly Black women, are disproportionately high.

Meanwhile, women's pulmonary issues are especially likely to go overlooked during pregnancy and childbirth, under circumstances in which women are least able to advocate for themselves (e.g., mid-labor), and most likely to be written off by doctors as overreacting. Dr. Sonali Bose, an associate professor of medicine and pediatrics, pulmonary and critical care medicine at Mount Sinai hospital, described how one pregnant patient was told for six full months that her shortness of breath was just a result of pressure on her diaphragm from her growing baby before doctors thought to do a work-up just to be sure—and discovered that she actually had asthma.

"A lot of our colleagues are almost afraid of taking care of pregnant women," Bose says. "But when fear stops us from asking questions, it stops us from solving treatable problems."

In critical care settings, these issues are often exacerbated by the fact that ventilators, which can be a lifesaving intervention for patients with severe pulmonary issues, are generally calibrated to male patients; when a woman is hooked up to one, it's hard to make sure she's receiving the proper volume of oxygen.

Today, awareness within the medical community surrounding women's unique respiratory health risks remains low, despite diligent efforts to turn the tide. Among the advocates for better care are Serena Williams, who nearly died from a pulmonary embolism after giving birth to her first child in 2017. Williams, like my patient

Sierra, battled with nurses to receive a lung scan after developing a cough so persistent it tore her Cesarean stitches.

"Lo and behold, I had a blood clot in my lungs, and they needed to insert a filter into my veins to break up the clot before it reached my heart," Williams wrote years later, in an essay for *Elle* magazine.

Unlike Sierra, Williams's story had a happy ending; she received the proper care within days, instead of waiting through a full year and multiple misdiagnoses only to find the truth too late. And yet their stories have eerie similarities: before they found the clot, a nurse dismissed Williams as she begged for a CAT scan. She just needed to calm down, the nurse told her. To rest. To breathe.

She said, "I think all this medicine is making you talk crazy."

◆ ◆ ◆

From urgent care clinics to emergency rooms, family practices to the ICU, the failure of doctors to ask women the right questions about their respiratory health inevitably leads to erroneous assumptions, to the wrong conclusions, and sometimes to fatal missteps. Some patients, like Sierra, languish without a proper diagnosis while the system fails them over and over. Others are misdiagnosed during cataclysmic medical crises in which every second counts.

The similarities between acute respiratory failure and panic disorders mean that women, and particularly young women, are too often assumed to be suffering from the latter when it's actually the former. In one harrowing case from my residency, a twenty-year-old woman named Tara arrived in the ER with acute shortness of breath. She'd been sent by her school's health office, who took one look at her and slotted her into a preexisting narrative: here was another high-strung perfectionist Ivy League athlete, having a panic attack during finals week. In the emergency room, still gasping for air, Tara told the intake nurse the same thing the school's health office had told her.

Here, the system began to break down. Proper emergency room triage means never taking a statement like this at face value. So many serious conditions can mask themselves as something more mundane, and diligence and curiosity are required to rule out the possibility of a true emergency. Every medical education includes warnings about the danger of pattern matching, of making assumptions, of thinking you know without having to ask.

But amid the chaos of the ER, things can too easily fall through the cracks. And so instead of asking Tara about her family history of clotting disorders, whether she was on birth control, and whether she'd experienced any pain in her extremities within the past week, the nurse nodded, took her story at face value, and told her to take a seat. And when someone asked her about the girl in the waiting room—the one whose head was hanging between her knees, the one who couldn't breathe—she repeated that same narrative, which by now had acquired the gloss of accuracy simply by virtue of being so familiar, and having been repeated so many times.

Perfectionist.
Finals week.
Panic attack.

It was a story they'd all heard before.

It wasn't until Tara collapsed in the waiting room that anyone thought to ask if the story, familiar as it was, might not be true.

Tara was experiencing a saddle pulmonary embolism brought on by deep vein thrombosis, a condition in which a blood clot forms in the deep veins of the legs, then breaks free and travels through the body, eventually getting trapped in the main pulmonary artery and cutting off the blood supply to the lungs. One in four people who develop this condition die instantly; of those who don't, another 10 percent die within weeks of diagnosis. Tara, who had multiple risk factors—a genetic clotting disorder, a recent history of leg pain, and a prescription for hormonal birth control—should have been identified immediately as at risk for something far more serious than a panic attack. Instead, she fell through the cracks and ended up in the ICU, fighting for her life.

Fortunately, Tara's story, unlike Sierra's, has a happy ending. She survived. She was lucky. But if someone had just asked the right questions, she wouldn't have had to be.

As it is, Tara's experience is not unique, nor is it confined only to cases in which an acute medical emergency is written off as neurosis, anxiety, or a panic attack. Myriad risk factors for women go overlooked by doctors in this field, owing to continued ignorance within the medical system about the interaction between cultural and occupational gender norms and women's pulmonary health. The conversation about workplace hazards to respiratory health almost invariably centers on industries dominated by men: construction, manufacturing, agriculture, fighting fires. But women in service industries like housekeeping and hairdressing are also exposed to harsh chemicals that can compromise a person's ability to breathe—and, unlike the men working in a sawmill or construction zone, their workday uniform doesn't include protective equipment. According to one recent body of research published by the American Thoracic Society's *American Journal of Respiratory and Critical Care Medicine*, women who work as housekeepers—or who regularly use cleaning sprays in the upkeep of their own homes—are at risk for a dramatic decline in lung function as compared with women who aren't regularly exposed to these products.

That female-coded labor, including household labor, comes with a risk of incurring chronic lung damage is a poignant and grossly overlooked part of the contemporary cultural discourse surrounding women's workforce participation and their disproportionate shouldering of the burdens of housework and childcare. It's also an enormous blind spot for medical professionals: for women with heavy and continuous exposure to cleaning products—which is to say, either working-class women who clean for a living or women in traditionally gendered arrangements that leave them responsible for the bulk of the household upkeep—the harm caused can be equivalent in its effect on the lungs to smoking a pack of cigarettes a day, every day, for twenty years.

And yet, while every medical form includes a question about your history of tobacco use, we never ask women about how many hours per week they spend cleaning their homes with chemical products or caution them on how to avoid damaging their lungs. We don't talk enough, generally, about the way that women's daily lives bring them into contact with things that may compromise their respiratory health. Cleaning chemicals. Salon products. Cooking fumes.

And then, of course, there's the matter of men.

◆ ◆ ◆

It's Saturday night in the hospital ER just outside a major east coast city, and the waiting room is a madhouse. Burns and scrapes wait alongside broken bones and concussions. A young mother holds a red-faced, feverish toddler whose screams rise in tandem with the undulating wails of an approaching ambulance. A grimacing teenage boy, bleeding from a gunshot wound to the leg, is rushed on a stretcher past the reception window, where a weathered old man is shouting at the intake nurse that he was bit—no, *B-I-T*, bit—by a horse. But even in the midst of the chaos, it's impossible not to notice her. She's standing very still, her eyes cast downward, her slender arms wrapped around her own body like she's either frightened, cold, or both.

She is so pale, so frail, as precious and breakable as a china doll. Her eyes are bright, her lips a blushing red, only slightly marred by the swelling at one corner, where a bruise is beginning to form. She's clutching a tissue in one hand, not to dry her eyes but to dab at her mouth—at the place where her lip split when he hit her.

When the people noticing her notice this part, they look away.

Unlike the consumptive girl, coughing gently into a lace handkerchief at the end of her short and tragic life, nobody will write any poetry about the girl in the emergency room. There will be no sonnets or songs about her otherworldly loveliness, about the way the dribble of blood from her split lower lip contrasts with the pale cream of her skin. There is no beauty or meaning in her suffering, and the thing that brought her to the hospital tonight will never be described, by anyone, as "a flattering malady" from which it would be very romantic to die; indeed, her ability to live day in and day out with the thing that's killing her confers no status, no respect, only shame.

As the clock passes midnight, she leans back against the wall, her chin dropping toward her chest. Her breathing is ragged and shallow, and her neck is beginning to bruise: a light purple striation in the place where, hours before, her boyfriend wrapped both hands around her windpipe and squeezed.

She lifts the tissue to her lips.

She coughs.

The intake nurse nods at her: "It won't be long now."

The girl nods back, knowing that it doesn't matter. She's been here before. She'll be here again.

She never tells anyone what he does to her—and for the most part, nobody ever asks.

◆ ◆ ◆

The signs of strangulation in women aren't always obvious. For every patient who presents with obvious ligature marks around her neck or a constellation of burst blood vessels on her cheeks or in the whites of her eyes, there is another who shows no signs at all—and many survivors suffer hypoxia-induced amnesia about the attack itself, owing to the effects of strangulation on blood flow to the brain.

This may be why strangulation assaults are underreported by victims; it is also why they too often go unrecognized by doctors in emergency room settings.

Tami Tiamfook-Morgan, an emergency room physician at Carroll Hospital Center in Maryland, still remembers the patient whose bruised neck they almost didn't notice, whose story came so close to being left untold. She had sustained a gash to her chest—her partner had assaulted her with a broken bottle—and was surrounded by police, EMTs, and nurses, all peppering her with questions she was too overwhelmed to answer.

"She wouldn't talk to anyone. I found out later that she was afraid that if she told the truth, they might take her children away," Tami says. It wasn't until she gave the patient an opportunity to speak privately—an opportunity that required time, space, and trust far beyond the prescriptive protocols of a busy ER—that the woman lifted her chin to show the marks where he'd strangled her. "You can still typically see the fingerprints in strangulation cases, but you have to know to look for it," Tami explains. "And once you see it, you still have to be gentle about asking what happened."

Although strangulation is not a medical disorder per se, it is impossible to discuss the broader issue of women's respiratory health without also discussing its intersection with domestic violence. Of all the injuries a woman may sustain at the hands of a violent partner, strangulation is the most dangerous, not because it is in itself lethal—a majority of women will survive being strangled—but because of what it signifies: it is a key marker for the type of violence that eventually escalates to murder.

Because emergency room doctors are in a unique position to help these women, it is especially tragic that a chaotic ER setting leaves little time for them to recognize the signs of strangulation or to persuade patients to disclose their injuries, which are devastatingly common: some estimates suggest that 10 percent of all women in the US will suffer a nonfatal strangulation incident in their lifetimes. And when doctors don't ask about strangulation symptoms, they also don't offer important information to women who may underestimate the ongoing risks to their health in the aftermath of being strangled, including hematoma, miscarriage, spinal injuries, and brain damage.

"This is on us," Tami says. "These women are traumatized, they're ashamed, they feel responsible. Sometimes they don't even know for sure what happened, because they were strangled until they passed out. If we as physicians don't create space for them to tell their stories, if we don't treat that as a priority in the same way we triage an open wound, we're failing them."

As is so often the case, things are better than they used to be while still not being good enough. When it comes to the broader issue of women's respiratory health, we should consider how the care we give to women is compromised by the lingering legacy of gendered narratives about who women are, or how they should be. Today's physicians do not romanticize domestic violence, for instance, in the way that doctors in the early nineteenth century romanticized tuberculosis. And yet we also do not treat it. In medical education, the harm caused to women's health by abusive partners is an afterthought. In practice, as we race from patient to patient in fifteen-minute increments, doctors are taught to ask after a woman's domestic safety—but only in passing, and only alongside a dozen other questions about a woman's health and medical history. I was sickened by what I learned about the prevalence of domestic violence while working on this chapter, and horrified at my own complicity: How many times have I asked a woman, "Are you safe at home?," never considering that this question in a medical setting leaves little room for any answer more complicated than a nod of the head?

The medical system holds victims of strangulation—and of domestic violence more broadly—at arm's length, in a way that is not entirely dissimilar from the way it used to treat the consumptive girl: as a doomed and beautiful creature, the nature of whose suffering is such that no medicine can cure her. We are, in some ways, still in thrall to the idea of suffering that confers status, that the victims of violence and consumption alike are both distant and captivating in their afflictions. So beautiful. So tragic. Such a terrible loss.

If only there were something we could do, we say. But what if there was?

guts

DIGESTIVE

THE PRICE OF GOING (AND NOT GOING) WITH YOUR GUT

The man said, "The woman you put here with me—
she gave me some fruit from the tree, and I ate it."
Then the Lord God said to the woman, "What is this
you have done?"

—Genesis 3:12–13

I look into myself to understand my infirmity and [the
goodness of] God who by a most singular mercy
allowed me to correct the vice of gluttony.

—Catherine of Siena, in a letter, 1373

It begins as an act of defiance. Catherine is sixteen years old when her older sister dies in childbirth, leaving behind a husband and children: a ready-made family Catherine is told it is her duty to step into. Her parents insist that she marry her sister's widower, and her objections fall on deaf ears—but this, this is a form of protest they can't ignore.

Catherine stops eating. Her meals are pushed away untouched. She cuts off her long hair, and between this and the effects of the fasting on her shrinking body, her womanly curves giving way to sharp angles and deep hollows, she takes back control: the less attractive she is to men, the more they leave her to live as she pleases.

By the time she enters the convent where she will live for the rest of her brief life before dying at the age of thirty-three, it is impossible to disentangle her lack of appetite from that sense of control: peace, purity, the absolute cleanliness of a body unadulterated by the presence of food. For years, the only sustenance that passes Catherine's lips is the body and blood of Christ himself, a single Communion wafer as light as air, a sip of dark wine to wash it down. Apart from that, she allows herself nothing but water and herbs, bitter ones, which she chews and spits out once she's wrung them of their flavor.

Even by the ascetic standards of the monastery, Catherine's refusal of food is extreme and unsettling; her sisters at the convent, and the clergy who mentor her, all encourage her to eat. But she won't. When they force her, she uses a twig to make herself vomit. Even as they stare and shake their heads, she senses the admiration, and maybe even envy, underneath their concern. This is something beyond chastity: a break from the bonds of her mortal body, a complete sublimation of her physical, animal needs. Faith fills her in a way that food never could. She has never been lighter, or cleaner, or closer to God.

Her last words, addressed to her creator, are "Father, into Your Hands I commend my soul and my spirit."

About her body, brittle and wasted from years of starvation, Catherine has nothing to say at all.

◆ ◆ ◆

The history of gastroenterology in women is not just a medical story but a biblical one. Ever since Eve succumbed to temptation by plucking and eating the forbidden fruit, women's appetites have been seen as particularly and inherently dangerous. Notions of purity, femininity, and holiness are inextricably linked to the idea of appetite: for food and, of course, for sex. Notably, eschewing one implied you could also resist the other.

The self-deprivation engaged in by Catherine of Siena in the fourteenth century was, in its less extreme iterations, a common practice within medieval religious communities—but also a gendered one. Men who claimed to be incapable of eating were few and far between; fasting was a woman's game, and, in medieval Europe, the best way for them to prove their spiritual bona fides. The less you ate, the holier you were. Catherine, who ate nothing at all, was canonized as a saint.

As the years passed, the idea of eschewing digestion as a form of religious purity eventually found purchase outside the church, and then inside the medical establishment. It made not just spiritual but logical sense that women should eat less, that they could rise above physical need and sensual desire in a way that men could not. At the table or in the bedroom, men were voracious; women were restrained. The ones who weren't, who openly hungered, were seen as odd and even suspicious.

Sugar and spice and everything nice: that's what little girls are made of.

—attributed to Robert Southey, 1820

By the time that gastroenterology emerged as a field of medical specialization in the late 1800s, the spiritual fasting of the medieval era had given way to a new consensus, more moderate but no less sexist, that women's diets should be restrictive in both quantity and quality. The medical thinking surrounding how, and how much, women should eat was characteristically unflattering to them: eighteenth-century doctors dug into the theory that women were more like children than adults, and that their appetites were hence similarly infantile, emotionally driven, and self-indulgent.

This idea of women as underdeveloped and childlike was prevalent across multiple fields within medicine, coming into vogue alongside Darwinian theories of evolution; depictions of the female skeleton from the same era speak to a similar conviction that women lagged behind men in the species' long march toward modernity. And in gastroenterology, as in most fields, doctors imagined that any treatment of female patients needed to begin by addressing these perceived shortcomings, unique to their sex.

One of said shortcomings was the location of women's reproductive organs inside, rather than outside, the body. The womb took up so much space, doctors noted, that women's digestive systems were necessarily impacted and more prone to irritation. Between that and their smaller teeth and jaws, the conclusion seemed obvious: women just weren't made to eat the same way that men were.

Alexander Walker, a Scottish practitioner whose ideas became influential in women's gastroenterology despite his predilection for pseudosciences, wrote decisively about female dietary needs in his 1845 tome, *Beauty*: "Women prefer light and agreeable food, which flatters the palate by its perfume and its savour."

Walker was mainly obsessed with the aesthetic implications of women's health, perhaps because it was an interest also shared by his wife, who wrote her own treatise on the subject four years later. (Like her husband, Mrs. Walker believed that women's inherent physical inferiorities meant they should eat only easily digested foods that "do not act too powerfully on their delicate fibres," and "only the quantity proportioned to the weakness of their organs, and to the trifling exercises in which they are occupied.") His conclusion, unsurprisingly, was that the most appropriate, natural diet for women was one that also coincidentally kept them thin:

"Hence it is, that women naturally and instinctively effect abstemiousness and delicacy of appetite. Hence it is, that they compress the waist, and endeavor to render it slender."

Meanwhile, the industrial revolution created an opportunity to reimagine the human body as its own sort of machine, while the scarcities of the era meant that fuel for that machine was often in short supply. Meat was set aside for men, whose energy requirements were greater owing to their physically demanding lives and work: the strong, vital male body required strong, vital food to sustain it. Smaller, sweeter foods were associated with women—a dainty diet for a dainty figure.

These gendered ideas surrounding diet eventually calcified into social rituals, including teatime, where women nibbled at delicate cakes and teeny-tiny sandwiches with the crusts cut off. (Women, frail as they were, could hardly be expected to eat anything that required energetic chewing.) Sugar was omnipresent, creating a paradox that persists today: women were expected to gravitate toward sweet foods but also to exercise immense restraint when it came to consuming them in order to remain slim. At restaurants like Schrafft's, a Victorian-era chain eatery that catered to women and advertised itself as "the daintiest luncheon spot in all the State," the menu was heaviest on two categories: salads and desserts. At the same time, the notion that these foods were insubstantial, frivolous, and not for men became culturally entrenched; one 1934 issue of *House & Garden* magazine includes a remonstrance from writer Leone B. Moates, who bemoaned that wives were attempting to make their husbands subsist on ridiculous "dainties" like "a bit of fluff like marshmallow-date whip."

In 1994, Australian sociologist Deborah Luton found that the gendering of foods had changed very little since the Victorian era: participants in her study identified feminine foods as "light, sweet, milky, soft-textured, refined and delicate," and specifically mentioned those tiny, crustless teatime sandwiches as a prime example of the type. The archetypal masculine food, meanwhile, was red meat.

A woman should never be seen eating or drinking, unless it be lobster sallad & Champaigne [*sic*] the only truly feminine & becoming viands.

—Lord Byron to Lady Melbourne, September 25, 1812

If the notion of diet as gendered began as something of a meme, it soon took on the sheen of medical legitimacy. The foods most appropriate for one sex were contraindicated for the other, always with scientific-seeming justifications. Women were warned that stimulating foods, especially salty, spicy, or acidic dishes, would overtax their sensitive nervous systems—or worse, increase their sexual appetites. The notion of food as a gateway drug to depravity, and hence ill health, was commonplace: a woman who overindulged in meat was considered just as debauched as one who drank too much. The medical edicts surrounding what women should and should not eat were in many cases a transparent proxy for controlling their sexuality.

The Victorian conflation of good health and good character make it difficult to untangle the medical conventions of this era from the moral ones, particularly when it comes to gastroenterology. The most influential health experts of the time, even the ones with formal medical education, operated more like modern-day wellness influencers when it came to the guidelines and treatments they promoted, and the dietary advice aimed at women in particular was designed less to improve health than to make their bodies and behavior conform to cultural norms. Women were discouraged from eating meat, or eating too much, not out of concerns that doing so might lead to bad health outcomes, but because appetite was a vice—one they were already considered congenitally less capable of controlling, hence the need for strict rules to contain it. Even a single piece of candy was imbued with all sorts of cultural baggage, depending upon the circumstances under which it was consumed. Food historian Michael Krondl, writing about the Victorian etiquette surrounding both candy and courtship, notes the potent interplay of dietary guidelines, etiquette, and the performance of femininity: "While a woman might favor a gentleman caller by nibbling a bonbon or two from the box he had presented her, the solo pleasure of consuming bonbons in private would only bring opprobrium."

In short, a woman with a dainty figure was, in her slimness, a portrait of self-restraint—which in turn advertised her as a person of culture, sensitivity, and elevated social class. And while the complex courtship rituals and specific dietary guidelines of that era have changed, the way that medical and commercial culture alike conceives of women's gastroenterology has not. Today we find a similar entanglement of health status with wealth status, of medical wisdom with pseudoscientific quackery and fad dieting, and of a struggle for control over women's lives that begins with controlling their appetites.

◆ ◆ ◆

The Battle Creek Sanitarium in 1910 is a monument to health—not as a bodily state, but as a luxury pursuit. It is part spa, part hospital, part fancy hotel; its thirty-acre campus boasts more than two dozen buildings outfitted with marble flooring, Persian rugs, glass greenhouses full of exotic plants. There are bespoke facilities for every imaginable type of therapy: water, light, heat, electric. There are eight indoor pools tiled in pristine white. The lobby is the size of a football field. There is a room just for enemas, complete with a patented machine that will pump a full fifteen quarts of yogurt into your anus if you fail to produce the doctor's prescribed four bowel movements per day.

There are, as one might imagine, a lot of enemas.

Most importantly, there is the doctor: John Harvey Kellogg, the country's greatest guru on the art and science of what he calls "biologic living." Kellogg is a ubiquitous presence, and an unmistakable one. While his staff wear crisp white uniforms, their lab coat collars and aprons stiff with starch, Kellogg favors a style more appropriate for church: impeccable suits, polished shoes, an accessory walking stick. Even with the lower half of his face hidden by an extravagant walrus mustache and a well-kept beard, he has a friendly demeanor—approachable as well as knowledgeable—and he often strolls the grounds of his institute with a pet cockatoo perched on his shoulder. (The cockatoo matches Kellogg's suits: pure white.)

More than one thousand patients might be in residence at the "San," as it's affectionately nicknamed, at any given moment, and Kellogg personally attends to all of them. He takes histories. He makes diagnoses. He prescribes treatments and regimens and extraordinarily strict diets that include not only specifications on which foods to consume, but also how many times to chew before swallowing. He also performs surgeries, sometimes, but what makes the San a destination for its health-seeking clientele is not Kellogg's medical expertise or skill in the operating theater—nor is it the lush grounds, the bathing facilities, the daily calisthenics, or the nightly entertainment.

It's the promise of control. Patients are not brought to Kellogg; they seek him out, from all over the country. And what happens at the San is not about what is done to you; it's about what you're doing for yourself. A hundred years before the term "self-care" enters the lexicon, before a cottage industry of influencers evangelizes about the joy, the fulfillment, of finding just the right combination of supplements to balance your gut biome, Kellogg invites the leisure class to perfect themselves at his health resort: with rest and relaxation, diet and exercise, and the purification of both body and mind that comes from resisting the siren song of your appetites. He will not heal you. He will empower you to heal yourself.

"Disease is cured by the body itself, not by doctors or remedies," he tells his patients, and they believe him. He has the cure, if you have the strength.

You need only come and take it.

Story books, romances, love tales, and religious novels constitute the chief part of the reading matter which American young ladies greedily devour. We have known young ladies still in their teens who had read whole libraries of the most exciting novels. The taste for novel-reading is like that for liquor or opium.

—John Harvey Kellogg, MD, *Plain Facts for Old and Young*, 1879

Although "taking the cure" at Kellogg's sanitarium resembled a lifestyle retreat more than a medical stay, Kellogg was among the best-known and most influential physicians in the country during his heyday at Battle Creek, where he served as director beginning in 1876. And while Kellogg treated both men and women in equal measure at the San, where he remained continuously occupied by the imagined link between dietary decadence and sexual depravity, he was especially convinced of women's unique susceptibility to corruption.

According to Kellogg, allowing women to enjoy spicy or even just flavorful foods was fraught with dangers both medical and moral: "Candies, spices, cinnamon, cloves, peppermint, and all strong essences, powerfully excite the genital organs and lead to the same result," he wrote in the 1880s. The ominous "result," of course, was masturbation, an act with which Kellogg was particularly obsessed. Not only did he believe that masturbation was the fearsome endpoint of eating too much peppermint, he also claimed it was the root cause of a litany of ills including epilepsy, warts, and acne.

Virtually all of Kellogg's dietary guidelines were designed with the goal of subverting sexual arousal in general and masturbation in particular, although to be fair, he didn't see this as only a problem for women, or even only as a problem for other people. One of the things that arguably made Kellogg such a cult figure at the time was that he practiced what he preached: eating a bland vegetarian diet, eschewing liquor and tobacco, and practicing complete sexual abstinence. His marriage was reportedly never consummated, and while he did raise forty-two children—all adopted—he and his wife slept in separate bedrooms all their lives.

But despite evidently having the courage of his convictions, Kellogg's myopic insistence on tracing so many medical problems back to the same source did not serve his patients well. As the proverbial man with a hammer to whom everything looks like a nail—or in Kellogg's case, a masturbator—he levied this diagnosis on an untold number of women, including many who were suffering from entirely treatable ailments with which their doctor should have been familiar. In one case, a female patient presented with a red and swollen breast, likely a condition called mastitis, resulting from an infected milk duct. Kellogg's diagnosis? "Hysterical breast," brought on by (what else?) masturbation. In another, a ten-year-old sexual assault victim's symptoms of "serious nervous disease"—which might well have been PTSD stemming from the assault itself—were chalked up to the girl's alleged masturbation habits, which Kellogg suggested she'd eagerly picked up from the man who raped her.

All told, there were few conditions in the human body that Kellogg didn't believe either stemmed from or led to sexual depravity. Even his fixation on bowel movements (remember, four per day!) ultimately came back to the quest to tamp down on any possible source of sexual excitement, as he believed that constipation would cause young girls to become dangerously and uncontrollably aroused.

Like many of today's contemporary wellness "experts," Kellogg boasted a roster of rich and famous clients who lent him an air of legitimacy no matter how ludicrous his ideas; residents at the sanitarium included Thomas Edison, Henry Ford, and even Amelia Earhart, who would visit the facility and take Kellogg's cure as part of preparation for her important flights. But Kellogg was also a doctor, with all the credibility that entailed. As a result, many of his methods seeped into the mainstream, where they were adopted not just by medical professionals who believed them to be on the cutting edge of dietary science but also by ordinary Americans. These were the people who could never afford a weeklong booking at the San, but who could buy the doctor's prescribed regimen to put on their own breakfast tables: a direct-to-consumer pipeline that entrenched Kellogg's nutritional mores—and with them, his convictions about the moral dangers of a spicy diet—in the public consciousness as much as inside the medical system.

Thanks to the influence of Kellogg and his contemporaries, including Sylvester Graham, the earliest versions of what we now understand as "diet foods" entered the mainstream beginning in the early twentieth century. Kellogg's bran flakes were among them; so was Graham's eponymous cracker.

Neither of these things much resembled their modern-day iterations, which contain sweeteners and preservatives that would no doubt have horrified their creators. (John Kellogg became estranged from his brother, William, after an intense feud over the latter's desire to make a flaked cereal that actually tasted good.) The original diet foods were flavorless—and intentionally so, as they were meant as an antidote to the spicy or otherwise stimulating flavors that these doctors believed were a cause of sexual corruption. They were also plant-based; Kellogg's promotion of a vegetarian diet stemmed in part from the belief that "flesh foods" (meats) left "undigested residues" in the bowels, which would linger inside the body and cause disease. (Kellogg called it "intestinal toxemia," but if you think this sounds a lot like "poop poisoning," you're not wrong.)

And while they were not contraindicated for men, it was women who put these products on their grocery lists, who served them at their tables, and who were told—in a way that men never experienced—that curbing their appetites was not just a matter of good health but moral urgency.

A century has passed since John Harvey Kellogg embarked on a quest to purify women's souls by boring their palates and cleansing their bowels, and Kellogg, along with Graham and his ilk, are generally dismissed as quacks by today's medical establishment. But this doesn't change the fact that for a period of decades—including some of modern gastroenterology's most formative years—America's best-known GI doctor was mainly concerned not with gut health, but with how to manipulate women's diets so that they might never become sexually excited. And, much like the putrid meat residues that Kellogg believed could linger in the bowels and poison the body, many of his ideas are still buried, unexpelled, in both the medical system and the public consciousness.

One can see Kellogg's fear of flesh foods echoed in the latter-day medical obsession with eliminating fat from the American diet. One can see the patients lining up for enemas at the Battle Creek Sanitarium echoed in the contemporary craze for colonics at beautifully appointed medspas—where someone like Gwyneth Paltrow might just be getting the same treatment in the next room. And while the flavorless cereals and crackers once hawked as a way for women to curb their appetites for food and sex alike have been replaced by a landscape of mass-produced, highly processed products that taste less like cardboard than their predecessors, they boast a similar nutritional profile—and a similar promise.

These foods, the advertisements claim, are ones you can enjoy guilt-free.

That dreaded enemy of loveliness and health . . . constipation.

—Ex-Lax advertisement, circa 1935

Girls Don't Poop

—novelty T-shirt, circa 2000

While John Harvey Kellogg's bran flakes were designed to satiate hunger without stimulating the palate (and, by extension, the genitals), there was another reason why they seemed tailored more to one sex than the other: they were an effective treatment for constipation, a problem that has always been more prevalent in women than in men.

Constipation was considered dangerous by doctors who shared Kellogg's mistaken belief that it led to "autointoxication": that unexcreted feces contained toxic by-products of digestion, which would seep into the bloodstream from the GI tract and poison the entire body from the inside out. And because constipation disproportionately impacted women, doctors increasingly became convinced that women must be doing something to cause it.

The reasons why a woman might be blamed for her own gastrointestinal distress ran the gamut: she was failing to exercise, or, barring that, she was overexerting herself. She was eating the wrong foods—or the right ones, but too much of them. She was either too sexual or too frigid. She was either unhealthily obsessed with her bowel movements or too distracted by frivolous concerns to pay them their due attention. Or, barring all that, she might be hysterical.

Perhaps needless to say, the notion that women were to blame for being constipated was about as scientifically legitimate as the notion that a person's blood, brain, and nervous system could be poisoned by the presence of unexpelled feces. (In other words: it was a load of, well, you know.) But among doctors, a portrait began to emerge of constipation not just as a woman's issue but a behavioral one.

In 1874, a London physician named Richard Epps kicked off the constipation discourse with a treatise titled, tellingly, "Constipation, Hypochondriasis, and Hysteria: Their Modern Treatment." Epps doubted the accounts of constipation as an issue rooted in women's anatomy or physiology. Instead, he hypothesized that women were spending too much time riding in carriages, attending too many parties, and neglecting to exercise, leading to sluggish bowels for which they were inexplicably reluctant to seek help. "[The] fair sex have a great (I had almost written invincible) repugnance to seek advice for this ailment," he wrote. "I have often noticed this repugnance in young patients."

"Consequently," Epps noted, young women suffering from constipation were "prone to the quacking of themselves with purgatives"—in other words, they would take laxatives to help themselves poop, but then they couldn't poop without them.

Incredibly, even as young women chose to relieve themselves with laxatives rather than seeking his help with their constipation, Epps seems not to have considered the possibility that bathroom issues might be uniquely embarrassing to his patients, uniquely laden with cultural baggage, and hence uniquely difficult to talk about. Indeed, he expressed bafflement that these same patients answered all his other questions about their health truthfully; it was only on the topic of their bowel movements that they dissembled. Their reluctance to open up, he wrote sniffily, "can hardly be therefore from a feeling that the query is indelicate."

Of course, the way Epps and other physicians of the era wrote about their constipated female patients leaves little mystery as to why these women might have preferred to keep this problem to themselves. "An Essay on Habitual Constipation," written in 1885 by Philadelphia doctor Samuel J. Donaldson, described the average constipated woman as privileged, lazy, negligent in her bathroom habits, and a victim of "nervous derangements"—right before he joined Epps in condemning her for relieving herself with laxatives.

Donaldson, a gynecologist, also theorized a connection between constipation and the reproductive system; perhaps unsurprisingly, he was among the doctors who believed that women's wombs simply took up too much space in their bodies to allow for a properly functioning GI tract. In 1893, New York gynecologist Andrew Currier joined Donaldson in lamenting the unsuitability of women's anatomy to digestion, while taking the allegations of neglectful pooping to another level. Bemoaning "the carelessness of young girls, especially schoolgirls" when it came to answering nature's call, Currier, proposed that "it would be far better for these individuals and for society if their intellectual culture were curtailed."

In other words, little girls were doing too much thinking, and not enough pooping, and these priorities needed to be reversed—not just for their sake but for the betterment of society.

Needless to say, the diagnosis of indifference, neglect, and laziness that doctors tended to direct at women with constipation was woefully inaccurate, and women who took this advice to heart, along with the chastisement not to use laxatives, did not see their condition improve. Meanwhile, an obsession with autointoxication, and its imagined relationship to GI ailments, was taking root in the medical community. While John Harvey Kellogg was pumping yogurt into the rear ends of his patients at the San, a Russian scientist named Élie Metchnikoff was arriving in Paris, along with yogurt cultures he had developed for promoting gut health. Metchnikoff was a step ahead of

Kellogg in his understanding of the gut biome, albeit still mistaken as to the effect of constipation on the body: he believed that probiotics would work inside the GI tract to combat the poisonous microorganisms that would otherwise seep into the bloodstream from a constipated person's colon and cause autointoxication.

Metchnikoff, who would win the Nobel Prize in 1908 for discovering phagocytosis, was something of a star in the scientific community, as was one of his protégés, a British physician named William Arbuthnot Lane. Lane was the closest thing in Victorian England to a celebrity surgeon—his patients included socialites, politicians, and members of the royal family—and one of the first and fiercest advocates of surgical intervention to alleviate constipation (which he termed "chronic intestinal stasis") due to its perceived danger as a precursor to autointoxication. These surgeries could include the complete removal of the colon—and the patients who required this intervention were, of course, mostly women.

Ironically, it is thanks to Metchnikoff and Lane, who were giants in their field and considered the foremost scientific thinkers of the time, that a misguided fixation on autointoxication became so thoroughly entrenched in the medical community—and with it, needlessly aggressive surgical interventions for constipation that disproportionately impacted women. Even Kellogg, who admired the work of these men, was nevertheless disturbed by their predilection for colectomies, a procedure which many patients did not survive; in 1917, he cautioned that "a more thoroughgoing trial of all other possible means, especially dietetic measures, should be made before resorting to so formidable a surgical procedure."

But the influence of physicians like Kellogg and Graham was waning at this moment; even as they had achieved the status of cultural icons, their morally obsessed, lifestyle-oriented approach to wellness was beginning to lose them the respect of the international medical community, where they were seen as "health faddists" rather than true scientists. In another world, someone might have realized that autointoxication was itself a concept unfounded in science; instead, scientists like Lane decided that Kellogg was right about the problem but wrong about how to cure it.

By the time that the idea of women being poisoned by their unevacuated bowels was finally debunked, it had spawned not just countless unnecessary colectomies but another, even more destructive medical theory known as "focal infection," which centered on the idea that all diseases, including mental illnesses, stemmed from a single, often invisible, highly localized infection somewhere in the body. Here, too, doctors agreed that the only course of treatment was surgical; here, too, the results were barbaric. Patients who were unlucky enough to encounter one of these doctors frequently had all their teeth extracted, owing to a widespread conviction that they were harboring hidden toxins. (You'll meet one such patient, Agnes, in our Urology chapter.)

Ultimately, both autointoxication and focal infection fell out of fashion; by the time Lane died in 1943, the medical community had come to view these theories as junk science. So had Lane himself having concluded that most gastrointestinal ailments were the fault of modern life and modern diets. He was, in fact, more right about this than he was about the wisdom of curing constipation by removing the colon, but by then it was too late. Lane's pivot to believing in a more holistic model of gastroenterology cost him both his reputation and his medical practice. In this, he serves as a cautionary tale about how easy it is for mistaken beliefs to become entrenched in medicine, and how difficult they are to correct. And as for the colectomies that Lane first popularized, then died having disavowed? They're still performed today.

The gut has a very complicated nervous system, just like the brain. The gut and brain send signals back and forth constantly. In disorders of gut-brain connection, these signals are like crossed wires; the gut nerve endings can be amplified such that patients feel things a lot more intensely than others.

—Daniela Jodorkovsky, MD, excerpt from interview, 2022

The patients are self-centered and often much worried about mucous stools.

—Sir William Osler, MD, 1912

The year is 1938. The field of gastroenterology is still riddled with misconceptions and strange prejudices, but then, so is society as a whole.

Dorothy, a trained nurse in her early twenties, knows this better than anyone. She comes from old New England stock; she is a daughter of Plymouth Rock, of proud Puritans, of the oldest Protestant tradition in the United States. And now she's in love—with a doctor, a handsome Italian Catholic, who wants to marry her.

Her family is furious. An Italian?! They say that if she goes through with it, they'll never see her again. They'll disinherit her, cast her out; she will be barred from entering their home. This is what her parents told her after she sent a letter to tell them about her engagement. They've been telling her ever since, as often as they can. The letters arrive like clockwork every few days, full of remonstrance and venom.

A joke: the letters are the only thing that's regular.

In the two months that follow the first of the vicious letters, Dorothy suffers from diarrhea, all day, every day. The worst part isn't the discomfort but the humiliation, the fear of finding herself too far from a toilet when an attack comes on. Her doctor prescribes medicine, which doesn't help. She changes her diet; it doesn't help, either. Dorothy's guts keep churning, and the letters keep coming, until finally, it's her wedding day. She and her doctor say their vows at the courthouse; he wears his best gray flannel suit, double-breasted. Hers is blue, to match her eyes.

When they get home, a new letter is waiting.

Dorothy's stomach twists.

She opens it.

She laughs.

After all of this, her parents have decided to accept her engagement. They're sorry to have missed the wedding—they're sorry for everything—and they hope she and her husband will come to visit them soon, at Dorothy's childhood home, where they will always be welcome.

It's such wonderful news, such a welcome change of heart, that it's several days before Dorothy realizes: after two months of agony, the terrible twisting and grinding inside her belly has completely disappeared.

◆ ◆ ◆

In 1912, Sir William Osler made one of the earliest known investigations into the phenomenon that was then called "mucous colitis" and is now referred to as "IBS"—and in doing so, embedded a stereotype in the medical system that still persists today. Then, Osler noted that mucous colitis had become "the fashionable complaint," increasingly prevalent in recent years, and mostly among women. And more than a hundred years later, the female gastroenterology patient is conceived of by contemporary doctors just as she was in Osler's time: anxious, difficult, emotional, and challenging to treat.

These patients, Osler noted, were "nervous in greater or less degree." They suffered from a litany of gendered ailments: hysterical outbreaks, hypochondriasis, melancholia. They were irritatingly obsessed with their health: "patients are self-centered and often much worried about mucous stools." His greatest sympathy, meanwhile, was not for the patients, but for their doctors: these cases were "the most distressing with which we have to deal, invalids of from ten to twenty years standing, neurasthenic to an extreme degree . . ."

The use of the word "neurasthenic" is especially telling. Doctors of the time used it to describe patients suffering from lethargy, fatigue, headaches, and irritability—which is to say, the way most people would feel if they had spent twenty years suffering from chronic and incurable diarrhea. But because the patients were mostly women—and because women, per the medical wisdom of the time, were weaker and more neurotic—Osler posited that IBS was a fundamentally female disease. In women, he deemed it the product of hysteria, while the rare, male patient was diagnosed as being emotionally weak, effete, *feminine*.

"Drugs are of little value," he wrote. "First the basic neurasthenic state is to be dealt with, and this may suffice for a cure."

In fact, Osler wasn't entirely off base about the interplay between an unhappy mind and an unhealthy gut. But without a more contemporary, nuanced understanding of how stress and stress hormones act on the GI system, Osler and doctors like him all ended up drawing similar conclusions—and suffering from similar frustrations, which they turned back on the patient. These women

weren't just difficult to treat, physicians decided; they were difficult, period. They were making themselves sick and miserable.

Nearly thirty years after Osler, the notion of the gut-brain connection was becoming accepted in the field of gastroenterology but
also still largely misunderstood. A tract titled "Mucous Colitis: A
Psychological Medical Study of 60 Cases" noted that "diarrhea as
a symptom of nervousness has been recognized for centuries. It is
only recently, however, that the reaction as a whole has been recognized and given the status of a syndrome."

This booklet, which included the case of the nurse whose stressful engagement coincided with a two-month case of IBS, was published by three physicians in 1939. The writers were top men in
their field: Dr. Chester Jones was employed by Massachusetts General Hospital as well as at Harvard Medical School, where he specialized in "disease of the nervous system." Dr. Benjamin White
was a recent graduate of Harvard Medical School and a gastroenterologist; he would eventually practice at the Hartford Hospital
in Connecticut for over thirty-five years. And then there was Stan-
ley Cobb, an army veteran and Harvard Medical School professor
whose belief in treating patients holistically was genuinely ahead
of its time. Unlike many of his peers, Cobb rejected the framework
that attempted to draw bright lines between the mental and the
physical, and between organic ailments—the ones with an identifiable cause—and functional ones, whose origins were a mystery
and were often treated dismissively by doctors as all in the patient's
head.

"What I wish to emphasize is that there is no problem of 'mind'
versus 'body,' because biologically no such dichotomy can be made,"
he wrote in 1943. "The dichotomy is an artefact; there is no truth
in it, and the discussion has no place in science in 1943 . . . The
difference between psychology and physiology is merely one of complexity. The simpler bodily processes are studied in physiological
departments; the more complex ones that entail the highest levels of
neural integration are studied in psychological departments. There
is no biological significance to this division; it is simply an adminis-
trative affair, so that the university president will know what salary
goes to which professor."

Cobb's inquiries alongside doctors White and Chester into the roots of mucous colitis were part of a long history in which his work as a neurologist continually revealed a powerful connection between the brain and the GI tract. He already knew that what happened in the stomach could manifest as remarkable results in the brain: in 1922, Cobb was tasked by Harvard with unraveling why starvation worked as an effective treatment for epilepsy, with his findings leading to the development of the ketogenic diet. But he still didn't quite understand the interplay of neurology with gastroenterology, or why such an issue should impact women so much more than men.

Instead, he and his coauthors ultimately posited that IBS was a function of personality type. The diarrhea these patients suffered from was a manifestation of their emotional brokenness: loose stools to counteract a rigid, terrible personality.

"The authors believe that the commonest source of parasympathetic overstimulation in patients with mucous colitis is emotional tension," they concluded. "The three emotions, anxiety, guilt, and resentment are the most commonly associated with tension in patients with mucous colitis."

Even at the cutting edge of medical inquiry, even with a more open mind in the mix than most physicians of the era had, this was the consensus wisdom when it came to women's GI issues: IBS is a bitch . . . and so are you.

Doctors are often handicapped by the mere fact that when treating the diseases of women, they suggest and insist on "examinations" and "local treatment." A great many of them do not know that this is absolutely unnecessary.

—Ray Vaughn "R.V." Pierce, MD, 1896

As much as the history of women's gastroenterology is a story of medical missteps, it is also a story of charlatans and snake-oil salesmen who knew all the right moves. Between the embarrassing nature of GI problems, the adversarial stance many doctors took toward patients who presented with them, and the natural tendency of people disenfranchised by a given system to seek ways around it, it was only a matter of time before a shadowy direct-to-consumer medical model sprang up in response to the shortcomings of the official one: a system that made patients, and especially women, feel like they were in control and getting the care they needed.

Doctors like R.V. Pierce, who advertised their cures via traveling medicine shows and mail-order catalogs, were not formally trained. Ray Vaughn Pierce was an 1862 graduate of the Eclectic Medical Institute of Cincinnati, a nineteenth-century center for alternative medical training; after he graduated, he founded the Buffalo-based World's Dispensary Medical Association, from which he dispensed tonics, elixirs, and nostrums including the "Extract of Smart Weed" that was advertised as "Dr. Pierce's Favorite Prescription." At the height of his success, advertisements for Pierce's products were ubiquitous—you might encounter one in the newspaper while you drank your morning coffee, another plastered twelve feet high on the side of a building on your way to work—and his dispensary was raking in the then-astronomical sum of half a million dollars per year.

Pierce's lack of formal medical credentials hardly mattered to the patients—mainly women—who flocked to purchase his wares. If anything, these practitioners of fringe medicine were better than the real thing. Those men who had been to medical school would doubt you, dismiss you, even blame you for making yourself sick. Dr. Pierce didn't do that. Dr. Pierce listened. His advertisements didn't just target women; they spoke to them, taking them into confidence, making them feel seen and respected.

"Many women lie to the doctor," reads one such advertisement, which was printed in newspapers all over the country in 1896. "They know that if they admit certain symptoms that the doctor will inevitably insist on an 'examination.'"

A woman reading this advertisement would have understood instantly the "certain symptoms" in question—constipation—as well as the fearful insinuations of the quotes around the word "examination": something invasive, something embarrassing, something any self-respecting woman would tell a lie to avoid. Yet rather than chiding her for failing to tell her doctor the truth, this advertisement takes an approving view of this small act of rebellion. Not only is it understandable, it's correct: "Quite often the doctor is too busy and too hurried to make the necessary effort to obtain the facts. He frequently treats symptoms for what they appear to be on the surface, when the real cause and the real sickness is deeper and more dangerous. A derangement of the distinctly feminine organs will derange the whole body."

The ad goes on at length, but you get the message—as did the woman for whom it was intended.

THE DOCTOR DOESN'T BELIEVE YOU, BUT I DO.

THE DOCTOR CAN'T HELP YOU, BUT I WILL.

THE DOCTOR DOESN'T KNOW WHAT'S WRONG WITH YOU—BUT YOU DO, AND YOU DON'T NEED HIM, BECAUSE WITH THIS PRESCRIPTION, YOU CAN CURE YOURSELF.

Even as they flattered women that they understood their own medical needs better than a dismissive doctor, the makers and marketers of supplements also spoke to something that women wanted even more than a well-oiled digestive system: beauty. "Girls, be Attractive to Men—Nature Intended You Should Be!" reads one ad; "The Girl the Men Admire . . . Is the one with sparkling eyes—a clear, radiant, youthful complexion!" says another, above an image of a blushing beauty caught in the respectful embrace of a young suitor. Even the Kellogg's company—the one founded by John Harvey's estranged brother, William—got in on the action: an All-Bran advertisement from the same era as Dr. Pierce's prescriptions proclaims that constipation "poisons the whole system" and "steals the charm and beauty of women."

As always, the conflation of health with beauty was a powerful marketing tool. Here women were offered a way to indulge their more base, and basic, desires—to be pretty, to attract men—under cover of simply making themselves well. And as quaint as these printed narratives seem, their message, and method, is timeless; it's why, in 2024, everything from colonics to Botox injections is marketed to women under the heading of "self-care."

Dr. Pierce, meanwhile, was a pioneer not only of the direct-to-consumer business of dietary supplements but also the alternative-medicine-to-politics pipeline. After making a fortune hawking his miracle cures, his name recognition from the "Favorite Prescription" days helped him win elections to the New York State Senate and then the House of Representatives, where he served for less than a year before resigning due to ill health. As for those prescriptions, it's unclear whether they ever had the promised effect on women's digestive systems or complexions, but there was another reason why his customers would have kept coming back for more: most of his elixirs, including the famous "Extract of Smart Weed," contained opium.

The patriarchy has seeped into women's intestinal tracts. Let's call it the pootriarchy.

—Jessica Bennett and Amanda McCall, "Women Poop. Sometimes At Work. Get Over It.," *New York Times*, 2019

Irritable bowel syndrome, constipation, gallstones, a delayed emptying of the stomach known as gastroparesis: these are among the many gastrointestinal ailments that still plague women disproportionately, as most GI conditions do. The reasons why are a complicated tangle of medical bias, cultural mores, entrenched pseudoscience, a lingering sense that digestive functions are unfeminine and embarrassing—and then, on top of all that, physiological differences that make the female gut more complicated.

On the latter front, hormones have a lot to do with it. The female body contains higher levels of estrogen and progesterone, and both of these inhibit the contraction of smooth muscles like the ones that line the GI tract. Food moves more slowly through a woman's gut than a man's. It also has farther to go, because women's colons are longer.

The anatomical differences in a female body make colonoscopies— a necessary procedure for diagnosing many GI problems—more difficult both for doctors to perform and for women to endure. It's a particular problem in a medical system where success is defined as seeing the maximum number of patients in the minimum amount of time: a gastroenterologist can perform fewer colonoscopies in a given day if the patient base includes women, which reads to a volume-based system as the doctor being less productive. This not only presents a challenge for women who may struggle to access the care they need but also creates professional obstacles for the few female gastroenterologists in the field (fewer than one in five practicing gastroenterologists are women), since most women prefer to receive this type of treatment from a doctor of the same sex.

Dr. Susan Lucak, a gastroenterologist who mainly treats IBS patients, explains the catch-22 of performing these important diagnostic procedures on women in a system that doesn't want to allow her the time to do it safely: "They are technically more difficult, and they're also riskier," she tells me. Ordinarily a colonoscopy takes her half an hour; on a female patient, she says, it may take twice that: "I have to allow an hour. Because they just take much longer, and they're riskier, and I have to be more careful."

But when it comes to those anatomical differences—the same ones that doctors in the 1800s chalked up to the inherent inferiority and weakness of the female body—there's more to it than pure biology. We don't have to call it "the pootriarchy," as *New York Times* writers did in a much-ridiculed 2019 article (title: "Women Poop. Sometimes At Work. Get Over It."), but they were undeniably onto something with the general thrust of the piece, which documented the ubiquitous anxiety women experience about pooping in public.

"We may be living in an age where certain pockets of the corporate world are breathlessly adapting to women's needs—company-subsidized tampons, salary workshops, lactation rooms," the article reads. "But even in the world's most progressive workplace, it's not a stretch to think that you might have an empowered female executive leading a meeting at one moment and then sneaking off to another floor to relieve herself the next."

As Dr. Lucak explains, women aren't born with the longer, more circuitous colon that makes their colonoscopies so much riskier to perform. At the age of twenty, a woman's digestive tract is anatomically indistinguishable from a man's, more or less. But all those years of holding it in—or not taking enough time to let it out— takes its toll.

"Guys, they go to the bathroom, they take their newspaper, and they sit there for forty-five minutes, right? In peace," Lucak says. A woman, on the other hand, doesn't have the luxury of spending nearly an hour in the bathroom: because her kids are screaming outside the door, because the boss will wonder why she's not at her desk, or just because she doesn't want anyone to figure out what she's doing in there. Women learn early and often that their bodily functions are embarrassing and should be kept hidden. They learn to either hurry up in the bathroom or hold it in until they can use one at home. And while the unexpelled feces in a woman's system won't cause brain poisoning, as John Harvey Kellogg once suggested, constipation does trigger changes in the body. An overstuffed colon has two choices: to explode, or to expand, and so expand is what it does. Multiply that expansion over the course of a lifetime, and the changes are profound.

The irony is that constipation begets constipation: the more a woman holds in her stools because it's not a convenient time to defecate, the more the colon grows to accommodate them. The more the colon grows, the longer it takes for waste to move through the system. The longer it takes, the more she suffers from constipation by default—and on, and on. And despite many advancements in GI medicine, very little has changed for women who develop the condition known as megacolon as a result of chronic constipation: even as William Arbuthnot Lane lost credibility in his own time, today's doctors still perform the partial colectomies he pioneered (albeit as a last resort).

Meanwhile, constipation remains such a constant and intractable issue for women that even non-GI doctors can't help but be aware of it. In the course of treating women for breast cancer, I often find myself warning my patients that one of the medications they'll be taking has a side effect of diarrhea.

I'm no longer surprised when their response is, "Great!"

My understanding of women's GI disorders has changed over the years. People have to be understanding and sympathetic and not just assume women's own anxiety and neurosis are to blame. I don't think it's the whole story. They weren't born like this.

—Gil Weitzman, MD, gastroenterologist, excerpt from interview, 2022

The doctors of yore believed that IBS was a disease with neither cause nor cure, the physical manifestation of a rigid and unpleasant personality, and even more miserable for doctors to treat than it was for patients to suffer from. When I did my own medical training in the early 2000s, the only difference was that doctors were slightly more hesitant to say all of this quite so candidly, or quite so loud.

IBS was still believed to be an anxiety-driven disease, a hallmark of psychological issues whether they had been documented or not. It was also a disease that nobody wanted to see listed in a patient's chart; the general consensus was that the stereotype of these patients as draining and difficult was based entirely in truth. That stereotype has proved extraordinarily intractable, in spite of advancements in the field of gastroenterology generally: even this year, when I mentioned to a colleague that I was interviewing a provider (Dr. Susan Lucak) who treats IBS patients exclusively, he went wide-eyed.

"I can't imagine taking care of IBS patients full-time," he said. "It's completely draining."

Medical history is full of moments in which a woman suffering from a functional illness—that is, an illness with no apparent cause—was told that her condition was psychosomatic, all in her head. IBS is perhaps the greatest example of one of these illnesses, but also a prime example of how doctors could be incredibly wrong even when they were a little bit right.

The existence of a gut-brain connection has long been established fact—it was via this same connection, after all, that Cobb observed how changes to an epileptic patient's diet could improve brain function. And yet, researchers are still discovering daily just how complex that connection is. The lining of the human GI tract, from esophagus to rectum, contains more than one hundred million nerve cells comprising the enteric nervous system (ENS), which operates both independently and in communication with the central nervous system in the brain and spinal cord. And that communication, despite what many physicians once believed, is a two-way pipeline within which either system might issue commands. A patient's anxiety can show up in the gut as IBS—or, an IBS-afflicted gut can send signals up the chain that manifest as anxiety. The ENS, which is sometimes referred to as "the second brain," means that the roots of IBS and other gut ailments are thoroughly tangled up with a patient's emotional state, mental health, and stress levels.

The mistake doctors made, and continue to make, is imagining that a disease that's in the patient's head must therefore, in some sense, be a fabrication over which the patient has control.

Consider the flow of hormones that regulates a woman's menstrual cycle. It begins with the brain, the hypothalamus, which sends a message to the pituitary gland, which responds by releasing gonadotropic hormones that trigger ovulation, menstruation, and so on. But those same hormones also impact the GI tract—and make certain IBS symptoms worse. In other words, the root of a patient's bloating, pain, and diarrhea may well be all in her head, in that it literally originates there. But is she imagining it? Responsible for it? Is it her fault that stress manifests in her body in the form of a disease that's extremely difficult to treat?

Additionally, the fact that IBS continues to be primarily a woman's disease—and more than that, a *young* woman's disease—means that a certain amount of soft sexism continues to surround it. Doctors are less versed in the gendered issues that may contribute to IBS; they're more likely to have been taught that the disease is psychosomatic and intractable; they're more likely to become frustrated with the patient, who they've been warned is probably a miserable, difficult person. (It doesn't help that IBS is, in fact, a truly miserable condition to have. A 2017 article in the *New England Journal of Medicine* notes that the impact of IBS on a patient's quality of life is so profound, "it has been estimated that patients would give up 10 to 15 years of life expectancy for an instant cure of the disease.")

Dr. Lucak's patients usually come to her after years of fruitless struggle to manage their symptoms. They've been shuffled from doctor to doctor, endlessly tweaked their diets, bought every supplement that someone on Instagram promised would perfect their gut biome. Many describe being sent home from previous doctors with a shrug and the same rote advice. More fiber, more water, less stress—and sometimes a more specific and galling recommendation: "You know, honey, why don't you get yourself a boyfriend?"

◆ ◆ ◆

If the history of gastroenterology is tangled up with issues of control, oncology is about making peace with the limits of it. Cancer comes not just with the fear of death but the horror of losing control: your disease isn't the product of a foreign invasion, a virus, or a bacteria but one of your own cells suddenly gone rogue and spreading sickness from within. For many of my patients, the sense of being betrayed by their own bodies manifests as a fixation on diet: What did I eat or drink that caused this? What can I put into my body now to fix whatever went wrong?

Sometimes, that quest to take back power over the body does yield positive results—less alcohol, more sleep, a more balanced diet—that promote better health and a better chance of tolerating the difficult path to healing ahead. But I also see too many women falling prey to the illusion of control offered by expensive supplements and endless marketing that feeds on their fear, and the medical system's weaknesses, with a series of familiar messages:

> The doctor doesn't believe you, but I do.
> The doctor can't help you, but I will.
> The doctor doesn't know what's wrong with you—
> but you do, and you can cure yourself.

In the best cases, this manifests in the form of a patient who submits to a traditional course of treatment but also spends a fortune, on the side, for expensive colonics and detox diets; it's as though she believes she won't get well unless she has also been purified. But one of the most heartbreaking things I have seen in my medical practice—and a stark reminder of the dangerous mistrust that lingers in a system where women feel doubted, dismissed, and disenfranchised—is the patient with a curable cancer who chooses to put her faith in supplements instead.

My last one was Sophia, a thirty-five-year-old HR professional and immigrant from Central America who bore the psychic scars of having lost her mother to breast cancer twenty years earlier. For a cancer patient, Sophia was lucky: her disease was not only curable but could be treated with minimal, mild side effects. But her mistrust of the medical system, owing in part to cultural barriers and in part to the dismissive treatment of her mother by doctors in the late 1990s, was all-consuming—and our efforts to persuade her were only further evidence, to her mind, of a systemic conspiracy to hospitalize her. Instead, she turned to alternative therapies, as scammy as they were ineffective: vitamin C tablets from Amazon and weekly IV infusions at a medspa that promised "immune-boosting" benefits.

By the time she returned, a year later, her cancer wasn't curable anymore. Within months, she was gone.

This is the dark legacy of charlatans like Dr. R.V. Pierce, but it is not only theirs: it also belongs to the medical doctors who doubted their patients, or blamed them, or shamed them, until the man selling opium-laced snake oil seemed like the best option. And while the chasm of mistrust that has existed between doctors and patients since the days of Dr. Pierce's Favorite Prescription may be shrinking, it's still one into which too many women end up throwing their time, their money, and sometimes even their lives.

Hot girls have IBS.

—Los Angeles billboard, 2021 (first attributed to Connie Shepherd, circa 2019)

Today, the landscape of women's gastroenterology is different but no less complex than it was when John Harvey Kellogg was pumping people full of yogurt at Battle Creek. The public conversation about women's GI health is still as much a product of popular science (or sometimes pseudoscience) and cultural mores as it is medical wisdom—but the wellness influencers of today are more likely to be patients than doctors, and even more likely to be young women, driving the conversation from the perspective of personal experience. It's on this front that things have undeniably changed for the better: the upcoming generation of women does not share the same sense of shame around these issues, and they're not afraid to talk about poop, including on social media, where entire communities have sprung up around the sharing (and sometimes over-sharing) of what used to be considered personal and embarrassing medical information. It's too soon to know how these young women might change the way that doctors approach GI health—but it's interesting to imagine that Gen Z might usher in a new era of gender parity when it comes to the length of their colons.

At the same time, the miasma of medical and cultural anxieties surrounding women's appetites—and the complex intersection of food with sex, and with sexual attraction—is undergoing a fascinating transformation. In its present form, it can seem almost empowering: a subversion of the stereotype of the IBS patient as an anxiety-ridden control freak, a celebration of GI problems as an identity unto themselves. Being uninterested in eating—or unable to eat at all—is still in certain senses a mark of femininity, but the vibe has shifted. Two centuries ago, the embodiment of femininity was a bonbon-nibbling coquette; today, she's an e-girl dancing on TikTok beneath a glittering digital marquee that reads, *HOT GIRLS HAVE IBS.*

Connie Shepherd, the twenty-five-year-old originator of the now-ubiquitous "hot girls have IBS" meme, is a self-diagnosed sufferer of the disease. In an interview with the website Stat, she said that it was just a factual observation: "The prettiest, tiniest girls that I knew . . . were always complaining about tummy problems," she said. "These are the same girls with food sensitivities, irregular bowel movements, girls and women who experience bloating, dietary restrictions, all of the same breed."

There are good things about the way that IBS has become an identity around which a community has sprung up: here women can find support, information, and the crucial knowledge that they're not alone. There are good things about the way that sufferers of GI disorders can find an outlet, safe from shame and stigma, to talk openly about what's happening to their bodies—or even find ways to make their suffering sexy. There are also good things about the holistic medicine boom that has sprung up online, where the spirit of experimentation can promote increased awareness of promising but peculiar treatments. (Among the potentially promising gut medicines whose visibility has been improved by social media: fecal transplants that aim to populate a volatile GI tract with microorganisms borrowed from another person with a stomach of steel.)

The only thing that remains is for this social, cultural, digital transformation of the conversation surrounding gut health to also work its influence on a medical system that has not yet fully caught up. But here, there's reason to be hopeful: when it comes to gastrointestinal medicine, scientific breakthroughs have often been downstream of social ones. And in this moment, perhaps more than at any other time in history, women are hungry for change.

CHAPTER 7

bladder

URINARY

A THOUSAND YEARS OF HOLDING IT IN

The young wife of the pharaoh has been in labor for more than seventy-two hours when her bladder finally ruptures.

She doesn't know it's happening. She feels nothing but the fierce, immediate, ceaseless agony of her contractions, as her body fruitlessly attempts to expel the child she's carrying. She labors with no purpose now except to relieve her own suffering. The baby is dead and has been for many hours, crushed against the bony confines of her pelvis, which is too narrow for it to pass through. She will never know this child, never nurse him, never hear him cry, and even knowing this, the cruelest part is yet to come: when the young woman's labor comes to an end, when they pull the baby free in a gush of blood and fluid, it will only be because the tiny corpse has decayed enough to allow its skull to collapse.

And what should have been a moment of great joy, the birth of a son to Pharaoh Mentuhotep II by his priestess consort Henhenit, is instead marked by tragedy: not just the death of the baby but the ruin of the woman who carried him. Her vagina has collapsed, crushed between her rectum and her distended bladder. Her large intestine has been forced out of her body by the pressure of childbirth; a nearly four-inch section of it protrudes from her anus. But the most destructive of her injuries is a fistula, a massive perforation between the wall of her ruptured bladder and her vagina.

For the rest of Henhenit's short life, she will be tormented by the unstoppable flow of urine that runs out of her bladder, down her vaginal canal, and onto her legs, her clothes, her bedding. Bacteria will breed in her now-useless urethra, causing ceaseless urinary tract infections that eventually move into her kidneys. The pharaoh will abandon her, sending her away from the palace to live in seclusion. It's not that he doesn't care; it's just that not even the most potent spices and incense can mask the way she smells.

At the end, Henhenit will die alone, in shame, having never again slept in a bed that wasn't damp and soiled. The physicians who attend her will agree that it's for the best—not because they didn't know what was the matter with her but because her condition was one for which there was no cure. Thousands of years from now, researchers will unearth two remarkable artifacts. One is Henhenit's mummified corpse, in which the damage to her body caused by traumatic labor is still visible: the crushed vagina, the prolapsed bowel, the ruptured bladder, have all been perfectly preserved.

The other is the medical wisdom of the time when it came to women who suffered from incontinence, not so much a solution as a helpless shrug:

[I]f the urine keeps coming . . . and she distinguishes it, she will be like this forever.

—The Papyrus Kahun, 1825 BCE

The condition is incurable and remains so until death.

—Avicenna, eleventh-century physician, on incontinence, 1025

Much as Henhenit's fistula could still be observed on her mummified corpse thousands of years later, the stigma and shame surrounding her condition—and the insouciant helplessness of the doctors who treated her—became calcified within the medical conscience, defining the approach to women's urinary issues for years to come. Even at the time, doctors would have found Henhenit's incontinence uniquely frustrating; the ancient Egyptians were skilled in pharmacology, dentistry, even surgery, and yet here was a problem about which they knew nothing, for which they had neither treatment nor cure.

But if their choice to write the problem off as unsolvable seems callously incurious from a contemporary perspective, they were hardly alone in it—nor in preferring to focus on ailments that they could actually treat. The history of women's urologic medicine is in many ways a history of unasked questions, unprobed possibilities, and unexplored territory, owing to the early and persistent perception that nothing could be done. Women, ashamed of their incontinence, tended not to talk about it; doctors, frustrated by their inability to help, tended not to ask. The medical literature that does exist on the topic is often permeated with despair. Writing about fistulas in the eleventh century, the Persian physician Avicenna could land only on a preventive and highly impractical, solution: women could avoid developing the condition, he said, if they never got pregnant in the first place. Johann Friedman Dieffenbach, a nineteenth-century German physician who specialized in skin transplantation and plastic surgery, similarly bemoaned the plight of incontinent women in 1845: "A vesico-vaginal fistula is the greatest misfortune that can happen to a woman, and the more so, because she is condemned to live with it, without the hope to die from it; to submit to all the sequelae of its tortures till she succumbs either to another disease or to old age," he wrote. Dieffenbach understood that the tragedy of incontinence wasn't just about physical torment but the social side effects of being constantly wet, constantly smelling of urine. "The Husband has an aversion for his own wife; a tender mother is exiled from the circle of her own children. She sits, solitary and alone in the cold, on a perforated chair."

Meanwhile, physicians in the "four humours" school of medicine—the one that believed health was tied to the balance of the bodily substances blood, phlegm, yellow bile, and black bile, and which remained in vogue from the time of Hippocrates until the mid-1800s—took it a step further, advancing the notion that incontinence stemmed from a natural female predilection for leaking. Menstrual blood, breast milk, vaginal discharge, urine: to be a woman, it seemed, was to be constantly discharging fluid, particularly from one's genitals. It's not hard to understand why, in the face of such an intractable problem, the idea that women were just naturally moist would have a certain appeal for doctors: if the patient's incontinence was a constitutional matter, simply part of the natural feminine condition, then surely it wasn't anyone's fault if they couldn't cure it.

At this time, we can see the beginnings of a trend that would only be exacerbated by the rise of organized medicine in the 1850s. Women's urinary issues went from being intractable to being invisible, a dark-matter universe of conditions that there was increasingly no way for women to talk about—even with each other. The problem of incontinence after childbirth was surely common knowledge among the midwives who attended to women during and after pregnancy, but midwives were about to be pushed out: as medicine began to evolve into a formal practice with multiple fields of study, a rivalry began to percolate between the physicians who practiced modern medicine and the "irregulars" who didn't. Naturopathy, osteopathy, homeopathy, and other "fringe" forms of medicine were officially out of vogue, and medical societies took steps to sideline those who practiced them.

Needless to say, the quest to push out the irregulars wasn't entirely unwarranted. Many of these doctors were not only not formally educated but often peddled worthless if not actively harmful treatments like phrenology or toxic (and noxious) herbal concoctions. But the medical gatekeepers didn't just bar the door to the con artists and medical misfits with their snake-oil tinctures and head-measuring calipers; they also shut women out of the profession entirely. The midwives, who had long been the primary custodians of knowledge about the medical issues that impact women specifically, found themselves relegated to the fringes. Medicine began to fracture into the system of specialization that still exists today, as doctors began to conceive of patients less as whole people than as an amalgamation of systems and body parts.

And as the system fractured, some of this ancient knowledge simply fell through the cracks.

By the 1870s, pregnancy and childbirth and all its attendant complications were suddenly no longer the purview of the female midwives who had been dealing with them for centuries, but of men, in the newly specialized field of modern gynecology. Not long thereafter, in 1902, the field of urology sprang up as gynecology's male counterpart—and if you'd asked one of these doctors at the time, he surely would have told you that they had everything covered. Boys have a penis, girls have a vagina, and each has a doctor, so what's the problem?

And that's how the medical profession just sort of forgot that women need to pee, too.

You can't say happiness without saying "penis"!

—urology novelty card, 2022

The William P. Didusch Center for Urologic History is the world's preeminent museum dedicated to the field of urology. It is also, not to put too fine a point on it, absolutely full of dicks. It's not just that virtually every historical figure in the field is male, although it is that, too (a list on the website of "doctors, inventors, educators and researchers who helped shape urology" includes exactly one woman out of eighty-one listings). It's that urology is widely understood, by both the general public and its practitioners alike, to be a place for penises.

Those who visit the Didusch Center will find no shortage of dick-based content to enjoy. The permanent collection includes all sorts of tools designed for use on male genitals, from an antique catheter made by Benjamin Franklin as a gift for his brother (thoughtful!) to circa 1900 anti-masturbation devices that look like bear traps and were supposed to prevent wet dreams (ouch!). A library of medical illustrations depicts every variety of penile affliction from curvature, to tumors, to gangrene. At the gift shop, you can pick up a pack of novelty cards replete with penile puns ("Urologists make a vas deferens!"), a set of surprisingly tasteful "phallus socks" with little penis silhouettes on them, a truly disturbing collection of bottle stoppers and corkscrews (use your imagination), or a "Hopping Willy" windup toy that looks like a penis with red plastic feet.

There's one piece of merchandise, just one, that mentions women at all: a toddler-sized T-shirt depicting a little boy getting walloped in the crotch by a tree branch. It says, *IT'S OK, MY MOM'S A UROLOGIST.*

The notion that a woman might not just be but also need a urologist is simply not considered—not by the purveyors of dick-themed novelty items, obviously, nor by anyone else. Urology is a male-dominated field in general—about 90 percent of urologists are male—but it's hard to overstate just how absent women are from urological medicine at a conceptual level. In the eyes of the history, the literature, the textbooks, the drawings, and, yes, the urology gift shop, the patients are men, men, men. It's not that the Big Dick Energy of urological medicine is off-putting to women; it's that it leaves no room for them to imagine themselves as patients. If urology is about dicks, and gynecology is about sex and babies, where does a woman suffering from incontinence seek help for her condition?

Death would have been preferable. But patients of this kind never die; they must live and suffer.

—James Marion Sims, MD, 1894

It is 1819, and James Marion Sims is trying not to cry.

Two hundred years later, Sims becomes known as one of the most influential figures in the history of women's medicine—and also one of the most controversial, a man with a fraught and complicated legacy. His likeness, a nine-foot statue cast in bronze, will stand for three-quarters of a century at the northeast corner of Central Park across from the New York Academy of Medicine on 103rd Street, until 2017, when someone spray-paints the word *RACIST* across its granite base and the city votes to remove it. Countless articles will be written both defending and decrying him; no consensus will be reached as to how he should be remembered.

But in the year 1819, James Marion Sims isn't controversial. He's not a doctor. He's not even a man. He's a six-year-old boy, bent over the knee of his schoolmaster, Quigley, a man with one eye and a face ravaged by smallpox scars. The one-eyed man is whipping Sims's legs with a hickory switch, and Sims is struggling to hold back his screams. He'll succeed for a while, until he doesn't, and, really, it doesn't matter. The man with the switch will keep whipping Sims no matter what noises he makes, or doesn't. He'll whip him until he either vomits or pisses himself from the pain. And then he'll stop, but only because it's another boy's turn, and only until tomorrow.

Tomorrow, he'll whip him again.

The violence the boardinghouse master inflicts on a six-year-old Sims is not unlike the indignity that Sims will inflict upon the enslaved women who come to him for treatment, and upon whom he will develop the techniques that define his legacy. It is brutal. It is degrading. And it is, perhaps most horrifying, utterly typical for its time.

It's 1840 when Sims sets up his practice in Montgomery, Alabama, in a modest two-story building made of red brick. Enslaved people make up nearly two-thirds of the population of Montgomery at this time, and they are the majority of Sims's patients; he treats them in a makeshift hospital installed in a corner of the yard. Like most doctors of the era, he's a general practitioner and surgeon. Gynecology as a medical specialty does not exist, and women's reproductive medicine holds no particular interest for Sims. Indeed, he seems to find it repulsive, and women who arrive at his office seeking treatment in this area are promptly turned away: "If there was anything I hated," he writes in his autobiography, "it was investigating the organs of the female pelvis."

Like so many doctors before him, Sims is also convinced that vaginal fistula is an intractable, incurable condition. He laments the tragedy that afflicted women endure—it is, truly, a fate worse than death—but he still turns them away, so thorough is his conviction that nothing can be done.

And that's how it goes for years—until, with an epiphany, it doesn't.

The patient who changes everything doesn't have a fistula, and she isn't a slave; she's a white woman, forty-six years old, whose uterus has been knocked out of position after falling from a horse. Despite the fact that her affliction resides in Sims's least favorite place—those loathed organs of the female pelvis—she's in too much distress for him to turn her away, and unlike the women suffering from fistulas, he thinks he knows how to help her. Placing her on her knees and forearms with a sheet thrown over her for modesty, he then approaches her exposed rear end from behind and inserts two fingers into her vagina. From this position, he is supposed to be able to press his fingers against the walls of the uterus, thus forcing it back into its proper position. But then something peculiar happens: he can't feel a thing. Where he had been touching the walls of the woman's uterus, now there's nothing—"As if I had put my two fingers into a hat." At the same time, the woman cries out with relief: the agonizing pain and pressure she had been experiencing since her fall is suddenly gone.

It's not until the patient tries to roll over—and releases a sonorous blast of air from her vagina—that Sims realizes what he's done . . . and what he could do, for those other women.

The ones who were supposed to be incurable.

The ones in the tent in the backyard.

That was before the days of anesthetics, and the poor girl, on her knees, bore the operation with great heroism and bravery.

—James Marion Sims, MD, 1894

Lucy. Betsy. Anarcha. We know the names of the enslaved women upon whom Sims operated, but their voices are silent; no first-person account of their experience survives, in all likelihood because none was ever made to begin with. As a result, we can never know what these women felt, or thought, about the conditions from which they suffered—and as for the experimental surgeries they endured at Sims's hospital, we have only his version of events to go on, one colored by prejudices of all kinds. Even his glowing account of Betsy's bravery raises uncomfortable questions, when doctors have long labored under the misconception that Black patients, and particularly Black women, suffer less from conditions that are excruciating to white patients. This problem persists today in contemporary medical settings, in the form of discrimination against Black patients when it comes to rating and medicating pain; in Sims's time, it is entirely possible that his willingness to perform experimental surgery on enslaved women—repeatedly, without anesthesia, and with nothing but opium to help them manage the pain as they convalesced—stemmed from the predominant wisdom of the time that they wouldn't really feel it, not like a white woman would.

For all of these reasons and more, Sims's legacy as a medical pioneer is among the most fraught, the subject of more controversy than that of perhaps any other practitioner in history. But he did operate on Lucy, Betsy, and Anarcha—and he did, ultimately, figure out how to fix the vesicovaginal fistulas that doctors had been dismissing as hopelessly incurable since 2000 BCE.

The problem with fistula, the reason why it had confounded so many physicians over so many years, was not just that it was impossible to fix but impossible to see, buried inside the dark interior of a woman's body. But Sims's patient with the prolapsed uterus had given him an idea: "If I can place the patient in that position, and distend the vagina by the pressure of air . . . why can I not take the incurable case of vesico-vaginal fistula, which seems now to be so incomprehensible, and put the girl in this position and see what exactly are the relations of the surrounding tissues?"

It would be some time yet before Sims developed the techniques and instruments (including the vaginal speculum, which he is widely credited as having invented) that allowed him to surgically correct a fistula, and even more time before one of these operations was truly successful. One of his patients, Anarcha, endured thirty surgeries before Sims successfully closed the abscess in her vagina—and there is perhaps no better story than Anarcha's to illuminate the tortured path of medical progress when it comes to asking the unspoken question, and treating the incurable condition. Even accounting for Sims's various biases in describing his work, there's no question that Anarcha was desperately in need of medical help. She was a petite seventeen-year-old—a "poor little girl," in Sims's notes—and a protracted labor had left her small, young body in ruins: she had a massive fistula through which "the urine was running day and night, saturating the bedding and clothing and producing an inflammation of the external parts wherever it came in contact with the person, almost similar to confluent small-pox, with constant pain and burning," Sims wrote. "The odor from this saturation permeated everything and every corner of the room; and, of course her life was one of suffering and disgust." In addition, Sims noted, there was a second perforation between Anarcha's vagina and her rectum, through which foul-smelling intestinal gas was continually leaking. Surrounded by the twin stenches of urine and feces, tormented by weeping sores on her legs and vulva, plagued by the constant flow of urine that saturated everything she touched, Anarcha was in agony and in anguish, trapped in a body that was repulsive to her and everyone around her.

But if Anarcha's condition made her life a living hell, her misery was a boon to the doctor who needed her as a test subject. Indeed, if she hadn't been so desperate, Sims might never have been so cele-brated: the only patient who could endure thirty surgeries' worth of experimentation, who could be expected to endure it, was one who had already been robbed of her agency, dignity, and happiness in every possible way.

Was it worth it, after all that, for Anarcha to be made whole again? Of course we know that Sims believed the answer was yes. Perhaps his patient would have said otherwise, if anyone had asked. What we do know for certain is that Sims ultimately did what many other doctors not only couldn't but didn't even attempt. We know he chose to confront what others turned away from: a condition that caused abject misery, shame, and stigmatization for every woman it afflicted until someone finally found a cure. We know that what-ever Sims's beliefs about the suffering (or lack thereof) of his en-slaved patients, he did ultimately perform fistula surgeries on white women and continued to eschew anesthesia, having concluded that the procedure was "not painful enough to justify the trouble." Such is the nature of so much medical progress: at the intersection of ex-perimentation and exploitation, healing and harm, desperation and innovation, a solution suddenly breaks through.

For James Marion Sims, the development of surgery to cure vesi-covaginal fistula made him a legend. For the women who were re-stored by the procedure, it was nothing short of miraculous. For gynecologists, it was an epiphany that would permanently change the field.

But for the field of urology, and the vast majority of women whose urinary issues stem not from fistula but another cause, it was barely a blip on the radar. For those women, the shame, the stigma, and the suffering would continue. For many of them, it never stopped.

Incontinence is often not considered among the patient's complaints because it is so prevalent among women that it is considered normal.

—Joshua Davies, MD, 1938

James Marion Sims is a controversial figure. He's also an outlier: most physicians, throughout most of history, took no interest in the female urinary system. Not only that, but the discovery of a cure for fistula arguably stole the spotlight, taking the focus away from all the other, less exciting things that might go wrong with a woman's urinary tract. The biggest, most intractable problem finally had a solution; all those miserable women with their weeping sores, their wet clothes, their isolation from family who couldn't stand the way they smelled, could finally be helped.

And yet, everything that made fistula so difficult to talk about and treat—the silence, the shame, the perception among doctors and patients alike that there was nothing to be done—remained true of other urinary issues, many of them incredibly common, many virtually invisible. If a woman had chronic urinary tract infections, or interstitial cystitis, or if she was just plain old peeing on herself because her pelvic floor had been weakened by age, childbirth, or both, she was hardly likely to mention it—and very few doctors considered it their responsibility to ask. Unlike fistula, these issues were neither obvious nor obviously meant to be addressed by a gynecologist. And as no one field of medicine stepped forward to address female urinary issues, these problems slid ever further out of sight and out of mind.

For this reason, the doctors who did take an active interest in the female urinary system from the late 1800s through the mid-twentieth century were a motley crew, with a diverse variety of backgrounds and motivations. Some of them, to their credit, knew that they were addressing problems that had gone egregiously overlooked by the medical establishment at large, and had enormous sympathy for the women afflicted—although even these men, the good guys, were something of a mixed bag. Take T. Gaillard Thomas, a later contemporary of Sims and a president of the American Gynecological Society, who bemoaned the lack of attention paid to women's incontinence in 1880, writing, "There are few diseases to which woman is liable, which have received so little notice at the hands of the ancients . . . this one, so annoying, so destructive of happiness and so urgent in its demands for relief, has received scarcely any mention." However, Thomas's supposed magnum opus, titled *A Practical Treatise on the Diseases of Women* was hardly a holistic text; like not only most gynecologists but most doctors of the era, Thomas conceived of women's ailments as originating exclusively below the belt and above the knees. And like most men of his time, he held highly offensive racialized beliefs about Black women, who he saw as both less susceptible to incontinence and less tormented by its symptoms if they did suffer. White women, Thomas insisted, could never tolerate the same pain: "How differently would the refined woman of a higher sphere be affected by a similar condition, and how utterly wretched!"

Or take Alexander Johnston Chalmers Skene, another gynecologist and contemporary of Sims, whose claim to fame is the discovery of twin glands in the female urethra that secrete a lubricating, antimicrobial substance that helps prevent urinary tract infections. Skene named the glands after himself—apart from his massive, broad-chested physique, it's the thing he's best known for—and he has been lionized as one of New York City's greatest contributors to advancements in women's medicine. And yet, when it came to bladder issues like interstitial cystitis or stress incontinence, he was undeniably a man of his time, with all the bizarre prejudices and fixations that implies. In what should by now be a familiar refrain, Skene firmly believed that these problems were either self-inflicted by his patients—brought on by masturbation or sexual deviance—or psychosomatic, the product of hysteria. In 1878, Skene noted a disagreement among physicians over the "retention of urine" suffered by "hysterical patients": some doctors believed that a hysterical woman might struggle to urinate owing to her constant sexual excitement, which caused the "chronically erect" clitoris to compress the urethra. Others believed that the women were only pretending they couldn't pee, because they found it sexually exciting to be catheterized. Skene, ever the diplomat, declared a tie: "I am satisfied that both kinds of cases occur." (Lest we take Skene too seriously, he also believed that he could tell the difference between a woman who masturbated and a woman who didn't by smelling her; the odor of the masturbating ones, he said, "cannot be described, but when once experienced is easily remembered.")

The notion of women's urinary issues as either psychosomatic, sexual, or both, is a recurring theme in the medical literature. As a result, actual treatments were often slow to be developed. In 1903, president of the American Gynecological Society C. Dudley lamented that the profession continued to overlook incontinence: "a commonplace though troublesome malady about which the literature, so far as I have been able to examine it, is not altogether satisfactory." Doctors had begun to experiment with some treatments, including massage, electric therapies, and the injection of paraffin into the urethral region—essentially a filler that narrowed the urethra in hopes of giving women better bladder control—but it wasn't until the late 1930s that both the prevalence of urinary problems as well as the psychological distress they caused began to be more widely acknowledged.

And even then, doctors continued to believe that all these misery-causing bladder issues were the result of female hysteria, neuroses, or otherwise all in women's heads. In one peculiar report from the 1953 *American Journal of Gynecology*, a doctor named L.R. Wharton described prescribing pelvic floor exercises to women whose incontinence was due to a "nervousness of psychic instability"—a physical treatment, despite his conviction that their condition was entirely psychological. But when many of the women failed to improve, he chalked it up once again to psychology: they were "too lazy or disinterested" to do the exercises, he scoffed. "They would rather be wet than weary."

And these are the doctors who cared.

This brings us into the mid-twentieth century. It's been a hundred years since James Marion Sims and his breakthrough fistula surgery, a hundred years in which so many more advancements could have been made, so many more questions asked. But then, the suffering of Sims's patients was never in doubt, nor was the question of whether there was something really, physically wrong with them.

These women, though, the ones whose bladder complaints have no clear cause, no obvious surgical solution? Nobody knows what to do with them, and the litany of familiar accusations begins to pile up. They're hysterical, neurotic, masochistic. They're imagining it or they're making it up. They're fabricating their symptoms: for attention, for sympathy, for the . . . erotic thrill of being catheterized? Sure, why not. Women could pee if they wanted to; or, they could hold it in if they just tried harder. Whatever it was, doctors agreed, women were probably doing it to themselves.

◆ ◆ ◆

It's 1956. The chronic cystitis patient clicks her dentures and shifts in her seat, eyeing the doctors, who are eyeing her in turn. She is twenty-nine years old, dressed in her best clothes, and nervous: she has emptied her urostomy bag nearly a dozen times today, but she's afraid it might already be full again, and the painful urge to urinate is overwhelming. She feels it all the time, even though they've long since removed her bladder, even though she hasn't sat on a toilet to pee in three years.

There is no way she can fail to see the judgment in the eyes of the men who are here to examine her. In their notes from this meeting, they will describe her as obese and ill-smelling, albeit attractively groomed, with fine features. If she were thinner, perhaps, they'd think she was pretty. She used to be slender, back in high school, back when she still had the kind of hopes and dreams that gave her a reason to care what she looked like. A husband, a home, a family. But at the age of twenty-nine, with a bag full of urine on her hip and a body scarred by multiple surgeries, with her bladder gone and half her teeth, too—they were extracted by a doctor who told her that they were making her kidneys bad—Agnes isn't in the business of caring what people think anymore. All she wants is to be left alone, including by these men, who are looking at her like she's an exotic animal in a zoo. She wouldn't even be here except that her favorite doctor, Dr. Leon, asked her to answer their questions. But Dr. Leon isn't here.

There are two of them. The urologist is Bowers. The psychiatrist is Schwarz. It's Schwarz who takes the lead, who asks the questions, looking at her all the while from under his thick eyebrows. Schwarz has an extravagant mustache and a massive head of hair, both of which will have thinned and turned white by the time he dies in

2010. Today, he's a young man, with a dark, intense look. He gazes at Agnes as if she's a mystery he intends to solve.

He asks her if she hated her parents.

When she says no, she can tell he doesn't believe her.

It would seem to be a reasonable hypothesis that in this patient the bladder served as a good pathway for the discharge of the unconscious hatreds and, together with the infection during puberty, a vicious cycle of hate, repression, enuresis, superimposed infection, inflammation, and iatrogenic traumas might have been sufficient for the development of chronic interstitial cystitis.

—Berthold E. Schwarz, MD, 1958

Although the objective reality of the alleged UFO accounts can neither be proved nor disproved, the data are entirely similar to many published experiences and seem to be authentic.

—Berthold E. Schwarz, MD, 1988

When a medical field goes underdiscussed and unexamined the way that women's urology has, the resulting knowledge vacuum attracts all sorts of peculiar theories to fill it, and peculiar people to go with them: doctors who are less concerned with healing patients than in using them to support a pet hypothesis about, say, the physical manifestation of female masochism as urinary complaints. Berthold Schwarz, the psychiatrist who attended chronic cystitis patient Agnes in 1958, was one such person: he was convinced, along with his case study coauthor Bowers, that her condition was largely psychosomatic—that her bladder was discharging not only urine, but "unconscious hatreds" stemming from her abusive upbringing.

To be sure, Agnes's childhood was a nightmare: her mother died when she was less than two years old, and she suffered from chronic bed-wetting, for which she was brutally mocked and punished by

her family. Her father, an absent alcoholic who had little involvement in her upbringing, joked that Agnes's bed-wetting would "float
her husband right out of the room"; the aunt who raised her, a cruel
and cleanliness-obsessed woman, would punish the little girl for her
nighttime accidents by forcing her to eat cardboard. Schwarz hypothesized that Agnes's lack of bladder control began as a subcon-
scious expression of her hatred for her aunt—or perhaps a way to
get her attention—which then manifested in her young adulthood
as the cystitis that would plague her all her life. The fact that Agnes
continued to experience symptoms even after the surgical removal
of her bladder was just further evidence, per these men, that her
ailment was psychological in nature.

In reality, Agnes's cystitis was almost certainly tied to the dys-
menhorrhea (severe, painful periods) that she'd experienced since
the onset of her menses at the age of thirteen. It's also not unlikely
that Agnes had endometriosis, which is strongly linked with—and
sometimes mistaken for—interstitial cystitis, since endometriosis
can create cell buildup on either the inner or outer wall of the bladder, causing pain, inflammation, and urinary issues. But the doctors who examined Agnes wrote off her painful periods, which were
so debilitating that she spent several days per month in bed, as a
"psychosexual" problem rather than a medical one, and wholly un-
related to her bladder troubles. When they mention it, it's casually
lumped in with her messed-up family relationships and her "lifelong
inability to make friends with members of either sex" as evidence
of her sexual, social, and emotional stuntedness. Agnes's real problem, they concluded, was masochism, and this was the source from
which everything flowed (or didn't, as the case may be).

That Agnes might have had a profoundly tragic life, and, sepa-
rately, a medical problem in need of treatment, seems not to have
occurred to these men. Instead, Schwarz and Bowers—two Ivy
League–educated doctors—held up her case as evidence that interstitial cystitis in women was primarily psychosomatic. She was, in
the end, not a patient but a curiosity. They poked her, questioned
her, gawked at her, and came up with a story they insisted was true,
even as Agnes insisted it wasn't. ("She dissociates from any apparent
awareness of hostility towards significant members of her family
or any of her physicians," they wrote.)

And then they left, not having helped Agnes, but having used her to confirm that the things they already wanted to believe were true.

Not long after the publication of "Masochism and Interstitial Cystitis: Report of a Case," Berthold E. Schwarz would pivot away from medical analysis to focus on his true passion: UFOs. His most famous publication is not the case report he wrote about Agnes, which was published in a relatively obscure medical journal, but a three-volume study of "UFO experiences" titled *UFO Dynamics: Psychiatric and Psychic Aspects of the UFO Syndrome*. Schwarz interviewed countless people about their alien encounters, including not just UFO sightings but abductions, alien autopsies, and encounters with the notorious "men in black." Perhaps most curiously, Schwarz does not seem to have approached his paranormal investigations with the same skepticism as he did the cystitis patient with a bladder full of hate.

"These reports are neither conscious nor unconscious fabrication," he wrote in 1968. "What they say they saw they think they saw!"

It makes a thoughtful physician wonder about the possibility of a mildly masochistic woman, i.e., destructive need in the female to suffer and "have trouble with" her genitourinary apparatus . . . the condition merits the physician wondering out loud as he alleviates symptoms, "Why do you suppose you have to have bladder pain and discomfort?"

—Oliver Spurgeon English, MD, 1970

Hunner's lesions, sometimes known as Hunner's ulcers, are a real and observable symptom of interstitial cystitis. They can be observed on the inner wall of the bladder and look like a road map of inflamed capillaries, or sometimes an ant bite, a white point surrounded by angry red tributaries that bleed when touched with a scope. Guy LeRoy Hunner, the gynecologist for whom they were named, warned that they were "elusive" and difficult to spot when he first identified them in 1916: "The ulcer area may be easily over-looked and the attention may first be arrested by an area of dead white scar tissue . . . In none of the cases has an individual ulcer area been more than a half centimetre in diameter, although two or three such ulcers have at times been grouped in a larger inflammatory area."

The fact that Hunner's lesions are both difficult to see and rel-atively rare (only 5 to 10 percent of cystitis patients have them) might explain why they weren't taken more seriously by the medical establishment in his lifetime. In 1929, Hunner noted with disap-pointment that doctors were still in the habit of writing off patients with bladder issues as head cases: "unfortunately for the patient," he wrote, they were being misdiagnosed as "neurotics or neurasthenics with the mind centered on the bladder."

Instead, it was the theory about women with interstitial cystitis being closet masochists—the same one favored by Berthold E. Schwarz—that ended up not just catching on but being taught to medical students, as if it were at least equally as valid a cause of cystitis as physiological factors. In 1970, ten years after Hunner's death, the main teaching textbook in the field of urology not only dismissed the lesions as overrepresented in urology literature but suggested that they were a useless distraction when it came to diag-nosing female patients:

"A medical entity as confusing, poorly understood, baffling etiologically, and taking up as much space as it does in the [text-books] on urology should merit a few words from the psychiatrist," wrote psychiatrist Oliver Spurgeon English in the third volume of *The Urology Textbook*. "The elusiveness of the actual visualization of the lesion, the vagueness of its response to any specific medication, its predominance in females (so often in conjunction with men-struation), makes one ask, 'Why does an individual need (or get) a bladder infection of this kind: an infection that is almost not an infection, a lesion that has a hard time being a lesion but which gives bladder discomfort?' It makes a thoughtful physician wonder about the possibility of a mildly masochistic woman, i.e., destructive need in the female to suffer and 'have trouble with' her genitourinary ap-paratus."

English was one of the most celebrated psychiatrists of the

twentieth century, and for good reason: he was one of the first doctors to recognize a link between mental and physical health, a proponent of therapy and family counseling, an advocate for fathers being more involved parents at a time when many men still balked at the idea. But when it came to women's urology, his ideas were the opposite of progressive.

English's section of *The Urology Textbook*, which focuses on the psychiatric valences of the field, reiterates the idea that women develop cystitis out of either masochistic impulses or a desire to punish themselves for "sexual adventuring either in the form of sex play or masturbation." He also suggested that cystitis was not just psychosomatic but a form of social contagion, so that even a case of "genuine cystitis" will likely be accompanied by several accessory cases of attention-seekers claiming to have the same condition. And as for the existence of Hunner's lesions, English threw all the way back to the ancient, discredited notion out of "four humours" medicine that women are just constitutionally leaky: "Just as some women tend to 'leak' somewhere in their bodies with colds, sinus infection, vaginitis, uterine bleeding or discharge and colitis, so they also tend to have genitourinary discomfort and other diseases. Hunner's ulcer seems to warrant suspicion of being in that class."

Perhaps most remarkable is that English didn't just believe women were causing their own urological problems by way of being neurotic; he also thought they were responsible for causing them in other people, particularly their children. If a child was struggling with toilet training, he wrote, it was because he "has not formed an emotional bond to his mother of sufficient strength to enable him to exert the necessary control. If he loves the mother enough, which means the mother must have loved him enough, usually he can accept this responsibility."

This text, which would have been required reading for any aspiring urologist of the time, paints a vivid portrait of how women's urology was considered (or, more often, not) by the medical establishment. Women were still treated as an afterthought; the typical patient, per both the literature and consciousness, was a man. When they did present with urological problems, they were treated suspiciously by doctors who thought they were masochists, attention-seekers, or channeling their emotional issues into their bladders. Imagine working up the courage to tell your doctor that you're suffering from the constant, painful urge to pee, only to be pointedly asked why you think you have to have this problem—the insinuation being that you're not really sick but rather feeling guilty about masturbating too much.

Even the recent history of urology demonstrates how women remain invisible as patients. Doctors still aren't asking. Women still aren't telling. And it's still, to an infuriating degree, all about dicks.

Your man spending too much time in the bathroom? Weak urinary flow can be an early warning sign for prostate cancer. GET HIM CHECKED.

—advertisement posted on the interior door of a women's bathroom stall, Maimonides Park, 2022

A couple of weeks before I speak to Dr. Angelish Kumar, I take my kids to see the Brooklyn Cyclones, a minor-league baseball team, at the Maimonides Park in Coney Island. When I go to the ladies' room during the seventh-inning stretch, I notice the advertisement above posted opposite the toilet I'm sitting on. As a marketing tactic, it's brilliant: toilet stalls are an especially good place for medical ads, a chance to reach a captive audience in a private moment. But this one enraged me: even when they're literally peeing, women are still being trained to think about urinary issues as not just a man's problem but one they're somehow responsible for.

It's no wonder we don't talk about it.

And this ad isn't an isolated incident; it's part of a long tradition in which women's urology has been not just medically but socially sidelined. The examples range from the extreme—the complete ostracism experienced by women with fistulas—to the mundane, as women have always had to pay more to pee, both figuratively and literally. Where men have always enjoyed the free use of public urinals (not to mention the ability to quickly duck behind a tree or a dumpster to relieve themselves), women's toilets were designed with locks that only disengaged if you put a coin in them. In the US, the campaign for equal access to public toilets is one of the earliest examples of women fighting back against the "pink tax" that imposes gendered costs on everything from tampons to razors; in 1969, Congresswoman March Fong Eu smashed a porcelain toilet with a sledgehammer in front of the California state capitol to protest. Historically, the lack of a safe, free place to pee has often served to keep women close to home and out of the public sphere; in some countries, particularly India, it's still a major concern.

It's not hard to see how the social invisibility of women's urinary issues creates a cone of silence around them, even today, and including at the doctor's office. Given the prevalence of these issues, this is a serious problem: 25 percent of women experience urinary incontinence; only a tiny fraction of these patients ever tell their doctor, and those who do often take years to mention it. The problem is even more prevalent among elderly patients, and these women are the most likely to be told that there's nothing to be done—that incontinence is an unavoidable outcome of childbirth or old age. Millions of women suffer from interstitial cystitis, which remains so overlooked that it takes the average patient between four and seven years to receive a diagnosis. And because of the persistent gender imbalance in urology—and the persistent notion that urology is a place for penises—women who seek help for urological issues often change their minds when they realize that they'll have to discuss a painful, personal, embarrassing problem with a male stranger.

◆　◆　◆

Her name is Sarah. She's forty-five, with three kids and a job as a waitress at an upscale chain restaurant. Ever since the birth of her third child she's suffered from stress incontinence, the type that happens when physical activity like coughing or laughing puts stress on the bladder, causing leakage. Her job requires her to lift things. Lifting things makes her leak.

She's lived for months in terror of the moment when someone at work realizes what's happening to her, when someone notices the wet patch where she's soaked through a pad or smells the odor of urine that seems to follow her everywhere. If only she could get another job—but she can't. So she's here, sitting on a table, trying to show the doctors what's wrong. If they can't see it, they can't help her. She knows this. She's trying.

"I won't be able to treat you if I haven't seen what the problem looks like," says her doctor. She says it gently, but Sarah shakes her head.

"I can't. I'm too embarrassed."

The doctor tells her it's okay. She says she just needs to see. She says it happens all the time—it's a urologist's office, after all. And Sarah knows this. She knows that if there were ever a place where it's okay to piss yourself, it's here, just as she knows that she has to show the doctors just how her body is betraying her, how urine flows down her leg every time she bends over, or coughs, or sneezes. She knows.

The doctor tells her again that it's okay.

Sarah starts to cry.

◆ ◆ ◆

"I can't imagine how they feel in an office where they've spoken with the urologist for a few minutes, and have not established a good rapport yet, and then they're expected to have their vagina examined and leak in front of this person," Angelish Kumar tells me. "I think that even just going through that in a doctor's office is enough of a barrier to prevent women from getting care for this problem."

Sarah, the waitress who burst into tears at the humiliation of having to demonstrate her incontinence in front of strangers, is Dr. Kumar's patient—and Kumar is one of a growing number of physicians who's trying to fix all the things that have long been wrong with the way the medical system approaches women's urology, starting with the lack of women working as physicians in the field. Although urology isn't remotely close to achieving gender parity, it's definitely getting better: the percentage of female practicing urologists saw a steady increase from 7.7 percent in 2014 to 10.3 percent in 2020. And having more women in the field appears to be beneficial to all patients, male or female: women urologists spend almost three minutes more on average with patients in a typical office visit than their male counterparts.

Kumar started out seeing both male and female patients, but pivoted to focus exclusively on women after realizing the unmet need—not just in the lack of female urologists but in the way urology signals to women that it's not for them. "It's really hard for women to find female urologists who they can come to with these problems, which are often quite bothersome and embarrassing," she says. "My website is designed specifically so that when women look at it, they say, this looks like the place that I want to go for help with this problem—as opposed to the urology websites for other practices where the first thing that pops up on the page is like, 'No scalpel vasectomy.'"

The legacy of silence, shame, and stigma around women's urology is a continued source of frustration for doctors like Kumar, who see every day how the contemporary medical system is set up not to serve her patients. The treatment algorithms for urinary tract infections, which more than half of all women will experience in their lifetime, have been outdated and underresearched for years. Patients will show up with chronic cystitis stemming from undiagnosed recurrent UTIs that could have been resolved years ago but went overlooked by doctors who didn't think to ask about urinary symptoms. Maternal health, including pelvic floor therapies to help prevent incontinence (a treatment regimen that is de rigueur for all new mothers in countries like France), is continually overlooked. The total dearth of conversation about things like postpartum incontinence leads women to believe that there's nothing to be done—"Women are expected to just live with these issues, and, you know, wear the pad, or don't go on the trampoline," she says.

It's a vicious cycle: women don't bother to seek urological help because they think there are no treatment options, a misconception they'll never be disabused of unless they seek urological help. This problem is only exacerbated by a medical system that often treats female urology patients as though they literally don't exist: the diagnostic codes that serve as an industry-wide standard for doctors still do not include entries for incredibly common ailments like genitourinary syndrome caused by menopause, or any specifically female pelvic pain or dysfunction. As far as we've come since the days when doctors dismissed fistula patients as hopeless and doomed to a life of misery, there are too many ways in which contemporary urology still renders women invisible.

I'm a mom of four wonderful kids—so, of course, I, like millions of other women, experience leaks every now and then.

—Brooke Burke, Poise spokeswoman, 2016

The way that women's urology has fallen so thoroughly through the cracks in the medical system is one part of the problem, and a big one. The stigma surrounding these issues—of losing control, of smelling like urine, of having to plan your life and restrict your activities around the possibility of wetting your pants—is another. But women's own complacency, and complicity, in staying invisible and undertreated: this is a problem, too, and one that no amount of institutional overhaul can fix. Too many women today remain woefully unaware that the urological ailments they suffer from can be effectively treated; too many women still think that urologists are dick doctors, full stop. And as we move away from the notion that these problems are too shameful to talk about, women must avoid falling into the opposite trap of imagining that they're normal, that something like stress incontinence is simply a woman's cross to bear because she chose to have children, because she had the audacity to get older, because there's simply nothing to be done.

This potent mix of shame and complacency is pervasive, even among some of the most empowered, independent, and privileged women in the world. During my research for this book, I was invited to the Hamptons home of some friends who were having a pool party to celebrate their son's tenth birthday. Amid the chaos of children laughing, splashing, and eating cake, the moms ended up clustered to one side, chatting. In this moment, we looked like a caricature of women having it all: a bunch of lawyers, doctors, finance girlbosses, and wealthy stay-at-home moms, reclining on the patio of a multimillion-dollar seaside mansion, a bottle of rosé chilling in an ice bucket at our feet, nary a stray hair to be seen on our collectively toned and tanned legs. If you'd asked any one of these women, they would tell you that they took their health seriously: They avoided processed foods, sugar, and the sun. They got plenty of exercise and regular mammograms. They were regulars at the medspa, the acupuncturist, the massage therapist. One of them, a financial consultant whose net worth was in the tens of millions, was sporting a diamond auriculotherapy cuff on her ear to stimulate her immune system. And yet, when I mentioned that I had spent the previous week researching women's incontinence in the 1850s—and how the shame and stigma surrounding urological issues has left many women convinced that it's normal to pee on yourself every time you sneeze, run, or laugh too hard—their faces dropped. Guilty looks were exchanged.

Finally, one spoke.

"Wait," she said, looking around furtively. "That's . . . not normal?"

In this moment, it was hard not to think of Oliver Spurgeon English, who believed that women developed urological ailments out of sexual guilt. His theory was woefully incorrect, of course, borne of offensive and paternalistic notions that have no place in contemporary medicine. But despite having all the wrong answers, English nevertheless managed to ask the right question, one that all women who are suffering in silence from incontinence, infections, or cystitis should now ask themselves: Why do you imagine that you have to live this way?

Because the answer is, you don't. None of us do.

defense

IMMUNE
SELF-SABOTAGE

Blame not the stars; 'tis plain it neither fell
From the distempered Heav'ns; nor rose from Hell,
Nor need we to the distant Indies rome;
The curst Originals are nearer home.
Whence should that foul infectious Torment flow
But from the banefull source of all our wo?
That wheedling charming sex, that draws us in
To ev'ry punishment and ev'ry sin.

—Girolamo Fracastoro, 1530

In 1847, a Hungarian physician named Ignaz Semmelweis was struggling to solve an infuriating and tragic problem. Women on the maternity ward in the hospital where he worked were dying in droves
from puerperal fever, a type of sepsis that occurs after childbirth.
Semmelweis tried and failed several times to determine the cause of
the fever, which seemed only to afflict women who were attended to
by the hospital's (male) doctors, but not those who gave birth under
the care of midwives—or even in the street. He wondered: Was it
the position in which they gave birth? (It wasn't.) Or perhaps the fever was somehow triggered by the presence of the priest who walked
the ward each time a woman died, followed by an attendant ring-
ing a bell? (This, too, was ruled out, although the other maternity
patients no doubt appreciated the cessation of this disruptive and

macabre ceremony.) But after the death of a colleague from puerperal fever—a colleague who had never set foot near the maternity ward but had been working in the autopsy lab—Semmelweis had a crucial realization.

The doctors were going from dissecting cadavers in one part of the hospital to assisting births in another . . . without washing their hands.

Fifty years before the introduction of germ theory into the scientific community, Semmelweis had stumbled onto what remains a key tenet of contemporary public health nearly two hundred years hence: the importance of hand hygiene to curb the spread of disease. But his campaign to persuade his fellow physicians to wash their hands with a chlorine solution before assisting births, while effective, was also short-lived and poorly received—in large part because nobody actually understood yet just how the immune system worked.

The immune system is first and foremost our body's defense against infection, springing to action in the presence of disease-causing microorganisms that don't belong. Everything that makes it such a misery to be sick—the pain and inflammation of an infected wound, the runny nose and rattling cough when you have a respiratory virus—is also evidence of the immune system at work, trying to expel the foreign invader. But contemporary immunology understands that this system exists in a delicate balance, one in which an overzealous immune response can be its own sort of problem. A deficient immune system is bad, but so is a dysfunctional one, in which the body's defenses go hyperactive and attack its own tissues as if they were foreign organisms. The latter scenario produces a variety of autoimmune disease—the body attacking itself—including multiple sclerosis, Hashimoto's thyroiditis, rheumatoid arthritis, diabetes mellitus type 1, and systemic lupus erythematosus.

In the scheme of things, and as compared with other systems, the immune system remained the least understood for the longest time. Before the invention of microscopes that allowed us to see the world of microorganisms that surround us, invisibly, at all times—and before the advent of germ theory that explained how those organisms interact with the human body—doctors had two reigning theories of what caused people to get sick. The first, which you've encountered already in the circulatory and urinary chapters, was the classic "imbalance of humors," which made infectious diseases just another one of the many conditions that were treated with bloodletting. The second was miasma, a theory predicated on the notion that illnesses like cholera or plague were caused by "bad air," which wafted like an evil cloud over the landscape, felling everyone in its path. More than two thousand years ago, the Roman architect Vitruvius warned against building a community too close to swamplands, lest the fetid exhalations of the local wildlife infect everyone:

"For when the morning breezes blow toward the town at sunrise, if they bring with them mist from marshes and, mingled with the mist, the poisonous breath of creatures of the marshes to be wafted into the bodies of the inhabitants, they will make the site unhealthy."

As was often the case with early medical theories, the notion of miasma was foundationally wrong while still containing a germ or two (so to speak) of truth. The common wisdom was that bad, disease-causing air originated from rotting organic matter and was identifiable by its foul odor—which, while technically inaccurate, did correctly surmise a connection between decay and disease. (Ignaz Semmelweis would make a similar calculation centuries later when he campaigned for handwashing protocols: his idea of using a chlorine solution stemmed not from an understanding that it would kill germs, but because it was the most effective at removing the scent and particulate matter of dead bodies from a physician's hands.)

Meanwhile, even once scientists developed the means to study microbiology, including microscopes that allowed them to see organisms too small to view with the naked eye, it took centuries for them to make the connection between bacteria and infection. In the late 1600s, a Dutch scientist named Antonie van Leeuwenhoek described with a state of wonder the "animalcules" he had viewed under a microscope: "Among all the marvels that I have discovered in nature," he wrote, "these are the most marvellous of all." It wasn't until the late nineteenth century when early pioneers of germ theory, including Louis Pasteur and Robert Koch, realized that the marvelous miniature world under the microscope also had implications for human health.

But if physicians managed to be partially correct even in their ignorance about how diseases spread, they were wildly wrong when it came to who they blamed for spreading them—which is to say, they blamed women. Much of the early medical advice on remaining disease-free is addressed to men and breaks down along a gendered binary that imagines men as sufferers, and women as contaminators. And the source of that contamination? The vagina, of course.

Given what doctors from the humorist school of medicine already believed—that women were particularly prone to a surplus of fluid and constitutionally leaky, and that menstrual blood was so toxic that it could poison a woman's body from within—it's not entirely surprising that these same doctors were deeply suspicious of vaginas. More to the point, they were downright terrified of what might happen if you stuck your penis into the wrong one.

This anxiety about the invisible nature of female anatomy was ubiquitous and reached well beyond the bounds of science (it's not a coincidence that so many cultures have their own version of the legend of a killer vagina equipped with teeth—the feared "vagina dentata"). But within the scientific community, it fueled the dire conviction that having sex with an "unclean" woman would cause men's dicks to fall off. In the early fourteenth century, French doctor and medical professor Bernard de Gordon warned his readers about the dangers of sexually transmitted diseases, writing that "diseases of the yard are numerous, following lying with a woman whose womb is unclean, full of putrid sanies, virulence." In the fifteenth century, the surgeon Petrus de Argelatta of Bologna (who would eventually become best known as the attending physician who examined and then embalmed the corpse of Alexander V) made a similar claim, stating that the vagina of a "foul woman" was full of "poisonous matter," which would lodge in the nooks and crannies of the penis, causing it to turn black and rot.

Remarkably absent from the literature is any sense that women might suffer from these diseases—or that men had any hand in spreading them. Indeed, the physicians at the time painted a vivid picture of women's vaginas as dark, fetid dens of terror, just waiting to destroy the pristine penis of some hapless paramour. When the Italian physician and poet Girolamo Fracastoro wrote his famous epic poem about syphilis in 1530, women were portrayed as wily temptresses who were ultimately to blame not just for the spread of venereal disease but also for virtually any misfortune that might befall a man, particularly those stemming from his own bad judgment:

> That wheedling charming sex, that draws us in
> To ev'ry punishment and ev'ry sin.

Fracastoro would eventually become renowned for a theory, "seeds of disease," which contemporary scientists view as an early precursor to the fully developed germ theory of the nineteenth century. But there are also seeds of something else, something more sinister, in Fracastoro's work—and in the work of every doctor who indulged in the notion that women were uniquely culpable in spreading sickness. Unlike humorism or the miasma theory, this suspicious view of women was not discarded by latter-day doctors in light of new advances and new knowledge. Instead, like a virus, it has persisted . . . and evolved. Over the years, variants of this line of thinking have continued to reinfect the collective medical consciousness with the insidious conviction that women are contaminators, harborers of infection, and inherently untrustworthy.

The result is a long history of women being treated as scapegoats for contagion—and a system that perpetuates said scapegoating not only in medical settings, but in larger society, often with the authoritarian force of the government's public health apparatus behind it. In the coming pages, we will explore the devastating impact of these ideas: in medicine, in research, in public policy, and in the lives of the individuals who dared to challenge them.

Many of those individuals were women, but not all. In 1865, an embattled and increasingly erratic Ignaz Semmelweis finally suffered a nervous breakdown. His insistence on handwashing, despite having virtually eradicated puerperal fever at every hospital where he insisted it be implemented, had only served to earn him the ire of the medical community. In part, this was a result of Semmelweis's own tactics; he was strident, combative, and prone to lashing out at critics (some scholars have hypothesized that these were symptoms of syphilis, which Semmelweis may have contracted from his work with afflicted patients). But doctors were also deeply offended by the notion that it was their own lack of hygiene, and not some constitutional flaw or error on the part of their female patients, causing the spread of disease.

Semmelweis was committed to an asylum, where he was beaten by guards and sustained severe lacerations which shortly became infected; within two weeks, he was dead. But not only did his passing go unmarked by his former colleagues at the Vienna General Hospital, his good work there had long since been undone. Years earlier, Semmelweis had moved on to a new position in Budapest, at which point the Vienna hospital promptly abandoned his handwashing protocols. Women were dying of puerperal fever again. Nobody could imagine why.

"Women catch cold by their criminal carelessness and wilful indifference to the simple rules of hygiene," said one physician, "then they come home to give it to their men folks."

—*The Daily Oklahoman*, January 6, 1916

The discovery of microbes and the introduction of germ theory in the late nineteenth century represented a huge leap forward in the field of immunology and spurred the advent of new scientifically driven public health interventions centered on reducing the spread of disease. Many of these solutions were civic: public health officials oversaw the draining of swamps where bacteria could fester, and the introduction of sanitation systems to keep human waste from contaminating the food and water supply. "Antisepticonscious" products made of porcelain made their way into kitchens, laundries, and bedrooms. The discovery of specific highly lethal germs, like tuberculosis, gave way to the creation of local and regional committees and health associations to sanitation and hygiene—and to the passage of local ordinances including, famously, a New York City law making it illegal to spit on the sidewalk. At the same time, a cottage industry of appliances and cleaning products sprang forth, empowering every household to take up arms against the threat of infection.

But when it came to matters of domestic hygiene, a familiar scapegoat reared its head. The development of germ theory quickly gave rise to an obsession with identifying those most responsible for preventing the spread of germs—and once again, a consensus emerged that women represented a particular health hazard. In the 1890s, at the same time as medical doctors were hotly debating whether or not corsets were causing women's skeletons to deform, bacteriologists were fretting over the dangers posed by women's fashions not just to the wearer but to the general public. Scientists cultured a variety of germs from the floor-dusting hems of ladies' dresses and sounded the alarm about the scourge of the "septic skirt," which would supposedly drag all manner of street-borne diseases over the threshold and into the home. One *New York Weekly* cartoon from the year 1900 depicts a maid beating the dust off her mistress's cloak, sending massive clouds labeled GERMS, MICROBES, CONSUMPTION, INFLUENZA, and TYPHOID FEVER into the air. The grim reaper, its skeletal hands clasped in grinning anticipation, lurks in the background—as do the unseen mistress's two small children. Women, terrified by the possibility that they were putting their families at risk every time they left the house, formed "Rainy Day Clubs" to advocate for raising hemlines in the name of health (only to be shamed a decade later for leaving their ankles exposed and hence making themselves vulnerable to the flu). Housewives were suddenly on the front lines of a war against microbes, expected to safeguard their families from dangerous contagion by maintaining a sanitary household. Even the American Medical Association weighed in, writing, "Medical men who know the value of a trained nurse can readily appreciate the value of a training which will not only make American wives prudent, economic and thrifty, but which will establish a sanitary regime in every room in the home as well as in the kitchen and dining room."

As has so often been the case where women are concerned, these medical recommendations surrounding home hygiene were bolstered by a new, corresponding set of social pressures and conventions. Making women masters of the domestic realm was a double-edged sword that also served to confine them: to keep house, you had to stay home. Meanwhile, the conflation of good health and proper hygiene with elite social class continued apace: a tidy house didn't just denote the upstanding moral character of the woman who lived there but elevated her and her family above the poor, nonwhite, and immigrant communities, who didn't even have ceramic toilets, let alone the time and money to devote to keeping them clean.

The class divide soon became fertile ground for the same anxieties that animated those fourteenth- and fifteenth-century texts warning of "foul women" with vaginas full of putrescent rot. Poverty, squalor, and sickness became inextricably linked in the public consciousness. The women in working-class families were engaged in labor outside the home; they had no time to play the domestic goddess inside it. And so it was in their homes where disease was imagined to take root and fester—and then to creep back out again, carried by the unenlightened, unwashed, and unclean, contaminating everything they touched.

I am an innocent human being. I have committed no crime and I am treated like an outcast—a criminal. It is unjust, outrageous, uncivilized.

—Mary Mallon, 1909

The girl from Cookstown, Ireland, is going to be a legend. Someday, people everywhere will know her name. Not the one her parents gave her, but the other one, the one that makes her infamous. A name given to her by strangers, pronounced by other strangers with a sneer. A name that will not only outlive her but take on a life of its own when she's gone, until it doesn't even belong to her anymore—until it's just the thing you call a person who callously spreads disease.

But in 1884, when she boards a ship and crosses to America in search of a better life, she is just a girl named Mary Mallon, fifteen years old and traveling alone. In her youthful face is the promise of the handsome woman she'll soon become: she has round cheeks; a small, upturned nose; and deep-set blue eyes that contrast strikingly with her thick, dark hair. Her plans are to make it to New York City, where she'll stay with an aunt and uncle, and hopefully find a job as a servant—a laundress, a housekeeper, maybe even a lady's maid in one of the mansions on Fifth Avenue, the part they call "Millionaire's Row."

Beyond this, Mary has no sense of what the future holds. She doesn't know yet that she's quite an excellent cook, so skilled that wealthy families will someday compete to place her in their kitchens—and that some twenty years from now, a rich banker named Charles Henry Warren will hire her to spend the whole summer at his grand home on Oyster Bay, Long Island, where she'll prepare meals for Warren's family and a rotating cast of guests.

Most importantly, she doesn't know that sometime in the years between her journey across the ocean and her arrival at Oyster Bay, she will begin carrying a passenger. Not a child—she will never marry and never become a mother—but a microbe, one that will intertwine its being invisibly with hers, poison everything she touches, and survive inside her like a curse for as long as she lives. Where Mary goes, disease and death will follow.

And eventually, so will doctors. The medical authorities of New York City will pursue Mary Mallon for years. They'll take away her livelihood and her liberty. They'll also tell her that perhaps she can have these things back if she allows them to take something else— her gallbladder—via an invasive surgery that she may not survive.

They will be mystified when she refuses, but then, most things about Mary are confusing to the men who place themselves in charge of her fate. She is unlike them in every way: An immigrant. A servant.

A woman.

Perhaps this is why, even after they hunt her down and eventually imprison her on a small island in the East River—where she will remain, in isolation, until her death—they never help Mary understand what is happening to her and why. They don't explain to her the remarkable new concept of asymptomatic carriers, who unknowingly spread disease without ever becoming ill themselves. They do not involve her in her medical care so much as instruct her, command her, and then punish her when she fails to obey. And when it comes to the Irish woman's legacy, her place in history, it is the medical system that determines this, too, stripping her of her identity as surely as it stripped her of her freedom. In a hundred years, nobody will remember Mary Mallon.

Everyone, however, will have heard of Typhoid Mary.

◆ ◆ ◆

In June 1909, two years after Mary Mallon's first arrest and imprisonment on North Brother Island off the coast of Manhattan, *New York American* magazine ran a story about her case. The headline, printed in block letters a quarter page high, was her now-infamous nickname—TYPHOID MARY—accompanied by an article spanning two full pages that described the "extraordinary predicament" of the woman who, "through no fault of hers . . . is a living, walking incubator of typhoid germs."

"Her case is the most remarkable with which we are acquainted," wrote Dr. William H. Park, one of the physicians responsible for Mallon's treatment, "because of the number of persons to whom she has communicated the disease."

While this may have been true as far as Park was concerned at the time, his assertion ultimately proved inaccurate. Mallon was not the most infectious typhoid carrier of the era; that dubious honor went to another food worker, Tony Labella, who was likely responsible for an estimated eighty-seven cases to Mallon's forty-seven. Yet it is her name alone—not Labella's, nor that of any other asymptomatic carrier—that remains synonymous with the wanton spread of disease. By the time Mallon died, having lived for more than twenty-six years in quarantine, she was one of several hundred known typhoid carriers to have been identified in New York City—and the only one ever to have been imprisoned as a threat to public safety.

Judith Leavitt, a historian and author of a book about Mallon's life, has identified a variety of reasons why she might have been both so uniquely mistreated and so thoroughly villainized by public health officials: she was Irish, an immigrant, a woman without a family. She was hotheaded, combative, and skeptical of the doctors who told her she was a typhoid carrier. But perhaps most importantly, Mary Mallon would have seemed the living embodiment of the archetypal contaminator, the "foul woman" who maliciously spreads disease while remaining seemingly untouched by sickness herself—a conclusion the physicians of the time seem to have drawn well in advance of ever meeting her.

Indeed, things might have been very different for Mallon if the men who sought to quarantine her had treated her with humanity and respect. Instead, in 1907, a sanitary engineer named George Sober stalked Mallon to her place of employment, told her he believed her to be diseased, and requested that she supply him with samples of her blood, urine, and feces—a demand that would have surely seemed preposterous to Mallon, however well-intentioned. When Mallon proved uncooperative, Sober and a male assistant followed her home and confronted her again—and then, proving unsuccessful, passed the case off to a public health official named S. Josephine Baker, whose colorful account of Mallon's capture sounds less like a public health initiative than an exhilarating big-game hunt. Mallon, who was by now convinced (and not unreasonably) that she was being harassed and persecuted by the authorities for no good reason, fled and hid from Baker and the five police officers who showed up to arrest her; when they located her and dragged her out, Baker described Mallon in the most dehumanizing terms while simultaneously expressing bafflement that she was not more receptive to her "sensible" demands.

"She came out fighting and swearing, both of which she could do with appalling efficiency and vigor," she wrote, noting that the ride to the hospital—during which she restrained Mallon by sitting on her—"was like being in a cage with an angry lion."

Although officials like Baker asserted at the time that Mallon was beyond reason ("She knew she had never had typhoid fever; she was maniacal in her integrity," she wrote), her own letters from quarantine suggest that she was less maniacal than righteously indignant, with a sophisticated understanding of not just the injustice of her situation but the way that the medical establishment was exploiting her.

"I have been in fact a peep show for everybody," Mallon wrote in a letter in 1909. "Even the interns had to come to see me and ask about the facts already known to the whole wide world. The tuberculosis men would say 'There she is, the kidnapped woman.'"

As for William Park, the physician who wrote in the pages of the *New York American* that Mallon was "a menace" who would require permanent imprisonment, she imagined giving him a taste of his own medicine: "I wonder how the said Dr. William H. Park would like to be insulted and put in the Journal and call him or his wife Typhoid William Park."

Some historians allege that Mallon's status as a villain—the notorious Typhoid Mary—was not cemented until 1915. Mallon had been released from quarantine under the condition that she never again work as a cook but was discovered working under a pseudonym in the kitchen of a Manhattan hospital where an outbreak of typhoid had recently occurred. She was recaptured and sent back to North Brother Island, this time remaining there until her death from complications of a stroke in 1938. An editorial in the *New York Tribune* pronounced Mallon the architect of her own demise: "The chance was given to her five years ago to live in freedom, and . . . she deliberately elected to throw it away."

And yet, the 1909 story about her case in the *New York American* suggests otherwise. It's not just that headline—*TYPHOID MARY*—but the illustration that frames the spread, a line drawing that runs the full length of the page. It's an unflattering portrait of Mary Mallon, her dark hair coiled atop her head, her face cast in shadow, gazing down dispassionately at the meal she's preparing. She has a pan in one hand, and in the other, a tiny skull—not tiny like the invisible typhoid microbes she unknowingly carried for years, but the size of an egg. It's death, tangible and unmissable, nestled in the palm of her hand.

She's tossing it into the frying pan.

If I were a judge, I would have such venomous, syphilitic whores broken on the wheel, and flayed, because one cannot estimate the harm such filthy whores do to young men who are so wretchedly ruined, and whose blood is contaminated before they have achieved full manhood.

—Martin Luther, 1543

If the advent of germ theory ushered in the archetype of the domestic goddesses, it also reinvigorated the notion of women as wanton contaminators, particularly when it came to the spread of sexually transmitted diseases (STDs). The early twentieth century saw an explosion in cases of syphilis and gonorrhea, which prompted a widespread moral panic as well as much consternation among public health officials who subscribed to roughly the same theory of STD transmission as espoused by an irate Martin Luther, ranting in the sixteenth century about "syphilitic whores." Once again, they believed, innocent young men were falling victim to the poisonous wiles of disease-ridden temptresses.

Having concluded that women in general, and prostitutes in particular, were responsible for the spread of venereal diseases, doctors began looking for ways to identify them—that is, the women, not the diseases. The research built upon a long-standing consensus within the medical community that a promiscuous woman could be identified by the size and shape of her genitals. One doctor, Horatio Storer, promulgated the theory in the mid-1800s that wanton women must be possessed of unnaturally large clitorises—although this did not stop him from diagnosing countless women with normal-sized clitorises as sexual deviants as well. Another, Dr. Robert Latou Dickinson, the gynecologist who we met briefly in the Muscular chapter, had a set of clay sculptures that allegedly displayed the labia of different "types"—"The Masturbator," "The Virgin," "The Homosexual," and so on—which resembled nothing so much as those twenty-first-century digital memes in which a ham sandwich with its meat spilling out is meant to represent the vagina of a sexually experienced woman. (They were also about as scientifically accurate.) Dickinson was particularly convinced that he could discern which of his patients were "erotic" women on sight: they walked with a "habitual rhythmic swing of the hips," exhibited "restless behavior" during examinations, and were prone to "unnecessary exposure (exhibitionism)"—a curious allegation coming from the man who habitually made his patients lie naked and spread-eagled on his table while he made detailed drawings of their genitals. (Note: both Storer and Dickinson are recurring characters in this book; keep an eye out for them in the Reproductive chapter.)

In late nineteenth-century Europe, doctors developed a sort of field guide for spotting alleged sex workers in the wild—what historian Mary Sponberg describes in her writings as "a kind of catalogue which allowed them to distinguish those women who appeared to have a particular aptitude for prostitution." Their efforts were mirrored in the United States by the formation of the American Social Hygiene Association, whose officials took a similar albeit far more energetic approach to stamping STDs out of existence. It was 1917, World War I was raging, and the alarming spread of venereal diseases among members of the US military had elevated the problem from a medical issue to one of national security.

What followed was one of the lesser-known and more horrifying public health initiatives in American history, one that flew bizarrely under the radar despite lasting for the better part of the twentieth century. It was called the American Plan, and under its auspices, vast numbers of women were essentially kidnapped, imprisoned, and forcibly treated with dangerous drugs in the name of the common good. In some ways, it was the saga of Mary Mallon all over again—but on such a massive scale, and with such an efficient government apparatus behind it, that its outrageous assault on women's liberties would not be fully understood for decades.

In his book about the American Plan, author Scott W. Stern describes how medical authorities stalked, arrested, and imprisoned women who were engaged in activities that marked them as likely STD carriers (said activities included sitting in a restaurant alone, changing jobs, or just looking suspicious). A positive test for gonorrhea or syphilis resulted in detention and treatment at a government camp, which could last for days, weeks, or months. In addition to being forced to accept mercury injections and arsenic-based drugs—the only available treatments for syphilis at the time—the women were subject to a strict code of conduct: "If they failed to show 'proper' ladylike deference," Stern writes, "these women could be beaten, doused with cold water, thrown into solitary confinement—or even sterilized."

What started as a program aimed at targeting prostitutes soon expanded to encompass the entirety of the nation. In theory, the law allowed the detention of any person, irrespective of sex, who was suspected of spreading disease; in practice, virtually all those impacted were women. The specter of the "foul woman" reared its head once again, this time with the imprimatur of both medical authority and the state behind it.

The skull motif that was used so effectively to imply conscious wrongdoing on the part of Mary Mallon pops up here, too, this time in official government documents; in one image, a voluptuous woman tells a soldier, "Two girls I know want to meet you in the worst way," as the two girls—with skulls for faces and the words "syphilis" and "gonorrhea" emblazoned on their skirts—lurk seductively behind her. Other advertisements functioned as a sort of anti-pinup-girl showcase, warning men that even the most beautiful, innocent-looking woman might be secretly harboring disease. "She may look clean," warns one, featuring a pretty girl-next-door type in a spotless white blouse. Another, featuring a Bettie Page look-alike with a cigarette dangling from her mouth, is even less subtle: "She may be a bag of TROUBLE."

And yet, despite the evocative image of women as ambulatory bags of germs, the notion that the women detained under the American Plan represented a genuine health threat was belied by the behavior of the authorities who targeted them: police and public health officers routinely forced these supposedly diseased women to have sex with them.

We all began to realize we needed a greater element of control over these girls. We needed to remove them from the community and control them so that they could not continue their promiscuous activity. We needed to control them so that we could be absolutely sure that they received every bit of the treatment that they so badly needed.

—PHS officer, circa 1940s

One possible reason why the American Plan went so under-scrutinized for so long was that one of its chief architects, Dr. Thomas Parran, became notorious for his involvement in a much more famous medical atrocity: the Syphilis Study at Tuskegee, in which Black men infected with syphilis were used as guinea pigs for observing the trajectory of the disease. The study lasted forty years and represents one of the most egregious breaches of medical ethics ever recorded; more than one hundred of its four hundred participants died from syphilis or related complications, and many of the patients' wives and children were infected.

Parran didn't originate the Tuskegee study—he inherited it from a predecessor in 1935—but it was under his watch that the infected men were cruelly lied to and deprived of treatment that would have saved their lives, even after the discovery of antibiotics in 1947 as an effective cure for syphilis. More importantly, though, Tuskegee was not Parran's first rodeo when it came to morally delinquent health initiatives: in 1918, when he was just twenty-six years old and a newly minted physician in the USPHS, he was cutting his teeth on the American Plan to effectively imprison women with STDs.

Parran was a controversial figure even in his own time, often sparring with the moral scolds who thought that preaching moral abstinence was the best way to rid the population of STDs, and once walking out of a scheduled radio appearance after executives censored the words "syphilis control" from his remarks. (This ultimately backfired spectacularly, as in the wake of the controversy, newspapers nationwide covered the story and printed Parran's remarks in full.) He also worked tirelessly to foment a frank, public conversation about controlling STDs, including authoring a study that appeared in the *Ladies' Home Journal* in 1937—much to the chagrin of those who believed that such topics were unladylike.

But Parran's passionate commitment to controlling the spread of disease led to the cutting of ethical corners when it came to medical consent, which he seemed to view as a nuisance rather than a necessity. During his tenure as surgeon general, Parran became aware of a US-run public health experiment in Guatemala, in which researchers were intentionally infecting incarcerated and mentally ill people with syphilis in order to study them. In 1947, a letter from Robert Coatney, a colleague of Parran's, was sent to Dr. John Cutler, one of the key figures in the Guatemalan study:

"As you well know, [Parran] is very much interested in the project," Coatney wrote. "And a merry twinkle came into his eye when he said: 'You know, we couldn't do such an experiment in this country.'"

What Parran could do, and did, was institutionalize the mistrust of women within the public health system. Under his watch, a powerful and toxic idea wove its way into the fabric of government, of medicine, and of American society: when it came to the spread of disease, women were always to blame, and never to be trusted—not with their freedom, not with their healthcare, not even as authorities on what was happening in their own bodies.

◆ ◆ ◆

The year is 1944. The United States is at war, and has been for the better part of four years; the Allied victory in Europe and Japan is still many months away. But on the home front, an entirely different battle is being fought—this one against a microscopic enemy that threatens the lives and livelihoods of countless Americans.

Much like the fighting overseas, this battle is captured in a newsreel, the kind that plays in movie theaters before the feature film begins. The setting is a Civilian Conservation Corps camp, a relic of the Great Depression that once housed young men in need of employment. Now, its barracks are full again, but its purpose and its population have both become something quite different, as becomes clear when the new residents come marching into view. Some of them glance at the camera; others keep their heads down. But these are not soldiers, or even men. They're women, one and all.

And they're all infected—or at least, that's what the government says.

Her name is Mary Lou, except that it almost certainly isn't, because she doesn't exist. She's the main character in this short film, "A venereal disease rapid treatment center," an avatar for every woman in the treatment camp for those infected with STDs. As an unseen narrator explains, this isn't a prison, but a hospital, one where patients of all ages live under the supervision of the state. "Young, old, city girls, farm girls, good, bad, average girls," he intones as they walk past the camera. As far as the government is concerned, there are no women here, no adults; only girls, girls of all ages, now under the control and supervision of the American Plan.

The actress playing Mary Lou is the living embodiment of the "average girl." Her age could be anything from late teens to early thirties; her face and body are so nondescript that she would be difficult to pick out of a crowd. Even the narrator identifies her only by the "rumpled dress" she's wearing as she arrives at the treatment camp, which she swiftly removes in order to be examined by the doctor. Other videos of this type, the ones for men, show the patients discussing their medical care ("I'd gone to this girl before," a guy named Jerry bleats when his doctor asks why he didn't wear a condom. "She looked clean!"). But Mary Lou never speaks; she is only spoken about, silent and compliant while the narrator details her fate.

Why is she here? To get well, certainly, but what is being depicted here is not medicine; it's a makeover, a redemption arc, from public menace to productive citizen. Mary Lou arrives rumpled, and diseased, and probably morally delinquent (it is implied though not stated outright that she's been engaged in prostitution). She leaves transformed, with a job offer—she's learned to weld during her confinement—and a new look. The rumpled floral dress is gone, replaced by a more modest, almost military garment, dark and stiff with large shoulder pads.

"And now she has a real job paying a decent living wage and a new life lands before her, thanks to the rapid treatment center," the narrator intones. This is the moral of the story: you, a fallen woman, can be made whole by the grace of the US government and the miracle of modern medicine. All you have to give up is your dignity, your freedom, your autonomy.

All you have to do is everything the doctors say.

The pity of it is, every wife can hold her lovable charm by simply using Lysol disinfectant as an effective douche.

—Lysol ad, circa 1950s

Although the national security threat represented by STDs—and the women who were allegedly responsible for spreading it—faded out of consciousness after WWII, the notion of vaginas as a source of sickness and putrescence was by now medically ingrained and culturally ubiquitous, even without the fear of a specific disease attached. The cult of cleanliness that had long surrounded women's domestic lives had also made its way into the boudoir, along with an entire cottage industry devoted to making them feel as bad about their unhygienic bodies as they did about their messy homes.

Sometimes, the same products were even recommended as cleaning agents for both. In the 1930s, advertisements for Lysol promoted its use as a douching agent, implying that women who didn't clean their vaginas with industrial-grade disinfectant would become sexually repulsive. The ad quoted above shows a distressed-looking woman attempting to embrace her husband, who is turning away and grimacing. The copy takes the form of a Q&A:

Q. What has she done? Is it really all her fault?
A. It is not so much what she has done as what she has neglected . . .
and that is proper feminine hygiene.

Needless to say, douching with Lysol is not just unnecessary but actively dangerous—but this wasn't the only product that women were sold to deodorize their vaginas at the expense of their health. Johnson & Johnson marketed talcum powder similarly to Lysol, as a necessary feminine hygiene product. Women were told that putting the powder in their underwear would reduce odor, only for a link to emerge suggesting that talcum powder could cause ovarian cancer. This information came to light in 2006, when the World Health Organization issued a warning—and in 2007, Johnson & Johnson agreed that they would stop marketing talcum powder as a genital deodorant . . . to white women. (In 2023, Johnson & Johnson settled a $8.9 billion lawsuit regarding talc as a carcinogen.)

Meanwhile, the conflation of these three disparate ideas—feminine hygiene, sexual purity, and good health—continues to find purchase in the medical system, even as it has faded out of fashion culturally. For all the impact of the sexual revolution, and all the work of feminists to eradicate the stigma from being a sexually active woman, the doctor's office remains a holdout: one of the few places left where a woman can be shamed for having sex, for being unclean, and all under the guise of it being for her own good.

◆ ◆ ◆

Rebecca is crying in my office.

She doesn't want to tell me why.

It's been four years since I first met her, shortly after her breast cancer diagnosis. That day, she was surrounded by family—her parents and brother had traveled thousands of miles to support her as we plotted a treatment plan, and she was determined not to let cancer derail her from the life and legal career she was just beginning to build.

But today, she's cancer-free. This is just a checkup, one I look forward to every few months because it's so wonderful to see how she's thriving. Once, our visits were about her survival; now, they're all about her life, and the psychological and physical strides she's made to no longer be defined by her illness. For a long time, one of her biggest fears was that she wouldn't be able to find anyone with whom to share the life she'd fought so hard to reclaim—that men would be turned off by her mastectomy, alarmed by her brush with disease. It was a joy and a relief, the last time I saw her, when she told me she was dating again.

And it's devastating to see her now, fighting back tears.

"I feel so stupid. I feel like you know everything about my life, but I'm too scared to tell you this. I'm still so embarrassed, even after six months."

I try to reassure her. I tell her she can tell me anything. I tell her nothing she says could possibly upset me.

I'm half right: when she tells me what happened, I'm not upset.

I'm furious.

Six months ago, after a year of struggling to meet somebody new, Rebecca finally had sex for the first time since her cancer diagnosis. But her new partner had not only ghosted her, he'd also left her with a morbid souvenir: genital herpes, a disease he'd known he had yet didn't disclose. But as upsetting as this was, it's not the lying ex-boyfriend who is the source of Rebecca's tears and shame. It's the doctor who she went to a few days after their encounter, who diagnosed her STD and then made a comment that shook her to her core:

"Perhaps," he said, "you should be having less sex, and focusing more on a monogamous relationship that will lead to marriage and children."

Through tears, Rebecca tells me how much progress she had made, how amazing it had been to finally see her body as a source of strength and pleasure rather than disfigurement. This doctor, in the blink of an eye, had taken away her confidence and left her feeling broken and shamed. It was worse, she says, than the day she was told she had cancer.

"He made me feel damaged," she says. "He made me feel like I was a threat. How could this possibly be?"

In this moment, I try to comfort my patient. I tell her she's not damaged, and not broken, and that she has nothing to be ashamed of. But when I think of her question now—How could this be?—I know the answer is that this is how it's always been. From Italy in the sixteenth century to a small-town gynecologist's office in 2021.

> *That wheedling charming sex, that draws us in*
> *To ev'ry punishment and ev'ry sin.*

◆ ◆ ◆

Rebecca's experience was the endpoint of centuries of misinformation, sexism, and fear that infected the medical system's treatment of women. How else to explain her doctor's instinct to shame her for her disease instead of offering treatment? His equation of better health with a life of traditional wifely domesticity, one in which she would presumably stay home to disinfect the toilet—or perhaps her genitals—instead of dating and having sex? The lopsided assignation of blame, such that the man who infected her vanished from the equation, leaving only the bizarre sense that she somehow did this to herself?

All those ancient anxieties about women as disease vectors, rather than disease sufferers, have a contemporary legacy, and not just in the experiences of individual patients like Rebecca. In 2006, the long-awaited release of a vaccine for human papilloma virus (HPV), an STD that is thought to be responsible for 90 percent of cervical cancers, was marred by the subsequent revelation that doctors were only recommending it for female patients—even though men spread HPV just as easily, and even though it's been linked not just to cervical, but also head, neck, and anal cancers.

And when women weren't being treated like contaminators, they were simply excluded altogether. Although the FDA's Office of Good Clinical Practice has been calling for gender parity in clinical trials since 1993, scientists have often been reluctant to follow those guidelines, owing to a misguided belief that female subjects and their variable hormone cycles make clinical trials too "messy."

The effort to make sure that science addresses the needs and unique biology of female patients has been a series of false starts. The 1993 FDA recommendation was followed in 2001 by a landmark report called "Does Sex Matter?," which also recommended prioritizing sex differences in biomedical research. In 2006, a group of researchers from the Society for Women's Health Research founded the Organization for the Study of Sex Differences, with the goal of aiding research and connecting specialists across a variety of fields. By 2016, the NIH had created a policy to encourage the inclusion of "sex as a biological variable" into research.

And yet, vital research continues to fall short when it comes to including women. In 2019, a key trial for a new HIV preventive studied the effects of the drug in thousands of male subjects while intentionally excluding women—despite the fact that 19 percent of all new HIV infections in the United States, and nearly half of infections globally, occur in female patients.

Notably, the bias against including women in clinical research is pervasive even in research that doesn't include human subjects. Immunotherapies, used to treat autoimmune conditions and, more recently, intractable cancers, were first studied in mice—but without sorting the mice (or their data) by sex, leaving a massive knowledge gap that was only uncovered much later, when they began testing the same drugs in people. As it turned out, women's bodies responded differently, not just in terms of efficacy but also exhibiting different and adverse side effects as compared with men's.

Here, too, the avoidance of research on female subjects stems from a belief that their fluctuating hormone levels make them too complicated to study, even though this same biological variability directly impacts the efficacy and effects of medicines in women's bodies as compared to men's. And often, the proposed solutions to women's lack of inclusion in biomedical research are hardly better than the original problem: in one case, researchers suggested doing experiments on male mice first, and then testing female mice only as a point of comparison to the male "default."

Somehow, even the concept of equality ends up replicating the same old paradigm that deems women's bodies, and women's biology, uninteresting in their own right. Women are the other, the variable, the weird and slightly defective riff on a norm defined by—and inclusive only of—men.

◆ ◆ ◆

The year is 1973. Leora smooths the dark fabric of her skirt and then folds her hands in her lap. She's waiting for the doctor to stop talking, which he's been doing for quite a while—slowly, carefully, sometimes pausing to make sure she's still listening.

Of course, she has no trouble following his explanation—she's a medical student herself, after all—but the doctor says it's important that she understand the seriousness of the situation, now that the test has come back positive. He says he knows it's difficult, but she must accept what he's telling her; it's simply too dangerous to do anything else. He says her husband will understand, when he knows how high the stakes are.

"But you must not become pregnant," he says somberly, looking her in the eye.

She looks back at him. She matches her serious expression to his.

"Prove it," she says.

The doctor sits up as straight as if she'd slapped him. He actually laughs a little, clearly not out of amusement but sheer surprise.

"I beg your pardon," he says.

Now she holds his gaze. Now she speaks slowly, taking her time. It is a serious situation. It's important that he understands.

She says, "When I got my blood test for the marriage license, they told me I had syphilis."

"You don't have syphilis—"

"Of course I don't. I told them I don't. That's why I came here, to prove it. Right?"

"Right."

"So here we are. The tests say it's not syphilis, it's lupus. But now you want to tell me lupus means it's too dangerous for me to ever have a baby." She takes a deep breath. "And I say what I said before: prove it."

◆ ◆ ◆

In immunology, as in medicine more broadly, women's perspectives are frequently overlooked—but it is with respect to immune system disorders that this blind spot can be especially catastrophic. Autoimmune diseases, in which the body's immune system mistakes its own healthy tissues for foreign invaders and attacks them, are among the trickiest to diagnose. For some, there is no blood test to detect them, no scans on which the disease will make itself known; there is only the patient's own knowledge of her body, her experience. Her voice is everything, and yet, too often, nobody listens.

Women are 80 percent more likely to suffer from autoimmune disorders than men, for reasons that scientists have yet to understand. They account for 80–95 percent of patients with primary Sjögren's syndrome, systemic lupus erythematosus (SLE), primary biliary cirrhosis, autoimmune thyroid disease, and systemic sclerosis; they make up 60 percent of arthritis and multiple sclerosis patients. In most cases, these gender disparities are acknowledged but never studied; doctors have long been prone to writing off the differences as hormonal without further inquiry. And when it comes to the patients themselves, women's perspectives go underrepresented for all kinds of reasons: lack of curiosity. Lack of research. Lack of trust from their doctors—and lack of confidence in their own abilities to speak up, ask questions, and demand answers about their health.

Leora, the patient who demanded an explanation after being told in 1973 that her lupus diagnosis made it too dangerous for her to ever become pregnant, was a rarity. But luckily, and crucially, her doctor was, too.

"I told her she should not become pregnant, because pregnancy was very dangerous for lupus patients," Michael Lockshin tells me. It's been fifty years since Leora sat in his office, and today he is the director emeritus of the Barbara Volcker Center for Women and Rheumatic Disease at the Hospital for Special Surgery in New York, but he still remembers the appointment vividly. "Well, that didn't sit well with her. She was Orthodox Jewish, and she was not going to tolerate that. She told me that I had to prove it to her. And so I actually started looking."

Leora's insistence on research to back up her doctor's orders didn't just change the course of her life—as of this writing, she has six children and seventeen grandchildren—but Lockshin's as well. Realizing that the common medical wisdom was incomplete or even inaccurate, he turned his attention to researching the interaction of lupus with pregnancy. It was an area sorely in need of better information: since the 1960s, the consensus among doctors had been that this was too dangerous to contemplate, full stop. So dire were the alleged outcomes of pregnancy in a woman diagnosed with lupus that it was one of the few circumstances, pre–Roe v. Wade, in which it was legal to procure an abortion.

But by 1983, research from Lockshin and others had revealed that there are ways to predict rare fetal complications in pregnancy with women living with lupus, and that women with lupus can safely have children with proper monitoring by a physician. The consensus wisdom, which doctors had been handing down as edict for years, was simply false.

For Lockshin, the realization of how wrong they'd been was unsettling—and instructive. After a tragedy in which another patient abruptly developed lupus during pregnancy and died, he attended a conference about the condition—"And basically, I ended up figuring out that no one knew what they were talking about," he says. "They didn't understand this disease. Here we were at Harvard, the best there is, and all we could do was shrug our shoulders."

And while the presence of remarkable doctors like Lockshin means incrementally less shrugging and more listening, it remains difficult for women with immune disorders to be heard. Many of these diseases are "undifferentiated," which is to say, not classifiable—and because of the way the medical apparatus currently functions, a disease without an official diagnosis becomes a patient without a path forward. Those who suffer from undifferentiated diseases are not included in clinical trials or other policy measures; these women, and there are millions of them, simply fall through the cracks of a system that has no means of registering their existence.

It's always blamed on, oh, well, you're just busy . . . It'll get to the point where a woman will come in and be like, I can't take care of my baby, I can't lift my baby anymore. And that's when someone finally says, Oh, well, let me look at your hands.

—Elizabeth Ortiz, MD, rheumatologist, excerpt from interview, 2023

After centuries of being held responsible for getting everyone else sick, it should come as no surprise that women are now also blamed—or taught to blame themselves—for their own immunological problems, whether they're accused of faking it, exaggerating it, or just making bad choices that leave them vulnerable to disease. Elizabeth Ortiz, a rheumatologist, has seen firsthand how a system that treats women with skepticism sets them on a path first to doubt, then to disillusionment: "People end up just kind of bouncing around between doctors, having things missed. Regardless of what condition we're talking about, there is suffering and damage that's being done."

One hundred years ago, Mary Mallon was stalked, arrested, and imprisoned by doctors who never explained what was happening to her in terms she could understand—who evidently saw her as too stupid and savage to meaningfully participate in her own medical care. Today, Ortiz says, she comes across cases every day of women who have spent years growing sicker and weaker while they desperately try to find just one doctor who will really talk to them. One patient, a woman in her thirties who had an autoimmune disorder called Sjögren's syndrome, had abandoned traditional medicine entirely after doctors diagnosed her disorder but failed to treat her most problematic symptoms.

"She had a pain syndrome that was brewing, that they weren't addressing. And they weren't discussing it with her either," Ortiz says. "She didn't even know she had fibromyalgia. All she knew is that she had Sjögren's, and she was taking medicine, and she wasn't getting any better."

By the time she saw Ortiz, the patient had developed such severe muscle weakness that she could no longer walk or feed herself. Ortiz says that when she began reviewing the woman's records, she started to cry: "You could just see in the record, how she had been failed. No one was talking to her. No one was explaining things to her."

It's not hard to see how women come to believe that being sick is not just their fault, but their problem to solve—or how this creates a breach into which unethical practitioners peddling self-help and snake oil can step. In some ways, it's a new riff on the old song about the carelessness of women who neglect their hygiene, only this time it's not your house or your vagina that needs disinfecting but your attitude. In the 1980s, a Yale physician named Bernie Siegel published a treatise on healing, *Love, Medicine & Miracles*, in which he suggested that a weak immune system was the result of its owner's emotional stuntedness. If you had the proper mindset, he argued, you would be able to heal yourself from within, no matter how lethal the malady: "A vigorous immune system can overcome cancer if it is not interfered with, and emotional growth toward greater self-acceptance and fulfillment helps keep the immune system strong."

In my own practice, I see women diagnosed with metastatic breast cancer who have been scolded that the most important thing they can do is maintain a positive outlook—as if survival is not a matter of medicine but proper mental hygiene. This toxic idea is pervasive across culture and class alike; I have seen women from religious communities told that they should pray their cancer away, while women from elite wellness circles try to manifest and visualize themselves into remission.

It is enraging, and it is also history made manifest: when sickness spreads, even through her own body, a woman will be blamed.

Yeah, my arm was really sore
And the side of my neck on the side that I got vaccinated

That's pretty normal

Yeah
This other thing though

                                                              ?

I'm having my period
And I have the WORST cramps and the heaviest flow I have
ever had, it's horrible

                                        Okay, that's weird

What?
The period thing?

                                                          Yeah
                                        Because . . . me too

—excerpt from chat logs between vaccinated women, January 2021

In some fields, the legacy of women's mistreatment or exclusion within the world of medicine expresses itself today only in subtle ways.

Immunology is not one of them.

In 2021, as vaccines for the Covid-19 virus made their way into the arms of Americans across the country, rumors began to circulate that the shots had a peculiar side effect: in addition to low-grade symptoms of soreness, fatigue, chills, or fever, women who got the vaccine were having disrupted or unusually heavy periods.

The response at the time, from public health officials and the press alike, was to call these women liars—and not just liars, but crazy science-denying conspiracists who were fueling anti-vaccine sentiments that would result in countless unnecessary deaths. Women who shared stories of menstrual side effects on social media were mocked, derided, and had their accounts suspended for "misinformation"; PolitiFact rated the entire controversy as "false," writing, "There is no data linking vaccines to changes in women's cycles or fertility."

PolitiFact was half right: there was no data as described. But this was not because the data didn't exist; it was because researchers had simply never bothered to collect it.

Here was a new wrinkle on the old habit of excluding women from biomedical research. In the case of the Covid vaccine trials, women were present as research subjects—but their unique concerns, the unique workings of their bodies, were still left out of the equation. Nobody asked women if the vaccine had disrupted their periods; indeed, researchers virtually never track the impact of treatments on menstruation unless the treatment is specifically fertility-related. The closest medical research can come to including women, even now, is to study them as if they were men.

It would take more than a year for the medical establishment to acknowledge what countless women already knew from experience: the Covid vaccine did, in fact, cause menstrual disruptions. A study spearheaded by female scientists who had observed such side effects early on revealed striking results, including in populations who weren't menstruating regularly: among respondents, 71 percent of women on birth control and 66 percent of postmenopausal women reported breakthrough bleeding within two weeks of getting vaccinated.

Katherine Lee, a biological anthropologist who led the aforementioned study, describes with frustration the months during which the vaccine's menstrual side effects were treated like some sort of wild conspiracy theory, including by journalists who should have known better.

"They would talk to some random infectious disease expert with no knowledge about periods, and they would say something along the lines of, 'There's no plausible mechanism by which this would happen. There's no biological reason why this would happen. There's no evidence that this is happening,'" she recalls. This, in combination with the dismissive (or worse) treatment of women who reported menstrual side effects post-vaccine, led to a staggering loss of trust in medical authorities at a crucial time: "People are like, 'No, but my period was weird. I know my body. I know what's happening. I know that what happened was weird for me.' They feel like their doctors are gaslighting them."

The historical parallels of this incident, not only to the incuriosity among researchers about the impact of treatments on female bodies but to the paternalistic attitude toward women on the part of public health officials, are hard to miss. As the menstrual side effects of the Covid vaccine became too obvious to ignore, says Lee, the conversation among doctors and public health officials took a distinct turn: "The fear was, oh my god, if we tell people their periods might be weird, they'll worry about fertility and be vaccine hesitant and blah, blah, blah."

In other words, faced with the realization that they had made a mistake—that they had mocked, dismissed, and suppressed the voices of women who had identified a genuine hole in the research— the response of medical authorities was not to admit fault and correct the error.

It was to worry that women, if they knew the truth about the impact of the vaccine on their bodies, wouldn't behave.

◆ ◆ ◆

The fear of disease runs deep in humans. At the heart of immunology is the terrifying truth that we share a planet with millions of invisible organisms that survive by infecting, sickening, and killing us—and a long history of scapegoating women for our vulnerability against an enemy too small to see.

The fourteenth-century specter of the foul woman with a womb full of deadly rot, which infected the imaginations of medical men at the time, has taken many other shapes over the years. She is Martin Luther's syphilitic whore. She is the immigrant cook, garnishing your dinner with teeming microscopic disease. She is the early twentieth-century fashionista spreading flu with her naked ankles. She is the 1940s good-time girl who looked so sweet, so clean—or the 1950s housewife whose neglect of "proper feminine hygiene" makes her husband gag. She's the cancer patient who couldn't visualize her immune system back to health. She's the derelict who let Covid into her house because she didn't wipe down the groceries with Lysol. She's the conspiracy theorist who wouldn't stop talking about how the vaccine altered her period.

She could be anyone. She could be you.

And the female body, so many of whose workings remain medically mysterious even in an otherwise enlightened age, and so revered for its ability to grow, nurture, protect, and eventually give forth new life, also remains a vessel into which we can place all manner of things: blame, ignorance, incuriosity, fear.

CHAPTER 9

nerves

NERVOUS

THE "BITCHES BE CRAZY" SCHOOL OF MEDICINE

No doubt exists that all women are crazy; it's only a question of degree.

—W. C. Fields, circa 1940

Frailty, thy name is woman.

—William Shakespeare, *Hamlet*, 1603

Receptionist: How do you write women so well?

Melvin Udall: I think of a man, and I take away reason and accountability.

—*As Good as It Gets*, 1997

Does any physician believe that it is good for a growing girl to be so occupied [with learning] seven or eight hours a day? or that it is right for her to use her brains as long a time as the mechanic employs his muscles?

—Silas Weir Mitchell, MD, 1891

We may also infer, from the law of the deviation from averages, so well illustrated by Mr. Galton, in his work on *Hereditary Genius* that . . . the average of mental power in man must be above that of women.

—Charles Darwin, 1896

Why are the pretty ones always insane?

—Chief Wiggum, *The Simpsons*, "Marge Simpson in: 'Screaming Yellow Honkers,'" aired 1999 on Fox

Wherefore women are more compassionate and more readily made to weep, more jealous and querulous, fonder of railing, and more contentious. The female also is more subject to depression of spirits and despair than the male.

—Aristotle, *The History of Animals*, Book IX: fourth century BC

The experience of this asylum did not differ, I found, from that of similar establishments, in proving that insanity is more prevalent among women than among men . . . Female servants are, as is well known, more frequently afflicted with lunancy than any other class of persons.

—Charles Dickens, 1852

Hysteria, like all neuroses, begins, among girls, with the cessation of their studies and the complete incapacity of learning anything.

—Pierre Janet, MD, 1913

As a general rule, all women are hysterical. And every woman carries with her the seeds of hysteria.

—Augustin Fabre, MD, 1883

[A woman] has a head almost too small for intellect but just big enough for love.

—Charles Meigs, MD, 1847

I respect a woman, but this bitch is crazy.

—Drake, "Bitch Is Crazy," 2007

The women are clearly hysterical.

Everybody knows this, even if no doctor has yet uttered the diagnosis out loud. They stand at a distance, hands stuffed deep into the pockets of their white coats, observing the patients with a mix of pity, fascination, and concern. Some of them scribble notes, considering possible treatment options; others just stare, a rapt audience for this medical sideshow that runs all day long.

One of the patients is crouched in a shower stall, where she's been for hours, clutching one mutilated hand to her chest. The bandages she was wearing this morning lie sopping at her feet, shredded where she tore them away with her teeth, answering the siren song of her compulsion. The mutilation is of her own doing: two of her fingers are bloodied and ragged, chewed down to the nub of bright white bone that peeks out where the flesh has been stripped away. A nurse stands over her, fresh bandages at the ready. She reaches for the patient's wrist.

"Come on, dear," she says, gently, but the woman snatches her hand away. She brings her fingers to her lips.

The nurse shudders as she begins to chew again.

Another is having a fit, one arm and one leg jittering uncontrollably, her jaw working with the effort to form words that never make it out of her mouth. She stares at her shaking hands as if they belong to somebody else, her eyes huge and pleading. The few sounds she manages to produce are garbled stammering. It doesn't matter; the doctors already know what's wrong with her—just as they know what's wrong with the woman in the shower, who will have her fingers amputated within the week. It's a nervous condition, the kind to which female bodies and female brains have always been understood to be tragically susceptible. Entire tomes have been written explaining that cases like these, shocking as they are, only reflect the weak constitution and latent capacity for madness that every woman harbors.

The doctors nod at one another. They stare. They sigh. Privately, they think that as terrible as the patients' plight, it could be worse: if this were another sort of place, like the infamous Pitié-Salpêtrière hospital in Paris, where Dr. Sigmund Freud penned his seminal lectures on hysteria, these women wouldn't be hidden away on a ward at all. They'd be paraded onstage in the operating theater, in front of a gawking, gasping audience who paid good money to stare.

But still, nobody says the word.

"Hysteria."

Indeed, nobody says that word anymore. Even if they wanted to, nobody would dare. Because this shocking moment in medical history isn't something out of the Pitié-Salpêtrière hospital, or Paris, or the nineteenth century. Sigmund Freud has been dead for eighty years.

This is 2023, in New York City.

But when it comes to the way the medical system views women, some things truly never change.

◆ ◆ ◆

While the *Diagnostic and Statistical Manual of Mental Disorders* (DSM) has not listed hysteria in its pages since the year 1980, the removal of the word from the medical lexicon has done little to diminish its influence. Indeed, few ideas have held more sway over women's lives—in medicine, in culture, in politics, and in society—than the pseudoscientific archetype of the hysterical woman.

For as long as doctors have treated female patients, they have also doubted and dismissed them as constitutionally unbalanced. Nervous. Hysterical. Anxious. The words change, but the song remains the same, and this is true even despite myriad other positive advancements in the medical system at large. Consider the patients you met in the preceding paragraphs, who were treated at a New York City hospital in 2023: even as the coronavirus pandemic had left the medical system in a somewhat chaotic state, these women had access to the best technology, to the most advanced treatments, and to compassionate physicians who could not be further in attitude or education from the men who, in the bad old days, would parade the female patients who had been diagnosed and institutionalized with nervous conditions in front of an audience, as if they were sideshow freaks.

And yet, when these cases tested the limits of a physician's knowledge and understanding, the specter of the hysterical woman suddenly appeared all the same, a ghost in the medical machine. These women had different backgrounds, different medical histories, and virtually no symptoms in common—but in the pages of each of their charts, the same diagnosis eventually appeared.

The problem, doctors said, was anxiety.

The truth was, they didn't have a clue.

Biologically speaking, the human nervous system is a communications network, conveying the signals that regulate everything from heart rate to organ function to feeling—not just physical touch but emotions, intelligence, mood. When it malfunctions, it's responsible for ailments like Parkinson's disease, epilepsy, ADHD, anxiety, or Alzheimer's disease. But when it comes to medical history, the nervous system plays a particularly unique role: it has been the scapegoat at the center of virtually every theory as to why women's brains were fundamentally different, deranged, and broken in comparison to the male "ideal."

As such, any consideration of women's neurology yields a dizzying amount of material, far more than I could ever hope to contain within a single chapter. Entire books could be written—and in many cases, have been—about every single one of the characters, settings, and theories you will encounter in the coming pages. But for our purposes, the nervous system is best understood not as one biological apparatus, but as a prism through which the medical community's entire understanding of women is refracted. This chapter, rather than attempting to sketch the history in its totality, zooms in on the biggest, brightest, and sharpest of those refracted points—and then zooms out to show how they connect to form the unmistakable shape of a larger, terrifying truth about what the scientific community saw, and still sees, when it looks at women.

It's a vision expressed not just in the medical literature but in philosophy, in literature, in stories and in songs—and once, by Jerry Stiller in the film *The Heartbreak Kid*, as he leads a despondent Ben Stiller away from the woman whose home he has just broken into in the middle of the night to confess his unrequited love. The line is the entire history of women's neurology distilled into a single phrase:

"Bitches be crazy. You know that."

Everything about her announces the hysteric. The care that she takes in her toilette; the styling of her hair, the ribbons she likes to adorn herself with . . .

—Désiré-Magloire Bourneville, MD, 1878

The first picture ever taken of Augustine, shortly after her arrival at the Pitié-Salpêtrière women's asylum in 1878, is striking in its ordinariness. She could be anyone: a young woman in a plain, dark dress, leaning sideways against a chair with her head resting lightly on one hand. The man who ordered the portrait will later describe her as a natural performer—an "active, intelligent, affectionate, impressionable, and capricious" girl who loves brightly colored ribbons, complicated hairstyles, and "being the center of attention"— but none of that is evident in this decidedly formal photograph, in which she gazes neutrally at the picture-taker with barely a hint of a smile on her lips. It's only her hair, pinned neatly atop her head in coiled braids, that so much as suggests the existence of this other Augustine, mercurial and coquettish and always craving the spotlight: if those careful braids might come undone, then so, too, might the woman wearing them.

From the outside, Pitié-Salpêtrière resembles a stone fortress, with the domed rooftop of its central chapel peeking up above a massive archway that is the only opening in its endless front facade. It has been months since Augustine first passed through that entrance, in the company of a mother who didn't seem to care if the doctors could cure her child, just as long as they would keep her confined within these walls. Out of sight, out of mind. Mother has rarely been back to visit since Augustine first fell ill, and then it wasn't out of love but self-interest. All she wants, all she ever wants, is to make sure her daughter never tells the police the truth about what happened.

As if they would listen. As if they would care. Mother doesn't understand that the truth about what happened to Augustine has already revealed itself here in this hospital, over and over. It happens every time, as the shimmering aura of an oncoming seizure clouds her vision, as her body begins to convulse. Her feet pedal helplessly against the mattress; her hands ball into fists. She screams and kicks against the air, fighting the invisible assailant who exists only in her memory.

The man had been her mother's employer. He held a razor blade to Augustine's throat while he held her down.

"Pig!" she shrieks. "You're hurting me!"

The doctors have witnessed this scene countless times and cannot fail to know it for what it is, but not one of them has ever suggested sharing the story with the police. Indeed, their notes explicitly describe Augustine's rape as "unfit for publication" in either legal or medical venues, instead worth documenting only insofar as an "inquisitive student of diseased and degraded human nature" might find her account illuminating. Inside the walls of Pitié-Salpêtrière, the hysterical girl is less a person than a point of interest, one who spends much of her time sitting or lying in a cast-iron bed that has been pushed up close to the windows—not so that she can see out but so that there's always enough light to take the photographs of her, which will eventually number in the hundreds. The camera stands beside the bed, always at the ready. It has captured her smiling and shrieking, weeping and laughing, or frozen on her back with her mouth open and gaping, like a snake that has unhinged its jaw. In one picture, Augustine poses looking over her bare shoulder, her hair loose and wild. She is gazing straight at the camera, her lips curled in a coy smirk, but this is a rarity; in most of the images, she doesn't seem to realize she's being photographed at all.

This is the attention they insist Augustine so enjoys. Does she? Maybe, or maybe they just need to believe that she does. Maybe this is the lie the doctors tell for their own benefit, to justify the endless hours they spend poking at her, pulling her hair, and pricking her skin. Hypnotizing her and shoving needles through the delicate webbing between her fingers while she sits insensible, or making her eat bits of charcoal, which they present to her as chocolate. Watching her, always watching her, not with the dispassionate eye of a diagnostician but the hungry gaze of the voyeur.

As for what Augustine truly feels, thinks, or wants, it is difficult to discern—for students of history looking back at her with pity, but also, perhaps, for Augustine herself. Under the spell of medical hypnosis, standing in front of the crowd that has gathered to watch her perform, it is not just impossible to say "no" or "stop"; it becomes increasingly impossible to distinguish the doctor's desires from her own. And what is the sense in knowing what you desire, when those desires have only ever been disregarded?

What does it matter, when people will take what they want from you, whether you want them to or not?

We found ourselves, in other words, in possession of a kind of living pathology museum whose holdings were virtually inexhaustible.

—Jean-Martin Charcot, MD, 1880

Historically, the "bitches be crazy" theory of neurology can be observed as much in absence as in evidence: not once, in the entire human history of medicine, has anyone ever advanced a competing theory that women are the smarter, saner, more sensible of the sexes.

"Hysteria," that catch-all term for female derangement that derives directly from the Greek word for "womb," is found described in substance if not by name in medical literature dating back to ancient Egypt. Papyruses from the second millennium BC describe how the movement of the uterus within a woman's body led to dangerous mental conditions, including tonic-clonic seizures and depressive disorders, which doctors believed could be cured only by forcing the wandering uterus back to its proper position—or sometimes, enticing it through the use of what can only be described as an absurd early precursor to aromatherapy. If the uterus had migrated upward, the medical texts instructed, acrid substances should be placed near the woman's nose, and pleasantly scented ones near her vagina, to lure it back into place. (Thousands of years later, this same notion of the uterus as responsive to olfactory stimuli would fuel the Victorian predilection for placing smelling salts under the nostrils of a woman who had fainted.)

Meanwhile, the actual term "hysteria" first emerged in the works of Hippocrates in the fifth century BC, again describing a disease resulting from the movement of the uterus—which by now was imagined not only to merely shift its location but to wander the entirety of the body like a sort of insensible animal, sowing chaos wherever it went. The Greeks blamed the wayward uterus for everything from obstructing breathing and blocking blood flow to poisoning other organs by pressing up against them; like the Egyptians, their standard cure for hysteria was to put something repulsive under a woman's nose to chase her womb back to the bodily south, although they also believed it could be forced back into place by sneezing. When humorism took over as the dominant medical theory of the moment, doctors declared that the cold, wet female constitution made a woman's uterus particularly prone to illness, especially if she had no male partner. In this iteration, the uterus is imagined as something closer to sentient, so dissatisfied with its lot in life that it ends up wandering around the body in a general state of disgruntlement.

Also in this case, unsurprisingly, the recommended cure for hysteria was marriage and sex.

Indeed, throughout history, a hysteria diagnosis proved remarkably adaptable to whatever medical and cultural mores happened to be in vogue at the time. Medieval physicians saw hysteria as a function of demonic possession, or perhaps the effects of witchcraft, although it also eventually emerged as a defense against accusations of the latter. Elizabeth Stover, a young woman who was accused of witchcraft in 1602, was spared at trial after a physician named Edward Jorden testified that her symptoms—including "suffocation in the throate, croaking of Frogges, hissing of Snakes . . . frenzies, convulsions, hickcockes, laughing, singing, weeping, crying"— stemmed not from dabbling in the dark arts but from the effects of a displaced uterus. In the 1700s, as the medical establishment became a venue for laundering various cultural anxieties surrounding female sexuality, hysteria was a go-to diagnosis for women suspected of being masturbators.

In short, anything and everything that was "wrong" with women could be attributed to hysteria—and was, with wild abandon. Every physician featured in this book accused his female patients of being hysterical in one way or another, and every woman who came into contact with the medical system would have done so under a cloud of suspicion. Hysteria defined the place of women in the world, as patients and as people: the consensus was that simply having a uterus put any woman at a biological disadvantage, as the temperamental organ could not help but impact the workings of the brain. In 1828, a psychiatrist and insanity expert named George Man Burrows articulated the medical consensus that uterine function was nothing less than the "moral and physical barometer of the female constitution."

"Yet the functions of the brain are so intimately connected with the uterine system, that the interruption of any one process which the latter has to perform in the human economy may implicate the former," he wrote.

By the time Louise Augustine Gleizes, the teenage girl who would become known by her middle name alone as the famous hysteric Augustine, turned up at Pitié-Salpêtrière hospital in the late 1800s, the medical wisdom surrounding hysteria had become an impenetrable tapestry richly interwoven with scientific and social influences alike. As always, the barrier between culture and medicine was permeable; nineteenth-century psychiatrists were particularly fixated on Shakespeare's Ophelia as a case study in hysteria brought on by a sexually turbulent adolescence. In 1859, Dr. John Charles Bucknill, president of the Medico-Psychological Association, wrote, "Every mental physician of moderately extensive experience must have seen many Ophelias."

So influential was Shakespeare's fictionalized depiction of female madness that even Ophelia's physical appearance was deemed medically salient. In the original First Folio publication of Hamlet, Ophelia's descent into madness was symbolized by her hair: neatly pinned up at first, then long and undone after she had gone insane.

Those cascading tresses soon became fully synonymous with the character of Ophelia—as in the famous nineteenth-century oil painting of a drowning Ophelia by John Everett Millais, which depicts her hair floating undone around her head like a halo—but also, in short order, with female madness at the conceptual level. It's no wonder that Augustine's doctors made so much of her propensity for complicated hairstyles, nor that so many of those famous photographs show her with her hair tumbling wild over her shoulders. Not only did Augustine's condition make for a sensational case study of hysteria, she even looked the part.

As for Pitié-Salpêtrière, it was here that the idea of hysteria as neurological in origin would fully take hold, under the leadership of chief physician Jean-Martin Charcot. Charcot, often cited as the father of modern neurology, ran his asylum as equal parts laboratory, hospital, and theater. Some of his work there was groundbreaking; Charcot was the first to identify and uncover the neurologic basis for a variety of diseases, laying the groundwork for essential advancements in the field and mentoring many of the famous doctors who would go on to shape it. But Charcot's deserved reputation as a scientist was bolstered by a public persona that was less medical doctor than circus ringmaster, particularly when it came to his work with hysterical patients. In Charcot's own words, the asylum was "a kind of museum of living pathology"—or, in other words, a freak show. And the inexhaustible supply of curiosities in Charcot's personal museum were not objects but people, mostly women, and many of whom had been committed to the asylum against their will.

At Pitié-Salpêtrière, Charcot paraded women like Augustine in front of a fascinated crowd, demonstrating the scope of their hysterical symptoms as well as his recommended treatments for relieving them, which were unorthodox and sometimes violent. Charcot claimed that a hysterical woman could be treated by applying pressure to parts of the body he called "hysterogenic zones," which sounds scientific enough in theory but translated in practice to punching his patients in the ovaries.

A painting of one of these performances captures the circus-like atmosphere: Charcot, wearing a dark suit and with his gray hair slicked back and tucked behind his ears, stands beside a swooning woman who is being supported by the arms of an assistant. Surrounding the scene is a rapt audience made up entirely of men. Many of the attendees at Charcot's sensational lectures were physicians and scientists—including Sigmund Freud, who would eventually leapfrog from Charcot's theories of a neurologically based hysteria to his own conception of the disorder as rooted in the psyche—but the public nature of the demonstrations attracted visitors with less wholesome motivations as well. One day, midperformance, Augustine looked into the crowd and spotted a familiar face among the onlookers, staring back at her and grinning. It was her mother's employer, the man who'd raped her.

He'd come to see the show.

It's important to note that Charcot was not unique in making a spectacle of his patients, nor in turning Pitié-Salpêtrière into a sort of tourist attraction. This was the Parisian Belle Époque, a boom time for artistic innovation and scientific progress alike—and a ripe environment for boundary-pushing physicians to lean into the theatrical. Hospitals for the insane were treated less like places of healing than human zoos where the public could enter and gawk at patients who had often been coached to behave in stereotypically crazy ways, and performances like Augustine's even became inspiration for art forms outside the hospital walls, including an entire genre of street dancers who incorporated seizure-type movement styles into their choreography. If the archetype of the female hysteric first arrived in mental hospitals out of Shakespeare, it traveled just as easily from hospitals like Pitié-Salpêtrière into the broader culture, entrenching the notion of women as unstable deeply into the public consciousness.

As for Augustine, she would stay at Pitié-Salpêtrière—as a patient, then an employee, and then a patient again—for five years altogether. She remained one of Charcot's pet subjects, even during the period when she was allegedly cured; after the doctor discovered that he could induce her hysterical episodes via hypnosis, he continued to summon her to the theater for public demonstrations. Perhaps unsurprisingly, things soon took a dark turn: Augustine relapsed and began to suffer from increasingly violent attacks during which she was subject to straitjacketing, ovarian compression, and electroshock therapy, all with little success. For all her fame as

Charcot's research subject, it is worth noting that he never actually managed to help her—and it should come as no surprise that eventually, Augustine became tired of being imprisoned within Pitié-Salpêtrière's walls. The details of her life thereafter have been lost to history, but we do know that she escaped. She wore a set of stolen clothes, perhaps left behind by a hospital intern; the long, beautiful hair that her doctors once found so striking was either hidden under a cap or shorn away. Nobody looked at her. Nobody chased her.

After so many years of performing for the public as Charcot's patient—the famous hysterical woman, the archetypal crazy bitch—Augustine stole back her freedom by disguising herself as somebody the hospital staff would never think to question: a man.

She had used as a weapon, though not with definite conscious purpose, for the gaining of her point in whatever quarrel came up, symptoms that are usually called hysterical; that is to say, vomiting, fainting spells and pains without definite physical cause.

—Abraham Myerson, MD, "Hysteria as a Weapon in Marital Conflicts,"
1914

The chief and primary cause of this development and very rapid increase of nervousness is modern civilization, which is distinguished from the ancient by these five characteristics: steampower, the periodical press, the telegraph, the sciences and the mental activity of women.

—George M. Beard, MD, "American Nervousness, Its Causes and
Consequences: A Supplement to Nervous Exhaustion," 1881

A hysterical girl is a vampire who sucks the blood of the healthy people about her.

—Oliver Wendell Holmes Sr., 1908

The lack of a known medical cause or even consensus definition of hysteria allowed for the proliferation of an enormous range of theories as to just what it was and how it should be treated. The women institutionalized at Pitié-Salpêtrière likely suffered from a range of ailments we now recognize as things like epilepsy, schizophrenia, or OCD—but these conditions were neither named nor understood at the time, leaving doctors trying to diagnose and treat a huge and varied array of conditions based on little more than the scientific trends of the time along with their own personal predilections.

Hence somebody like Charcot, who believed that hysteria stemmed from some sort of malfunction in the neurological interface between a woman's organs and her brain, focused almost exclusively on its bodily manifestations while giving little thought to whether the traumatic history of a patient like Augustine might also be a contributing factor to her condition (or, for that matter, whether it might be both in bad taste and medically inadvisable to punch a patient in the ovaries). By contrast, Dr. Désiré-Magloire Bourneville, one of Charcot's disciples, was both more politically progressive than his mentor and also more interested in how childhood experiences can come to bear on a patient's physical and mental health; he took an interest in Augustine's thoughts, not just her symptoms, and it is thanks to him that we have such detailed records of Augustine's history, her utterances during her attacks, her relationship with her parents, even her dreams.

And then there's Sigmund Freud, who was such an avid student of Charcot that he not only personally translated the doctor's work into German but named one of his sons after him—but who nevertheless decided that hysteria was not a neurological derangement of the female organs but rather a function of sexual repression. Which, of course, just happened to be a topic of greatest personal interest to him, one on which he would predicate his life's work.

Additionally, from the late 1800s through the early twentieth century, any discussion of hysteria was often laid atop the existing scientific consensus that women had evolved to be dumber, weaker, and more fragile. It was at this time that scientists were busy scrutinizing women's skulls for evidence of their inferiority, while none other than Charles Darwin mused that women were best appreciated as "[an] object to be beloved and played with—better than a dog anyhow."

Soon, doctors were in general agreement that hysteria in women was a function of this innate inferiority, one often brought on by their attempting to somehow subvert the passive, domestic, subservient role that was a woman's biological destiny. One favorite scapegoat on this front was women's education: in 1873, Dr. Edward Hammond Clarke of Harvard Medical School issued a dire warning to educators and parents alike that too much schooling would render women hysterical. There was, he said, no way a woman could receive the same education as a man "and retain uninjured health and a future secure from neuralgia, uterine disease, hysteria, and other derangements of the nervous system." Clarke was not only convinced that hysteria resulted from women's systems being overtaxed by too much thinking—the result of the body's energy and resources being redirected to the brain at the expense of her ovaries—but testified that one of his patients had literally studied to death: "Believing that woman can do what man can, for she held that faith, she strove with noble but ignorant bravery to compass man's intellectual attainment in a man's way, and died in that effort."

The notion that hysteria was the result of too much intellectual stimulation existed in tandem with treatment protocols that aimed to make women as uneducated, docile, and idle as possible, including the "rest cure" developed by Silas Weir Mitchell. Mitchell specialized in treating hysteria and neurasthenia (a hysteria-adjacent condition that literally means "weakness of the nerves") by confining women to bed for weeks or months at a time, force-feeding them rich foods, and depriving them of any creative or intellectual outlet whatsoever. The rest cure didn't actually cure women so much as break them, which Mitchell openly acknowledged: after months of being confined to bed with no one to talk to and nothing to do but stare at the walls, he said, women were "glad enough" to follow any orders he wanted if he would just let them get up. Ironically, Mitchell and his practices are most famous now for inspiring the 1892 horror story "The Yellow Wallpaper," in which a woman slowly loses her mind while being subjected to the rest cure by her physician husband. The author, Charlotte Perkins Gilman, was one of Mitchell's patients; she wrote the story in defiance of her doctor's orders after his so-called cure nearly drove her insane.

Here, a pattern begins to emerge. Women who were diagnosed with hysteria in fact suffered from a variety of illness, physiological and mental alike (except on the numerous occasions when there was nothing wrong with them at all). What they had in common was not a medical condition but something far more intractable: they were all frustrating to men.

Hysterical women didn't listen, didn't cooperate, didn't behave. Their symptoms often seemed rooted in defiance—of convention, of etiquette, of a husband's or doctor's demands, and of the inferior role that physicians had been so reliably assured was their evolutionary birthright. As such, it's not a coincidence that the preferred treatments for hysteria often involved restricting women's freedom, whether it was to pursue an education or even to get out of bed. But when these measures proved insufficient to curtail hysterical symptoms—which by this point had expanded to include anything from tonic-clonic seizures to being tired to reading too many novels—the medical establishment was all too happy to restrict these patients' lives even further . . . all the way into a squalid cell with bars on the windows, guards at the door, and the wails of fellow imprisoned women echoing down the halls all night long.

At the State Hospital at Trenton, N.J., under the brilliant leadership of the medical director, Dr. Henry A. Cotton, there is on foot the most searching, aggressive, and profound scientific investigation that has yet been made of the whole field of mental and nervous disorders . . . there is hope, high hope . . . for the future.

—*New York Times*, 1922

Helen, the woman in the room at the end of the hall, is pacing again. Her stockinged feet make no sound as she walks the perimeter of the room, but if you look down, you can see the restless movement of her shadow in the narrow space beneath the door. The doctors used to plead with her to stop, to rest, to try to control herself, but that was only at the beginning, in 1911, when she was first brought to the asylum by her father after a series of hysterical attacks. Now it's 1916, and they've all but given up; a note in her file identifies her as a "chronic demented patient."

If you asked Helen, she'd say that's funny: she used to be a nurse.

Next door to Helen, who can't stop moving, is Amelia, who can't move at all. The doctors bound her hands and feet after diagnosing her with violent psychosis—not because she hurt anyone, but because she kept removing her clothing.

Across the hall from Amelia is Elaine, who did hurt someone, or at least tried to: she went after her husband with a tire iron after she found out that he'd been spending fifty dollars a month to keep his mistress in a brownstone in Bensonhurst, one twice as large as the one where she'd lived with him, cooking his meals and mending his clothes, for fifteen years. Her husband dumped her on the asylum doorstep and left without a word. Her sister, who came to take care of Elaine's children, wrote last week to say that he'd taken his things and moved to Bensonhurst.

Next door to Elaine is Margaret, whose husband requested the doctors cure her of her penchant for reading novels. Next door to her is Ida, diagnosed with religious excitement. Farther down the hall are Rose, Wilhelmina, and Alice: hysterical, hysterical, psychotic.

◆ ◆ ◆

These are the residents of the New Jersey State Hospital for the treatment of the insane. None of these women are suffering from the same condition, and yet, they are all here for the same reason: because this is where a man wanted them to be.

And when they leave—that is, the ones who do leave, who survive to make it back to the other side of the asylum's high brick walls—they won't be the same women they were when they came in. The doctor, the one with the piercing gaze and heavy jaw, the one who waits behind the door of the operating room where patients are dragged, screaming, into surgery, will see to that.

This place, and that man, they take things from you. Your time. Your freedom. Your memory. Your dignity.

And your teeth.

Especially your teeth.

◆ ◆ ◆

Once a scientific consensus emerged that the best treatment for a woman with a nervous disorder was to commit her to an asylum, the number of woman diagnosed with such disorders skyrocketed— not because of anything the women themselves were doing but because of an explosion in inquiries from men, usually husbands or fathers, who were eager to take advantage of this medical corrective for women's "abnormal" behavior (that is: any behavior of which the men disapproved).

The cited reasons for institutionalizing women at the time were wildly varied, including depression, lacking a menstrual cycle, novel reading, spiritualism, vicious indulgence, hard study, menopause, religious excitement, domestic trouble, and sunstroke. In virtually all cases, however, the inquiry into a woman's sanity was initiated by a man close to her. The details of many cases are so outrageous as to beggar belief: women were committed for having postpartum depression, for being either too interested in sex or not interested enough, or even as a pretense for allowing a philandering husband to pursue affairs without worrying about being discovered. In one famous case from 1860, a sane and sensible mother of six named Elizabeth Packard was sent to an asylum by her husband for disagreeing with him—although this story, at least, has a happy ending. After being imprisoned for two years in a state mental hospital, Packard sued for her freedom and won (and immediately filed for divorce).

But if this moment presented a certain sort of opportunity for husbands who wanted to be rid of their wives, it was an even greater boon to doctors who wanted to test invasive, experimental, unproven treatments on patients who couldn't say no. And on that front, there are few physicians who did more—or who did more damage—than Dr. Henry A. Cotton.

Cotton, a Johns Hopkins–trained physician, was just thirty years old when he was appointed the medical director of the New Jersey

State Hospital at Trenton in 1907. At the time, he was seen as one of the most gifted, groundbreaking, and progressive physicians in his field, and rightly so: Cotton was a pioneer in the treatment of mental illness and spoke out fiercely against both the stigmatization of mental illness and the abusive practices that were de rigueur in asylums at the time, both of which he considered deplorable. Among the major changes he made at Trenton was to outlaw the use of mechanical restraints like cages and straitjackets on patients, along with hiring a staff of exclusively female nurses (men, he said, were too prone to treating the patients roughly). Most of all, he said, he wanted asylums to be run like hospitals, where people with mental illnesses would be treated and not just confined: "Is there any reason why these patients should be denied the physical studies, interpretations and general hospital treatment so profitable to the public at large simply because the infection to which they are subject happens to have affected the brain rather than the heart or joints?"

Unfortunately, there was a dark side to Cotton's activities, one that hinged on a key word in the aforementioned quote: "infection."

Cotton's tenure at Trenton coincided with the discovery and proliferation of germ theory, which he believed held the key not only to diseases like malaria or typhoid but to mental illness as well. And when it came to hysteria, Cotton argued that other doctors had gotten it wrong. The solution was not ovarian compression à la Charcot, or endless psychoanalysis à la Freud, but locating the hidden nest of insanity-causing microorganisms in the body: "a bacteriological model of madness." Remove the infection, he insisted, and you'd cure the patient.

It was, at the time, a revelation. Cotton was heralded as a hero by the press and within the medical community; his methods, which reportedly boasted an astonishing success rate of 85 percent, became a sensation. In 1922, the New York Times applauded his work as "the most searching, aggressive, and profound scientific investigation that has yet been made of the whole field of mental and nervous disorders," lamenting only that Cotton had not pushed his cures earlier and more aggressively. Patients themselves clamored to be treated at the Trenton asylum—or if they couldn't get there, demanded that their own doctors adopt Cotton's methods themselves.

There was just one problem: Cotton's theory of focal infection was almost entirely wrong. His groundbreaking methods, when other doctors attempted them, didn't replicate. And his miraculous cure for insanity, the one everyone wanted to try? It was pulling out his patients' teeth. Sometimes it was just a few; usually, though, it was all of them.

Cotton didn't only perform these barbaric (and, tragically, completely ineffective) treatments on women, but given the overrepresentation of women as patients—and particularly patients with whom, again, nothing was actually wrong—it meant that the worst of his brutality was reserved for them. Although the teeth were generally Cotton's first and favorite target, they were only the beginning. A woman who persisted in her hysteria even after Cotton had taken her teeth was liable to lose her tonsils next, followed by her gallbladder, her stomach, her spleen, her cervix, her colon, and, eventually, her ovaries—although Cotton was uncharacteristically conservative about this last one, advocating that it be done only under "extreme conditions." (Unfortunately for his patients, by "extreme" he meant "if she's not better within a few months.")

In some ways, Cotton had come full circle from the days when doctors attempted to cure hysteria by using aromatherapy to lure a woman's wandering uterus back into place. Only now, it wasn't just the uterus but any organ that could be making a female patient crazy. And thanks to advances in surgical techniques—not to mention the fact that he didn't require a patient's consent to use them—there was nothing stopping him from chasing suspected infections around a woman's body with a scalpel, cutting out pieces until she was cured . . . or dead.

Incredibly, Henry A. Cotton was not the first physician to posit a surgical solution to hysteria. The association between nervous disorders and female anatomy was a popular one in the mid-1800s, leading to suggestions from physicians like Isaac Baker Brown and Horatio Storer (who we'll meet in the Reproductive chapter) that removing a woman's ovaries, uterus, or clitoris could cure her of insanity. But even as populated as the history of neurology is by scandals of this type, the one perpetrated by Cotton is especially grotesque. His much-boasted-about 85 percent cure rate was a lie, of course; in fact, as many as 30 percent of his patients died, and none were actually cured. And yet he carried on extracting his patients' teeth and organs in the name of science for more than twenty years.

The duration of this scandal likely stemmed from the fact that Cotton's reputation as a groundbreaking scientist, along with his genuine, deeply held conviction that he was alleviating his patients' suffering where nobody else could, evidently captured the imagination of the scientific community, the press, and even the patients themselves so thoroughly that nobody wanted to consider the possibility that he—that they—were wrong. As for Cotton's critics, they were all too easy to dismiss—because they were going against the consensus view that Cotton was a genius, but also because they were mostly women. When a handful of fellow physicians and psychiatrists tried to sound the alarm, an investigation into the Trenton hospital was commissioned but promptly suppressed by one of Cotton's mentors when it became clear just how many of his patients were dying; the investigation was conducted by psychiatrist Phyllis Greenacre, a woman. A year later, another investigation was initiated, this time by the New Jersey State Senate, but again was scuttled by outrage from Cotton's supporters; as reported by the *New York Times*, "eminent physicians and surgeons" rushed to testify that Cotton's hospital "was the most progressive institution in the world for the care of the insane." And those who testified that Cotton had dragged patients screaming into the surgical suite and operated on them while they begged him to stop? They were former patients and nurses—which is to say, women.

As for Cotton, he passed away in 1933 and did not survive to see his work discredited. While he was alive, however, he refused to entertain the possibility that his so-called cure didn't work, let alone that he was doing harm. If anything, the State Senate investigation into his hospital—in which many of Cotton's former patients testified that they'd been mutilated by him without consent—only caused him to double down on his near-religious certainty in his own good works: "We must bear in mind that it is only by being persistent, often against the wishes of the patient . . . that we can expect our efforts to be successful," he said. "Failure in these cases at once casts discredit upon the theory, when the reason lies in the fact that we have not been radical enough."

In the end, even in the face of growing evidence that he'd made a terrible mistake, Cotton could only cling harder to his theories . . . and his forceps. In 1926, as the State Senate investigation unfolded, he performed another series of surgeries—but not in the hospital, and not on patients who had been diagnosed with hysteria or psychosis or any other ailment. These surgeries were different, a living testament to Cotton's unflagging faith that he was right, and righteous, in his methods.

He took his wife's teeth first. Then his two sons'.

And then, finally, defiantly, Henry A. Cotton put the forceps into his own mouth and began to pull.

Dr. Freeman: Do you have any of your old fears?

Patient: No.

Dr. Freeman: What were you afraid of?

Patient: I don't know. I seem to forget.

Dr. Freeman: Do you remember being upset when you came here?

Patient: Yes I was quite upset, wasn't I?

Dr. Freeman: What was it all about?

Patient: I don't know. I seem to have forgotten. It doesn't seem important now.

—conversation between Walter Jackson Freeman II, MD, and lobotomy patient, 1936

Walter Freeman shifts the car into fifth gear, urging it to go faster as the highway stretches long and empty in front of him. He has gone so many miles already. He has so many more miles to go. For all the patients he's visited in the past weeks, there are so many left still to see. Not to treat them, not this time—he is an old man now, long since retired—but to witness the legacy of his work, the way a man at the end of his life might linger contentedly in a garden he once spent his hours tending. Pausing beneath a tree he planted as a sapling thirty years ago, gazing awestruck at the solid trunk and sprawling canopy.

People are not trees, though; they don't stay where you plant them. And so Walter spends his days traveling, crisscrossing the country to reconnect with those whose lives he touched. Some of them he knew just where to find, having kept in touch with their families for years. Some, he's had to hunt down through changes of situation, employment, address—but he's happy to do it. More than happy. Determined. He needs to find them, because he needs to see for himself. To make sure. To be assured, one last time, that he changed their lives for the better.

◆ ◆ ◆

Not that he needs assurance. The very idea is preposterous. Of course he helped them; helping them was all he ever wanted.

His friends and former colleagues tend to shift in their seats when he shares these thoughts aloud. They look away or look at their feet; they look anywhere but into Walter's eyes. But they don't understand. They weren't there. They couldn't possibly know how beautiful it was, how pure, to witness the moment when suffering becomes serenity. They had never seen the look of absolute calm that came over a patient's face in that moment when the fine point of the surgical pick finally penetrated through her orbital bone and into her frontal lobe.

But Walter saw it. And from the first, he understood that this would be his life's work.

Now all he wants is to look back at that work with pride. He wants to look into the faces of all the people he helped and see the gratitude in their eyes. Because they are grateful, surely. They always greet him with a smile, he thinks, and surely that means something. And if there's something a bit odd in those smiles—something distant and vacant, like a house with the lights on but nobody home—well, Walter Freeman isn't thinking about that.

◆ ◆ ◆

In some ways, the rise and fall of the frontal lobotomy marks a turning point in women's medical history: this was more or less the last gasp of an ideology that advocated for surgical solutions to behavioral problems.

In its heyday, the lobotomy—in which doctors inserted a surgical pick through a patient's eye socket and into the brain to sever connections in the prefrontal cortex—was treated much in the same way as Henry Cotton's tooth pulling had been a decade earlier. From its introduction in the 1930s the procedure was hailed as a bold and innovative medical breakthrough, and the man who invented it, a Portuguese physician named António Egas Moniz, won the Nobel Prize for his work. There was even for a time a certain amount of overlap between the new enthusiasm for lobotomy and the old one for Cotton's practice of surgical bacteriology. Agnes, the patient with chronic cystitis who we met in the Urinary chapter, both underwent a lobotomy and also testified that a doctor had removed her teeth because it was "making her kidneys bad."

Mainly, though, lobotomy was positioned as a cure for mental problems: nervous disorders, hysteria, deviant thinking or behaviors. Unsurprisingly, they were disproportionately used on women, who would be recommended for lobotomies for all the same reasons they were committed to asylums. Indeed, the people most pleased with the effects of lobotomy on a woman were often not the patients themselves but their husbands. A case study from 1936, which features the chilling conversation quoted above between a doctor and lobotomized patient, ends with what is evidently meant to be a positive note: "Her husband said that she was more normal than she has ever been."

No doubt this was comforting to doctors, who could tell themselves that the memory loss, the lack of affect, and the dull look in a patient's eyes wasn't evidence of damage at all; it was just her abnormality, finally scrubbed away.

In the United States, the lobotomy was popularized by two neurologists, Walter Freeman and James Watts. A paper published in the *Southern Medical Journal* by the two men in 1937 stated that the procedure was a cure for all manner of psychiatric ills including insomnia, nervous tension, apprehension, and anxiety. Despite admitting that lobotomies caused personality changes—"Every patient loses something by this operation. Some spontaneity, some sparkle," they wrote—they nevertheless continued performing them to widespread acceptance, with Freeman being particularly evangelical about the procedure's purported benefits. By 1952, approximately fifty thousand patients in North America had undergone lobotomies, with some four thousand of those performed by Freeman himself.

Unlike Cotton, Walter Freeman was eventually banned from performing the surgery for which he'd been such a zealous advocate in 1967, after a patient died when he pushed the surgical pick too far into her brain—but lobotomies had long since fallen out of favor by then, owing to a growing recognition of the damage caused by the procedure. Megan McArdle of the *Washington Post* describes this turn of events as "a fact of which Freeman seems to have been acutely conscious," and his end-of-life quest to revisit his patients, as a search "for evidence for lobotomy's benefits, enough to salvage his legacy." Like Cotton, confronting what he'd done, how many lives and bodies he'd destroyed, was apparently more than Walter Freeman could bear.

The medical establishment, however, had long since moved on.

Although doctors had attempted to delineate a clear barrier between neurological and psychiatric medicine in the early twentieth century, the two fields nevertheless remained intertwined, especially as it became increasingly possible to treat problems through chemistry rather than surgery. Lobotomies fell sharply out of favor as a result of the introduction of a new drug, chlorpromazine, in 1954—but it wasn't long before the drug migrated beyond hospital settings and into the mainstream, where it was sold as a cure-all to the same women who, thirty years earlier, might have been institutionalized for failing to adhere to cultural norms. Only instead of inflicting docility on women at the point of a pick or a scalpel, now, you could get them to ingest it voluntarily in the form of a pill.

An ad from this era for the sedative Meprospan illuminates how companies sold women on gender-conforming domesticity dressed up as essential medicine: "She has enjoyed sustained tranquilization all day," the copy reads, accompanied by images of a dark-haired housewife shopping for groceries, cooking dinner, and attending a PTA meeting. Another ad for the same sedative, this from the 1960s after it had been rebranded as Miltown, is even more explicit: "Is anxiety and tension fast becoming the occupational disease of the homemaker?" it asks. "Some say it's unrealistic to educate a woman and then expect her to be content with the Cub Scouts as an intellectual outlet."

A full century after physicians warned that overeducated women would only make themselves hysterical, here was the same exact message, now repackaged for a modern audience. Women had ignored these warnings, sought equality and education, and paid the price: now, they couldn't be content with their lot in life, their domestic destiny, without the aid of consciousness-numbing drugs.

And unlike the surgical fads that preceded it, the notion of drugging women into complacency—or better yet, persuading them to drug themselves—has proved remarkably resilient in medicine, even as hysteria and nervous disorders were replaced in the popular lexicon by anxiety and depression, and even when society had long since recognized the benefit to women of getting an education and working outside the home.

Today, the same forces that once spurred the barbaric practices described in these pages remain subtly embedded in neurology and psychiatry. The normal range of human emotions in women may not result in a diagnosis of hysteria anymore, but it is still being pathologized in contemporary medical settings: one 2004 study found that women who were unhappy because of marital problems, motherhood, menopause, and the like were increasingly likely to be diagnosed as mentally ill and prescribed mood-altering drugs. Alzheimer's disease afflicts twice as many women as men, yet only 12 percent of the funding for research goes to projects focused on women. Multiple sclerosis, a debilitating neurological disorder that predominantly affects women, often goes undiagnosed for years as doctors dismiss women's symptoms as ordinary tiredness, a pulled muscle, or—in one infuriating case—a pinched nerve from wearing overly tight pants. And when it comes to pain management, women (and particularly poor and minority women) are categorically undertreated.

It's not hard to see how these shortcomings connect to a familiar litany of older, toxic beliefs: Women are drama queens (so don't treat their pain; it's not really that bad). Women can't handle the intellectual and emotional rigors of equal participation in society (so when they develop a degenerative disease that leaves them unable to think or even move, we don't need to be urgent about it). Women who behave in difficult or frustrating ways aren't just annoying, they're abnormal (so let's pump them full of mood stabilizers; it'll be doing us all a favor).

This is how we find ourselves, still, in a world where women who have nothing wrong with them are steered into medical solutions for ordinary human problems—while women in genuine crisis are waved away.

◆ ◆ ◆

At first, Miriam's case seems nothing short of miraculous.

An elderly woman is knocked down by a cyclist while crossing the street. She's propelled into a trash can—she hits her head on it, hard—and then crashes to the pavement, unconscious. Even before the ambulance arrives, a wave of palpable worry passes through the crowd that has gathered around her: she's so old, and so small, one of those birdlike women who look like a stiff breeze would blow them away. She's still breathing—thank God, there's that, at least—but someone mutters that the cyclist should be charged with attempted murder, and a murmur of assent goes up. This is serious. Even if she lives through it, she's sure to have broken a hip, a leg, any number of ribs.

But, no: later that night, Miriam leaves the hospital with nothing but a little road rash and a broken clavicle. The CT scan showed no head trauma, no bleeding in her brain; the X-rays showed no other broken bones. The ER doctors say she's unbelievably lucky—and everyone else nods along. So lucky. Miraculous, even.

It takes a month for the bruises to heal.

It takes slightly less than that to know that something is terribly wrong.

Nobody ever mentioned the potential risk of concussion, but it's increasingly clear that Miriam suffered one in that moment when her head hit the garbage can. It's also utterly impossible to find anyone who will treat it; worse, nobody even believes it. Her symptoms—she is uncharacteristically nervous, confused, and keeps misplacing her keys only to find them inside the bathroom medicine cabinet or on the top shelf of the refrigerator—are too easily dismissed, misunderstood, explained away by a system that is ill-equipped to recognize them for what they are. They say it's PTSD, or anxiety, or just the normal consequences of old age; they say she's just acting out because of emotional trauma, because getting knocked down was so scary.

They say they might be able to fit her in to be seen by a neurologist, maybe, on a date six months from now.

I hang up the phone.

I try not to scream.

Because I'm in charge of Miriam's care, but not because she's my patient.

She's my mother.

◆ ◆ ◆

In the months after my mother's accident, I could focus on nothing but trying to make sure she received the care she needed. But since then, I've come to understand how exemplary her case is of the systemic disenfranchisement that women with neurological issues experience within the medical system. Concussions are among the least understood and least studied neurological conditions in women, even as their impact among professional male athletes has become subject to a congressional investigation, millions of dollars in awareness raising and research, even a major Hollywood film.

Unlike NFL players, women who experience concussions often experience them alone—from accidents or, more tragically, at the hands of an abusive husband or partner. Reliable statistics on concussions in women are hard to come by, but given rates of domestic violence, it is reasonable to assume that millions of women have suffered concussions or other neurological trauma in this milieu, many of them repeatedly. And unlike NFL players, female concussion victims don't have the benefits of a team protocol or national awareness campaign that encourages them to heal. Many women never seek medical attention at all, and those who do often have their concussion symptoms overlooked or dismissed by doctors who don't understand what they're looking at, who don't even know what to look for. It's not unusual for first responders to assume women in domestic violence situations are drunk, high, or mentally ill, when they're actually suffering from head trauma.

In all these cases, the patient doesn't receive proper care or counseling about how to manage her injury, making it far more likely that she'll suffer long-term consequences. The tragedy is, this is one area in which women not only achieve but exceed gender parity: untreated, they are even more debilitating to women than they are to men.

◆ ◆ ◆

Within the first two months of 2023, a series of patients suffering from the same problem came to psychiatrist Allie Baker's office. All were women, and all had postural orthostatic tachycardia syndrome, a condition that results from dysautonomia (or a disorder of the parasympathetic nervous system) surrounding the regulation of blood pressure (per the Circulatory chapter, this condition is also known as Grinch syndrome because of its association with an undersized heart). All were experiencing classic symptoms: dizziness, fainting, heart palpitations, shortness of breath. But all of them, in what is more or less the contemporary iteration of the "bitches be crazy" theory of medicine, had been misdiagnosed: one was referred for an eating disorder, another for depression, and a third for panic disorder.

"It is staggering, actually," Baker says. "Not one clinician they encountered prior to me thought to check orthostatics [a measurement that compares a patient's heart rate and blood pressure while lying down, sitting, and standing]. Now, if you walk into my office, you have to prove to me that you don't have dysautonomia—before we even discuss meds and psychotherapy."

In one sense, Baker's patients were lucky: their true medical problem was identified before they'd started down a fruitless road of trying to medicate and counsel away a psychiatric condition they didn't actually have. But before that happened, each of them was riddled with guilt and anxiety at being so physically impaired by a problem that doctors wrote off as something of their own making: *It's all in your head.*

And while the medical establishment has rightly relegated the word "hysteria" to the dustbin, women with nervous system dysfunction are still habitually misdiagnosed—and needlessly medicated—for the nearest contemporary equivalent: anxiety. One of my patients, a fearless woman named Stella who had reported from the front lines of the war in Afghanistan before her successful battle against breast cancer, found herself being treated like a caricature of feminine fragility five years later.

"One side of my face fell. It lasted three weeks, and I went on a high dose of steroids and I did everything right . . . but then other symptoms started."

Stella's condition, known as Bell's palsy, had resolved. But now she was light-headed, exhausted, and experiencing numbness and tingling all over her body—all suggesting possible nervous system dysfunction. But when she called her doctor, a general practitioner she'd been seeing for ages, his reaction was astonishing: without a second thought, over the phone, he diagnosed her with anxiety.

"I said, 'You've known me for ten years. I've had cancer. I've had anxiety in my life. This is not it,'" she says, laughing at the memory. "I said: 'I'm not even anxious right now!'"

Ultimately, Stella spent months suffering from debilitating fatigue along with other symptoms—and being told by doctor after doctor that it was just anxiety, a mood disorder, or withdrawal from the steroids she hadn't taken in months. Finally, she asked for a referral to a female neurologist who almost immediately discovered an unusually high level of antibodies for Epstein-Barr, the virus that causes mononucleosis, in Stella's blood.

Her symptoms weren't anxiety, and they weren't all in her head; they were the result of a very real virus that she'd had a bout with in high school, and that had been inactive in her body ever since until something triggered its resurgence. Even though there was little to do but take an antiviral medication and hope it would eventually cause her symptoms to subside, just knowing what was wrong—and being listened to by a doctor who believed her when she said something was—was invaluable.

Bridget Carey, the neurologist who finally unraveled Stella's case, says that trust makes all the difference. Neurological disorders are nebulous, and express themselves differently in each patient. "You have to kind of go by the patient's subjective experience of what it feels like to be in their body," she says. But when it comes to who has their subjective experience listened to, a discrepancy emerges: "In my thirty years of practice, I'll just tell you, it's women a lot more than men who end up in my office with an incorrect diagnosis of anxiety alone."

The lack of trust in female patients to accurately or usefully describe their symptoms isn't even (or at least, only) about individual doctors with individual biases. As Allie Baker notes, contemporary medicine is designed to demand—and profit from—a quick and certain diagnosis that slaps a label on patients, dispenses the complementary treatment protocol, and scoots them out the door in fifteen-minute intervals.

"So many women are put on medicines for symptoms that, you know, they may help on the margins, but it's not addressing the primary issue," Baker tells me. "You can't even start to understand the primary issue or suspected primary issue neurobiologically, because our criteria are diagnostic." The digitization of medical records has only made this problem worse: not only are many of women's neurological problems difficult to diagnose but they're too complex to fit within the rubric of the available medical billing codes.

And so, even in the absence of any overt desire to dismiss and sideline women, a system that isn't built to accommodate uncertainty ends up doing it all the same. If you consult the contemporary literature to find out how best to serve women with neurological problems, it's as though these conditions—and the patients afflicted by them—don't even exist.

The great question that has never been answered, and which I have not yet been able to answer, despite my thirty years of research into the feminine soul, is "What does a woman want?"

—Sigmund Freud, MD

To Sigmund Freud, who believed hysteria was a psychiatric condition resulting from sexual hang-ups originating in childhood, women were a mystery he longed to (but never could) unravel. His mentor, Jean-Martin Charcot, thought the same condition was purely a neurological phenomenon—and treated women as though they were his own personal collection of curiosities, a spectacle to be displayed. It's easy to read accounts of these men's work, of the goings-on at a place like Pitié-Salpêtrière, and think that much has changed since then.

But then, one thinks of those women in the New York City hospital in 2023—the one who'd chewed her hand down to the bone yet still couldn't stop putting her fingers to her lips, the one stammering and twitching in a futile attempt to communicate with the doctors, who could only stare in confusion—and it's very hard not to conclude that some things haven't changed at all.

Both of the women in the opening pages of this chapter were failed by a system that found them curious, then mysterious, and then, finally, so frustrating that the only thing to do was dismiss them with a catchall diagnosis that meant they'd be treated for something, if not actually the thing that was wrong. Even if doctors no longer lump in patients with epilepsy, trauma, various psychotic disorders, and ordinary belligerence as all suffering from the same condition—and even if women are no longer subject to involuntary commitment to mental hospitals just because a husband or father considers them "abnormal"—the way the medical system responds to difficult women still holds echoes of those long-ago days.

And then there are the patients who echo the legacy of those difficult women.

Her name is Roxy. She's been suffering from epilepsy since the age of fifteen, the same age as Augustine in that first photograph from her early days at Pitié-Salpêtrière. Being alive at a more enlightened time, Roxy ended up in a neurologist's office instead of imprisoned in an asylum—but the neurologist himself turned out to be a practicing member of not only the "bitches be crazy" school of medicine but the one that believed a woman with a neurological disorder could be cured just by finding the right man.

"That shithead advised her mom to encourage her daughter to

have sex, which would thereby stop the seizures. A new low," says Saadi Ghatan.

Ghatan is the chief of neurosurgery at Mount Sinai West and a world-renowned expert in epilepsy. Roxy is his patient, having found her way to him after struggling with her condition for fifteen years. The neurologist who thought that sex would cure her was just the beginning. Her family was poor and couldn't afford to pursue treatment for the seizures that plagued her. The epilepsy made it difficult for her to hold down a job. She fell in with an abusive man, then fell pregnant. The relationship came to an end on the day her twins were born, several weeks premature—after her boyfriend stabbed her and threw her down the stairs.

But that was before. Now, Ghatan shows me a photo of himself and Roxy, taken in his office after her recovery from a successful implantation of a neurostimulator to treat her epilepsy. "Look at the light in her eyes," he says.

But he doesn't have to tell me to look. I see. It's impossible to miss. She is looking straight at the camera—again, not unlike Augustine in her most famous photo—but apart from this, the pictures have little in common. It's not just that Roxy is older, with darker skin and shorter hair. It's the look on her face. Not coy, but triumphant.

A hard-won victory.

Roxy began her medical journey with a harsh lesson in how much ignorance could still be found lurking within. It could have been worse, of course; she could have been alive at a time when women like her were institutionalized, lobotomized, robbed of their teeth and tonsils and organs until their spirits shattered or they died. But she ended with a new lease on life, thanks in no small part to a physician who broke the cycle. Who treated her like a person. Who saw her fierceness not as an abnormality to be corrected, but as a source of strength.

There's a tattoo on Roxy's right shoulder, beside the keloid scar from the day her boyfriend stabbed her. It's a harsh image: drops of red blood drip from the long-healed wound, and the handle of a knife emerges from one side. But the real kicker is the text that stretches below the wound.

It reads, *I'll slit your throat with the knife you left in my back.*

And this, perhaps, is where Roxy's path and that of her historical doppelgänger truly diverge.

Augustine, trapped for years in the Pitié-Salpêtrière hospital with doctors who saw her as a novelty to be displayed rather than a patient to be healed, only ever wanted to escape.

Just imagine how different things might have been if she'd wanted revenge.

CHAPTER 10

hormones

ENDOCRINE
THE HORMONE HANGOVER

I would cite your little screed (which I am sure you are now sorry for) as a typical example of an ordinarily controlled woman under the raging hormonal imbalance of the periodic lunar cycle—thus proving the point against which you rail.

—Edgar Berman, MD, American surgeon and author, 1970

Of all the organ systems we address in this book, the endocrine system is perhaps the least visible and hence the most mysterious. Inside the body, it functions as its own miniature, self-contained economy trafficking in just one product: hormones. These chemicals—there are more than fifty altogether—are manufactured by the body in a gland or organ, then transported through the bloodstream to another part of the body to work their magic (or wreak havoc, depending) on everything from mood to appetite to body temperature, as well as on processes like puberty or sexual reproduction. Insulin, which is produced by the pancreas to regulate glucose levels in the body, is a hormone; so are melatonin, which regulates sleep, and adrenaline, which causes heart rate and blood pressure to spike in moments of terror, excitement, or stress. And then, of course, there are the sex hormones: androgens, estrogens, and progestogens, which are manufactured in the testes or ovaries.

Every human body, regardless of sex, is internally awash in hormones; every human being, regardless of sex, produces the sex hormones associated with both male and female bodies. And yet, despite both the ubiquity of hormones and the breadth of the functions they perform, somehow only women have ever been saddled with the suggestion that their hormones make them unpredictable, incompetent, and unfit for certain types of work—and only women are commonly dismissed as "hormonal" when their emotions or behavior become inconvenient.

Like many medical breakthroughs, advances in endocrine medicine in the early twentieth century had unintended, and unfortunate, second-order effects on women. The same system of thought that led the scientific community to scrutinize women's smaller skulls for evidence of their innate intellectual limitations, or to bemoan the uterus as a putrescent vacuum full of darkness and disease, also begat similar conclusions when it came to the function of hormones in the body. It was a conclusion in search of a hypothesis: doctors already "knew" that women were inferior creatures, and so any biological or anatomical differences between their bodies and men's were assumed to be among the factors that made them that way.

In other fields, this mindset led to genuine horrors, including unnecessary and brutalizing surgeries in which doctors sought to cure their women patients by removing their offending (read: female) body parts. And yet, medicine's early and ultimately misinformed theories of how hormones worked in women's bodies may have been the more damaging when it came to women's equality, both in the eyes of the medical system and in society more broadly. An organ, at least, could be removed; the discovery of hormones, on the other hand, suggested that women were simply marinating at all times in a potent mix of chemicals that made them volatile, foolish, and emotionally unstable from the moment puberty hit.

The belief in a sexual binary between men's hormones and women's further entrenched not only a sexist mindset in medicine but a state of ignorance when it came to the reality of how the endocrine system worked. Early on and for too long, doctors believed that estrogen was both unique to women and uniquely deleterious in its effects on them. Male hormones were exalted while female hormones were maligned. A man with high testosterone, it was understood, was virile, a warrior, a stud. A woman with too much estrogen, on the other hand, was just crazy. And while science eventually came to understand that all hormones were present in all bodies, that narrative—the "bitches be crazy" theory of women's bodies, brains, and biology—wasn't so easily set aside. Not by doctors, not by society, and sometimes, worst of all, not even by women themselves.

In 2004, I was a third-year medical student doing my surgical rotation at Massachusetts General Hospital—whose acronym, MGH, was often jokingly said to be an abbreviation for "Man's Greatest Hospital," owing to its brutally demanding and militant approach to medical training. (In fairness, MGH has begun to make improvements on this front in recent years, but its reputation lingers on.) On the night that I was working with the trauma surgical team, a pair of EMTs burst through the emergency room doors wheeling a stretcher. There was a young woman strapped to it, and she was covered in blood. She had been in terrible car crash, hit dead-on by a drunk driver who had strayed over the center line into oncoming traffic. Her bones were broken. Her skull was fractured. Her spleen had ruptured. As the trauma team hurriedly but methodically assessed her condition to see if her body could withstand surgery, I could see on their faces the grim recognition that she was unlikely to survive.

As a student on my first clinical rotation, the only thing I could do was stand aside while the patient was wheeled into surgery—and try to comfort her mother, who had rushed to the hospital from her home several hours away, not sure whether her daughter would still be alive by the time she arrived. When the young woman was finally wheeled out of surgery and into the ICU, still unconscious, her body heavily bandaged and perforated by countless tubes and monitors, her mother pulled me aside to beg me for information: Did I understand what was happening? Was her child going to make it? She was in tears, and soon, so was I—which was against the rules.

When he saw me crying, my supervising resident called me away from the patient's bedside and leaned in, his voice low and serious.

"Pull yourself together," he said. "Now. You're never going to last in this line of work if you can't keep your emotions in check."

That's when I said it. Looking at my shoes, wiping tears from my face, I mumbled: "Sorry. Sometimes estrogen gets the better of me."

When I think of this moment now, I cringe. Not just because of how easily I sought refuge in the toxic stereotype of the hormonal, unstable woman, but because of the way my supervisor nodded in agreement.

It was the first time I allowed myself to be complicit in perpetuating a harmful narrative rooted in the medical system's ancient and insidious bias against women's bodies, but it wouldn't be the last.

Of the ovaric liquid I will only say that it acts with less power than the orchitic liquid. However, sixty old women in Paris have derived benefit from its action, according to an American lady physician.

—Charles-Édouard Brown-Séquard, MD, 1893

The year is 1889, and Dr. Charles-Édouard Brown-Séquard is feeling every one of his seventy-two years. It's not just the infirmity of age that he hates but the indignity of it. He misses that feeling of boundless energy, of insatiable curiosity, of lingering in the lab in the wee hours of the morning, teetering on the precipice of scientific discovery—until, eureka, the truth reveals itself.

It was this energy, this thirst to understand, that earned the doctor his reputation as an innovator (and, at his most extreme, something of an eccentric). The idea that this vigor might someday leave him used to be unimaginable. But here he is now: depleted.

Tired.

Old.

Far from rushing from place to place, or experiment to experiment, Dr. Brown-Séquard spends most of his time these days sitting: at home, in the lab, in the cabin of the horse-drawn carriage that transports him between both, where he feels as though his bones are jangling together every time the carriage hits a bump in the road. At night he eats very little and falls into bed exhausted, only to find he's unable to sleep—yet another of nature's ironic insults to those in the sunset of their lives.

Charles-Édouard Brown-Séquard doesn't know what hormones are—indeed, the word itself hasn't even been invented yet. But he knows what he's lost, and he thinks he knows why. Surely it's not a coincidence that a man's virility, his strength, his masculinity, always seem to dissipate at the same time as his sexual prowess begins to wane.

And surely, through the miracle of modern science, a man could find a way to turn back the clock, replenishing what has been depleted.

All he needs, Dr. Brown-Séquard thinks, is time and determination.

And guinea pig testicles.

Lots and lots of guinea pig testicles.

◆ ◆ ◆

While the term "hormone" would not find its way into the medical lexicon until 1905, science had been circling the idea of endocrine function for much longer without fully understanding what it was. Doctors were well aware that removing the sex organs had powerful effects over the behavior and characteristics of humans and animals alike, thanks in no small part to the practice of castration and the presence of eunuchs, the earliest records of which date back to the second millennium BCE. But here, understanding more or less stalled until the late nineteenth century, when Charles-Édouard Brown-Séquard decided to ask a different sort of question.

Brown-Séquard was a French physiologist and neurologist, known for being brilliant and curious but also something of a weirdo, especially when it came to involving himself in his own experiments. As a young scientist studying cholera during an 1853 outbreak of the disease on the island of Mauritius, he swallowed the vomit of one of his patients in an attempt to catch cholera himself—all in the hopes of dosing himself with an experimental treatment of his own design. Now, in the final years of his life, Brown-Séquard had another type of experiment in mind: Everyone knew what happened to men if their testes were removed. But what if you injected an intact but aging man with the secretions from a younger set of testicles?

In a sort of early prototype for hormone replacement therapy, Brown-Séquard spent two weeks injecting himself with a mixture of water, semen, blood, and secretions from the crushed testicles of an animal. (For this latter substance the doctor started with dog testes, but then, for unknown reasons, switched to using guinea pig testicles instead.) The results, he declared, were magnificent: "All I can assert is that the two kinds of animals have given liquid endowed with very great POWER," he wrote. Per his report, the injections improved his strength and stamina virtually overnight. He could run up stairs! He could lift heavy weights! He could project a stream of urine farther than ever before and poop with the vigor of a man half his age! "Even on days of great constipation," he wrote, "the power I long ago possessed had returned."

Although this book focuses mainly on the ways in which medicine has misunderstood and maligned women—and Brown-Séquard did wonder if his results could be replicated to a lesser extent in women by injecting them with ovarian secretions—this is one instance in which men were not spared from experimental medicine and snake-oil cures that tweaked at their deepest fears and anxieties. Brown-Séquard's research suffered from various flaws, and given the minuscule amount of testosterone actually present in a dog testicle (let alone a guinea pig's), the renewed vigor he claimed to achieve was almost certainly the result of a placebo effect. But that didn't stop doctors from distributing the "Brown-Séquard Elixir" to the droves of male patients who demanded it in hopes of becoming virile once again. Only Brown-Séquard's peers in the scientific community were unimpressed: when he presented his results, one medical journal cited them not as a groundbreaking experiment, but rather as proof that any professor over the age of seventy should be forced into retirement.

While Brown-Séquard neither discovered hormones nor managed to effectively harness them, the questions he was asking did presage the dominant, and gendered, cultural narrative surrounding their impact on the body—and they did spark something in the medical imagination at large. His research is credited by many as catalyzing the entire field of endocrinology; then, as now, the idea of turning back the clock on aging (and especially on the aspects of it that impacted men's penises) was a subject of great interest to the scientific community.

Over the following decades, the breakthroughs in endocrine research began to pile up. The word "hormone" was coined in 1905 by a British physiologist named Ernest Starling, after he identified and traced the digestive hormone secretin from its receptors in the large intestine to its origins in the pancreas. From there, scientists began conducting a flurry of experiments to identify different hormones and their functions, naming them along the way: Adrenaline. Insulin. Growth hormone.

And then, of course, there were testosterone and estrogen. The latter, which regulates the female menstrual cycle, was discovered—and named—in 1920. Its etymology is telling: it comes from the Greek *oistros*.

It means "mad desire."

[W]hen excessive sexuality, amounting perhaps to sexual insanity, exists in women we must look for an excessive ovarian secretion as the primary cause of the condition; and contrariwise we find the deficient ovarian secretion may lead to melancholia, perhaps indirectly.

—William Blair-Bell, MD, gynecologist, 1916

Even before the discovery of estrogen and its impact on the menstrual cycle, physicians had long been suspicious of women's periods. As detailed in previous chapters, menstrual blood was by turns considered toxic, unclean, a source of dangerous contagion. The humorists saw it as evidence of women's generally leaky constitution, which made them naturally prone to bodily imbalance. Medieval doctors believed that it was responsible for all manner of female ailments, a "filthy" substance that clogged up a woman's body and poisoned the other organs—not to mention putrefying the penis of any man unlucky enough to have intercourse with her.

Of course, not having a period was a hazard of its own: lacking a menstrual cycle was one of the dozens of reasons cited by doctors for institutionalizing women against their will.

The common thread through all of this is that menstruation made for a convenient medical scapegoat: over and over, doctors pointed to it as the fundamental root of women's unpredictability, infirmity, and instability. (None of this was helped by the cultural shame surrounding periods, including the religious edicts that declared menstruating women so dangerous that they needed to be exiled from their homes and kept away from other people until they were no longer bleeding.) Even as the movement for women's equality in medicine and otherwise began to pick up steam, the idea that women were enfeebled by their menstrual cycles remained so pervasive that it was cited by the Harvard Medical School as a reason not to admit them as students—a policy that persisted until 1945.

In 1876, Dr. Mary Putnam Jacobi, one of the first and most famous female physicians of the time, won the prestigious Boylston Prize at Harvard Medical School for a 281-page article addressing the medical community's ill-founded beliefs about the menstrual cycle. Her essay, an attempt to inject both reason and perspective into a conversation dominated by male physicians, also clapped back specifically at several men who appear elsewhere in this book, including Horatio Storer, a gynecologist who we'll meet in the Reproductive chapter. Storer had asserted that women could not be doctors as a result of their periods: the menstrual cycle, he wrote, "unfits them for any responsible effort of mind and in many cases of body also."

Jacobi thoroughly dismantled arguments like Storer's: she discussed the current physiological literature on the subject, performed surveys of more than 250 women, and charted their pulse pressure variations during menses to see if women really were stressed to the point of incapacitation by their periods (they weren't).

But it didn't matter. The male discourse leaders in the medical community had gone all in on the notion that there was something pathological about menstruation—and the more they learned about the substances that would eventually be called "hormones," the more convinced they became. Years before anyone knew what estrogen was, doctors were nevertheless quite certain that women's bodies and behavior were being controlled by their reproductive organs, specifically by secretions stemming from the ovaries. Among those spearheading this theory was William Blair-Bell, a British gynecologist and author of *The Sex Complex: A Study of the Relationships of the Internal Secretions to the Female Characteristics and Functions in Health and Disease.*

Blair-Bell, a lantern-jawed man with pale, close-set eyes and a passing resemblance to the actor James Cromwell, published his book in 1916, a moment at which the medical world stood on the precipice of discovering estrogen and its attendant functions. As such, his work is prescient in some ways, despite being downright ludicrous in others: Blair-Bell was convinced that women were internally controlled by an insidious substance produced in their ovaries, which he referred to as "ovarian secretions." An excess of secretions, he wrote, would result in "sexual insanity"; a deficiency, in melancholia. A chief symptom of the aforementioned sexual insanity was masturbation, which like many doctors Blair-Bell was obsessed with. To prevent masturbation, he recommended marriage as a prophylactic measure—ideally as soon as a girl hit puberty.

Needless to say, identifying the ovarian secretion that caused women to go mad with desire was a chief concern. In one case study, Blair-Bell described a patient who had confessed to having had multiple affairs, arguing that she had been induced into a temporary state of moral corruption by her overproductive ovaries: "[The] sexual stimuli were so great that until they were exhausted her sense of right and wrong was completely obliterated," he wrote.

When estrogen was finally discovered—scientists would identify and name it in 1920, and discern its chemical makeup after isolating it from the urine of both pregnant mares and pregnant women in 1929—Blair-Bell and others like him took it as vindication. All this time, he'd been saying that a substance produced in the ovaries was making women crazy! And now, here it was.

The chemical war between the male and female hormones is, as it were, a chemical miniature of the well-known eternal war between men and women.

—Paul Henry de Kruif, PhD, American biologist and author, circa 1940s

The discovery of estrogen, along with its counterpart, testosterone, initially fueled an erroneous but absolute conviction within the scientific community that men and women were utterly divided: biologically, anatomically, and chemically. That conviction would be complicated but never fully dispelled when endocrine research eventually revealed the truth: that so-called female sex hormones were also present in the bodies of males. Ernst Laqueur, who is credited with the discovery of testosterone, was aware as early as 1927 that estrogen could be found in the male testes, a fact of which he could barely begin to grapple with the implications.

"It is now proved that in each man there is something present that is inherent in the female sex. Whether we will succeed in determining the individual ratio of each man, in terms of a given percentage femininity, we do not know," he wrote—but note that even now, the cognitive association between estrogen and femininity remained unbroken. The next breakthrough came in 1934, when another doctor, named Bernhard Zondek, published an article announcing the presence of estrogen in the bodies of stallions. Zondek, too, was clearly bewildered by his own results, writing, "Curiously enough, as a result of further investigations, it appears that in the urine of the stallion also, very large quantities of oestrogenic hormone are eliminated . . . I found this mass excretion of hormone only in the male and not in the female horse."

Clearly, the scientific reality was more nuanced than a simple binary in which women were full of estrogen while men were full of testosterone, a fact that researchers were forced to confront as more information—not to mention the existence of the pituitary gland, the "master gland" that regulates sexual and reproductive development in all humans—came to light. But so entrenched was this gendered conception of hormones and how they worked that doctors could not imagine a world in which estrogen belonged in the bodies of men. Its presence was seen as an aberration, which soon gave rise to theories that it caused men to become aberrant, which is to say, effeminate. These theories didn't ultimately hold water—the tests doctors ran on "girly" men revealed no greater concentration of estrogen in their bodies than in those of their more conventionally masculine counterparts—but the scientific community's unshakeable belief in a male-female hormone binary made it all too easy to disregard results that contradicted it. And so, doctors continued to postulate that effeminate men must be suffering from an excess of the same hormone that rendered women so unstable, moody, or sexually deviant.

As the years passed, the breakthroughs of the 1920s and 1930s gave way to questions about how medicine might leverage all this new endocrine knowledge, particularly when it came to sex hormones. And while Charles-Édouard Brown-Séquard had been dead for years by then, something of his spirit—and the fascination that fueled his experiments—was beginning to find new purchase in a nascent but promising conversation about hormone replacement therapy. Doctors were beginning to ask: What if a man who had gone soft in some way, whether it was an effeminate disposition or the indignities of old age, could be reinvigorated through infusions of manly, masculine hormones?

But when it came to imagining similar solutions for women, something interesting happened: the notion of a cure was replaced by a vision of control. Not just over the bedeviling hormones that made women crazy, but over all the processes governed by those hormones. To manipulate a woman's estrogen levels promised control over her mood, her desires, her menstruation, her ovulation— and ultimately, over the one thing that did, and does, make women at once more vulnerable and more powerful than men: pregnancy.

Too many children, too much fighting, too much anger, have made of this woman a nagging bitter wife, and of the husband, a selfish bully.

. . . A wise man never plants more trees than he can care for.

—*Roots of Happiness*, Puerto Rican Health Department film, 1953

Twenty years before he made a scientific discovery that would become a linchpin of the sexual revolution, Dr. Gregory Pincus was something of a wunderkind: a Harvard professor and fearless researcher, known for pushing the boundaries of scientific progress and good taste alike when it came to endocrine science. His first brush with fame came in 1934, when he was just thirty-two years old, after he announced that he had produced a litter of rabbits via artificial insemination—and then again in 1937, when he produced another rabbit, this one bred via parthenogenesis without using a male gamete at all. The fatherless rabbit, born from an egg that Pincus "fertilized" with a mix of saline and the hormone estrone, appeared on the cover of *Look* magazine to great fanfare—but this was soon overtaken by controversy and condemnation after Pincus was misquoted in the national news as saying he intended to pursue similar research in humans. Reporters rushed to debunk the notion of women using Pincus's same methods to impregnate themselves, without the involvement of men.

"There is no likelihood, in other words, that women will take over the world completely, banishing the males, made wholly superfluous, to the battlefields where they might conveniently exterminate themselves," the *Santa Barbara News-Press* assured its readers in a report on Pincus's rabbit experiments.

Pincus, however, was undeterred: by 1938, he was an international authority on sex hormones and the author of nearly six dozen published papers. He was also more interested than ever in pushing the limits of endocrine science, harnessing the power of hormones to achieve an unprecedented level of control over the human body, and particularly over reproduction—which gave him something in common with feminist groups at the time, and particularly with women like Planned Parenthood founder Margaret Sanger, for whom reproductive autonomy was a key issue. At the intersection of Pincus's scientific curiosity and Sanger's activism, a singular goal emerged: the invention of a pill that would prevent pregnancy.

But here, there were obstacles: religious, cultural, and legal. In the United States, disseminating contraceptives—or even just information about how to use them—was banned by the government well into the 1960s. The National Institutes of Health refused to fund basic research in the reproductive sciences and was outright forbidden from funding birth control research until 1959. The only way to study this was through private funding, often under the guise of "fertility" studies, and so this is what Pincus did, teaming up with another biologist named John Rock to begin experimenting with manipulating the hormones of human women. Their funding, two million dollars, came from a philanthropist named Katharine Dexter McCormick, who they met through Sanger. McCormick's interest in birth control was not just political but personal, dating back to 1906, when she vowed never to have children out of fear they would inherit her husband's schizophrenia.

Like Sanger—and many other early advocates for birth control—McCormick was something of a eugenicist, and pragmatic to the point of indelicacy: "How can we get a 'cage' of ovulating females to experiment with?" she once asked. But she wasn't alone in looking for loopholes or for "caged" women to experiment on: Drs. Rock and Pincus circumvented government regulations by first testing their birth control prototype on inmates at the Worcester State Psychiatric Hospital in Massachusetts, under the pretense of studying fertility. And here, already, Pincus was thinking a step ahead—not just when it came to testing his drugs on patients who couldn't meaningfully consent but also in how to make the pill something women would one day take voluntarily. The progesterone contained in the pill would completely interrupt the body's normal menstrual cycle, a fact Pincus suspected women would find alarming. So, at his suggestion, they developed the regimen still in widespread use today, whereby women take the pill continuously for twenty-one days and then stop for one week to menstruate.

Creating an artificial "period" that came like clockwork every twenty-eight days allowed Pincus to sell an illusion, at once groundbreaking and insidious. What he promised was total freedom from pregnancy without any alteration to the body's "natural" cycle; what he was actually doing, however, was flooding the bodies of his patients with powerful hormones that fundamentally altered their biological processes—and came with serious side effects.

◆ ◆ ◆

Although many of the doctors profiled in this book were fueled by a sincere (albeit deeply paternalistic) desire to help their patients, and struggled to strike a balance between healing women and exploiting them, Pincus does not appear to have been troubled by the possibility that his groundbreaking research was coming at the expense of his subjects' health and happiness. By the time he moved his studies out of insane asylums and onto the island of Puerto Rico, where research could be conducted in relative freedom from the prying eyes of government agents and on a population that was often desperately impoverished, it was clear both that women in these studies were suffering, and that Pincus didn't particularly care. Women taking his prototype pills reported bleeding, blood clots, nausea, and migraines. They were required to submit to daily vaginal smears, and invasive monthly biopsies of their cervixes and uteri. In some cases, women were made to undergo laparotomies, in which the abdominal cavity is sliced open and pulled apart to expose the organs within, so that researchers could observe their ovaries in real time.

Unsurprisingly, women who initially volunteered for these studies often didn't want to continue—but those who objected or asked to drop out were scolded, shamed, and even extorted to continue serving as guinea pigs. In 1955, one of Pincus's research partners, a professor of pharmacology at the University of Puerto Rico School of Medicine named Dr. David Tyler, successfully recruited female medical students to participate in the trials, only to resort to blackmailing them with the threat of failing grades when they wanted to stop: "I have also told Garcia that if any medical student exhibited irresponsibility . . . I would hold it against her when considering grades," he wrote in a letter to Pincus. A year later, Dr. Edris Rice-Wray, a female medical missionary who was conducting Pincus's research on women recruited from the slums of Rio Piedras, wrote to Pincus with similar complaints: "We have some trouble with patients stopping the tablet. A few cases have had nausea, dizziness, headaches and vomiting. These few refused to go on with the programme. Two were sterilized. One husband hung himself, desperate over poverty."

The tone of these letters is remarkable and revealing: far from being horrified at the plight of the women they were experimenting on, researchers were mainly frustrated that the women wouldn't behave. By the time the trial had concluded, three of these patients were dead—reportedly from heart attacks, but with no autopsies performed, it's also possible that they died from blood clots or other side effects related to the pill.

Pincus did eventually come in for criticism from fellow doctors for his reckless treatment of patients, but only after he had published his results in the prestigious *Lancet* medical journal. (One letter to the editor read, "This use as guinea pigs of chronic psychotic patients who are not able to give or withhold valid permission in physiological research of this type must be as repugnant to many of your readers as it is to me.") He also does not appear to have taken any of that criticism to heart: in 1966, six years after the FDA approval of the pill, Pincus was quoted in the *New York Times* downplaying its related health risks. And the women who complained of side effects? All in their heads, he said: "Some of these side-effects are largely psychogenic. Most of them happen because women expect them."

Of course, if Pincus had any qualms about having been too hasty to rush the pill to market, he would likely have felt vindicated by the popularity of his invention. Two years after it became available, more than one million American women were using oral contraceptives. But these women were, in some ways, just as much guinea pigs as those recruited (or exploited) by Pincus for the medication's early trials. In the 1960s, the pill contained a whopping 100 to 175 micrograms of estrogen as well as ten milligrams of progesterone—enough to cause serious and sometimes deadly side effects. It wasn't until 1969, when medical journalist Barbara Seaman published her book *The Doctors' Case Against the Pill*, that doctors began to acknowledge that the high doses of estrogen in those early birth control pills put women at risk of blood clots, heart attacks, and strokes. Congressional hearings on the matter were held the following year.

Some of the technical problems with the pill have since been solved: today's formulations contain less than 50 micrograms of estrogen, and less than one milligram of progesterone, which largely allays the risk of deadly side effects. But no similar scrutiny has ever been applied to Pincus's original messaging surrounding the pill—or the way he persuaded women to manipulate their own reproductive cycles under the pretense that nothing unnatural was happening to their bodies. For all the incredible freedom it has provided to women for more than sixty years, the birth control pill still comes with this fraught legacy, one that obscures the truth about both its science and its side effects, and which sits uneasily on a landscape where reliable information about women's hormones is already so hard to come by. Too often, what little we teach young women about sex and reproduction is designed less to inform than to alarm; many sex education programs, especially those designed amid the teen pregnancy panic of the 1990s, are actively misleading with respect to the science of hormones and pregnancy out of a desire to scare young people away from having intercourse. The result is a world in which women are taught for years that their bodies are frightening, unknowable, and uncontrollable—but also that pregnancy is both their responsibility to avoid, as well as to be avoided at all costs—and expected to get on the pill almost automatically. Almost as a rite of passage. Almost as if it remains less important for women to understand their bodies than it is to keep those bodies under control.

A large percentage of [menopausal] women who escape severe depression or melancholia acquire a vapid cow-like feeling called a "negative state." It is a strange endogenous misery . . . The world appears as through a gray veil, and they live as docile harmless creatures missing most of life's values.

—Robert Wilson, MD, 1966

There's a man in the waiting room of Dr. Robert Wilson's Park Avenue office.

Already, this is strange. Not just the unexpected appearance of this stranger, late in the day and without an appointment, but the question of what he's doing here—a middle-aged man, sitting alone, in the office of a prominent gynecologist. The visitor himself seems aware that he's out of his element: he's the only one in the waiting room, but still looks as if he's trying to hide, sitting back uncomfortably in a corner with the brim of his hat pulled low so that his pale, pointed face is hidden in shadow. When Wilson calls him into the office, he's struck by the way his visitor moves. "Rather furtively" is how he'll describe it later—but of course, by then, he'll understand the reason why, just as he'll understand why the man can't seem to sit still, alternately glaring at the doctor and then looking at his feet with embarrassment.

Now, though, they sit opposite each other in silence until the visitor finally clears his throat.

It's his wife, he says.

"She's driving me nuts," he says.

He tells Wilson that this is his last stop, and his last hope: all the other doctors said there was nothing to be done, that this is just how things are for a man whose wife is going through what everyone refers to, euphemistically, as "the change of life."

That's when he reaches into his pocket. The object he brings out is a beauty, with rich, brown leather grips and a short, black, gleaming barrel, the better to be pulled free in a hurry without snagging on anything—or, God forbid, accidentally firing. Wilson flinches at the sound as his visitor lays the gun down on the desk and then sits back, leaving it there in between them. Allowing the doctor to see it, and to understand that he's serious.

"If you don't cure her," the man says, "I'll kill her."

◆ ◆ ◆

Years from now, Wilson will tell this story in the pages of a book about his life and work. By then, the stranger with the gun will be dead, and his wife long since out of danger, the doctor's treatments having proved effective. But when he thinks of this moment, he does not remember it as some might, as an interaction with a lunatic from which he was lucky to escape alive. Quite the opposite, actually. That stranger with the furtive gaze and loaded gun, who was ready to murder his menopausal wife rather than spend another minute by her side? Wilson might not have agreed with his methods (he would later discover that his visitor was a prominent figure in organized crime), but about his madness, there was no question.

"The man," Wilson's memoir reads, "was completely rational."

◆ ◆ ◆

Though the threatening stranger who visited Dr. Wilson's Park Avenue office sometime in the mid-twentieth century surely didn't know this, the way he felt about his wife's menopause—if not his intended method of dealing with it—was very much in keeping with the medical consensus about the condition. Until quite recently, virtually all the medical literature agreed that menopause was a serious problem. But it wasn't a problem because of the debilitating symptoms it inflicted on women; it was how it impacted their behavior in ways that were irritating to men.

In the nineteenth century, Charles-Édouard Brown-Séquard was among those who believed that aging women could have their vitality restored by injecting them with "ovarian secretions" after their own had dried up. But even when doctors didn't necessarily have any idea how to treat menopause, they were often obsessed with it—or at least, with how annoying it was to be around. In 1871, British physician Edward John Tilt hypothesized that menopause was to blame for everything from uncontrollable peevishness to kleptomania to "demonomania," or the conviction that you'd become possessed by the devil. "One patient, aged forty-six, thought the devil had placed a cord from the pubis to the sternum," he wrote. "Another, aged forty-nine, had been troubled by cerebral symptoms ever since cessation, at forty, and thought the devil lodged in her womb. A third, aged forty-eight, declared that he had taken up his abode in each hip-bone." The root of all these demonic delusions, Tilt concluded, was menopause—although he was also optimistic that his patients would be better off after their menstrual cycles had ceased entirely.

"When women are no longer hampered by a bodily infirmity periodically returning," he wrote, referring to menstruation, "they have more time at their disposal, and for obvious reasons they are less subject to be led astray by a too ardent imagination, or by wild flights of passion."

Those "obvious reasons," of course, were that if menopause made women crazy, then having a period made them even worse.

For equally obvious reasons, Tilt had little notion of how to actually alleviate the symptoms of menopause. But eventually, endocrine science advanced to the point where not only did doctors know what hormones were, they were beginning to understand their medical applications. Estrogen and progesterone were already being prescribed for menstrual irregularities or premature menopause long before the advent of the birth control pill, and hormone replacement therapy (HRT) was approved by the FDA in 1942. But it wasn't until twenty-four years later, when Dr. Robert Wilson and his book, *Feminine Forever*, entered the arena, that doctors began to conceive of menopause as a disease to be treated rather than an inevitable misery to be endured. At the time that Wilson received his unusual visit from the armed stranger, he was one of the only doctors using HRT to treat the symptoms of menopause.

Wilson didn't mince words when he first appeared on the endocrine scene in 1962, publishing an article about menopause in the *Journal of the American Geriatrics Society*. The article was coauthored by Wilson and his wife, Thelma, and opened with a bang: the first sentence reads, "The unpalatable truth must be faced that all postmenopausal women are castrates."

Although Wilson's descriptions of women in menopause as castrated, shriveled, sexually disinterested creatures floating through the world in a "vapid cow-like" state of dissociation read a bit like dispatches from a message board in one of the more misogynistic corners of the internet, he was more or less the first doctor ever to take menopause seriously as a medical condition—and he had nothing but contempt for those who didn't. "Even today, the many dangerous and agonizing symptoms that often accompany a woman's 'change of life' are still shrugged off by many otherwise-reputable physicians as nothing but 'a state of mind,'" he wrote, excoriating the medical community that had, in his view, abandoned women to suffer for no other reason than sheer sexism.

"Let us reverse the situation," he once wrote. "Suppose the man of medicine noticed his own genitals gradually shrinking year by year. Would he be as indifferent to genital atrophy as he now appears to be?"

And yet, even Wilson's fierce advocacy on behalf of women suffering through menopause was somewhat tempered by paternalism. *Feminine Forever* is dedicated to Wilson's wife, which led to this somewhat nauseating excerpt from the foreword by endocrinologist

Dr. Robert B. Greenblatt: "Like a gallant knight he has come to res-cue his fair lady not at the time of her bloom and flowering but in her despairing years; at a time of life when the preservation and pro-longation of her femaleness are so paramount."

To be sure, the notion that menopause represented not just the loss of her menstrual cycle but of her femininity was foundational to Wilson's work; to him, HRT represented nothing less than the restoration of a woman's womanhood. Unfortunately, the cour-age of Wilson's convictions was not matched by the diligence of his research. His 1962 article and 1966 book were both based off the same body of work, an uncontrolled study of just 304 women between the ages of forty and seventy. After that, Wilson seems to have been far more interested in evangelizing about HRT as a treatment for menopause than in continuing to study it: *Feminine Forever* describes the therapy as something akin to a magic bullet, all upsides and no drawbacks. And when it comes to those upsides, Wilson's arguments on behalf of women remain inextricably tangled up with other, more male-oriented concerns. With HRT, Wilson wrote, the menopausal woman "will be much more pleasant to live with and will not become dull and unattractive."

And then there's the matter of sex. On this front, much of Wil-son's praise for HRT centered on its ability to make a woman just responsive enough to keep her husband satisfied, but not so horny that she'd go looking for enjoyment elsewhere. In one section, he laments the patients who refuse HRT out of fear that it might turn then into nymphomaniacs: "No woman's morals were ever threat-ened by estrogen," he wrote—leaving it unspoken but implied that men whose wives were being treated with HRT also need not worry about them cheating.

Somehow, even in the hands of a truly passionate advocate, treat-ing menopause had once again become a question not of alleviating women's suffering, but of making them more pleasant company for men—including the "entirely rational" crime boss who planned to murder his wife if Wilson couldn't cure her.

"Outright murder may be a relatively rare consequence of menopause—though not as rare as most of us might suppose," Wilson mused, going on to explain that the side effects of meno-pause were so miserable to live with, for all parties, that they "often resulted in the psychological equivalent of murder in the form of broken family relations and hatred between husband and wife."

As for the crime boss—who, incidentally, was dying of tuberculosis—Wilson began giving his wife estrogen injections and reported that she responded well: "Her disposition improved noticeably after three weeks, and soon she was very busy taking care of her sick husband."

Note the wording, the description of what improved. Not her health, not her symptoms, but her disposition. Of course, Wilson would have been pleased that his patient was feeling better—but at the end of the day, the most important thing was what her husband thought.

And what mattered to him was that she was once again the type of woman he insisted she be: nurturing, caring, attentive to his needs. On her best behavior and under control.

◆ ◆ ◆

Today, the medical debate surrounding HRT is far more fraught, and more complicated, than it was in 1966. This isn't entirely Dr. Robert Wilson's fault, but he certainly had something to do with it, as his evangelical zeal for hormone replacement therapy almost immediately outpaced the available, limited research into whether or not it was truly safe—research that then acquired the gloss of settled science, requiring no further investigation. It's not hard to see why Wilson would have been reluctant to cast doubt on the treatment that he had almost single-handedly put on the map and used himself on thousands of women. Indeed, like so many of the men featured in this book, he had a powerful incentive not to keep asking questions. Wilson had accomplished something groundbreaking, something that would change the face of endocrine medicine forever, and something that seemed to be effecting a downright miraculous change in the lives of the women who tried it.

JoAnn Manson, a professor in the department of epidemiology at Harvard's T.H. Chan School of Public Health, recalls being surprised by the flimsiness of the science surrounding HRT when she first graduated from medical school in 1979. Women were being given the treatment at the onset of menopause almost routinely—"But there was no randomized trial," she says. "There was no really good understanding of the benefits and risks and health impacts of hormone therapy."

Manson was right to be concerned—if not about HRT itself, then about the lack of research surrounding it. Four years earlier, in 1975, an alarm had gone up in the medical community after studies showed that taking estrogen during menopause (the regimen favored by Wilson) was linked to a significant increase in the risk of endometrial cancer. The good news was that this problem was easy to solve: when doctors added progesterone, a hormone that inhibits the growth of endometrial cells, to a woman's HRT regimen, her risk of cancer was virtually eliminated. But to uncover this unknown risk now, nearly ten years after Wilson and *Feminine Forever* had advertised estrogen as a sort of silver bullet for all menopausal ills, was unsettling: What else didn't we know?

It took nearly thirty years for the other shoe to drop, but when it did, it was shattering. The controversy stemmed from the Women's Health Initiative, the largest women-only randomized clinical trial in history, which tracked health outcomes for 160,000 postmenopausal women across a variety of factors. In June 2002, a rumor began to spread within the medical community: part of the trial involving HRT had been prematurely suspended.

The abandonment of a clinical trial ahead of schedule is never a good sign. At a press conference, Jacques Rossouw, the acting director of the WHI, announced that the study had uncovered adverse effects of HRT that "outweigh and outnumber the benefits." Those adverse effects included a statistically significant risk of heart attack, stroke, and blood clots—as well as an increased risk of breast cancer.

Although the risk of any of these things to a given individual was in fact extremely small, the general response to this announcement was panic, including within the medical community. In a 2023 *New York Times* feature on the history and treatment of menopause, Manson describes how HRT went from miracle cure to medical pariah: "Within six months, insurance claims for hormone therapy had dropped by 30 percent, and by 2009, they were down by more than 70 percent."

And while further research eventually revealed that the truth about HRT is far more nuanced—for many women, the benefits of the treatment vastly outweigh the risks—the fear surrounding it has proved difficult to put back in the bag. (During my own medical training from 2000 to 2011, the prevailing dogma was that HRT caused breast cancer and that nobody should do it.)

Manson, along with another physician named Andrew M. Kaunitz, attempted to correct the record in 2016 with an article titled "Menopause Management—Getting Clinical Care Back on Track." It's an increasingly pressing issue, she explained: our population is aging, millions of women are entering menopause each year, and many of them continue to suffer from debilitating and entirely preventable symptoms that not only wreck their quality of life but also needlessly stress the healthcare system.

"There was huge confusion, misunderstanding, and some chaos ensuing at that point," Manson tells me. "The pendulum had swung to the complete opposite side: hormone therapy is bad for all women, toss your pills and patches, don't even think about taking this poison. That was the impression that women were left with, and clinicians were overwhelmed. They were not given a really clear understanding that the absolute risks were low, especially in younger women."

The continued reluctance of doctors to prescribe HRT for menopause symptoms, in combination with a lack of awareness among younger physicians about the newer, better research into HRT's efficacy, has created a devastating hole in the medical system. Within it is not just an immense amount of unnecessary suffering but also quacks and snake-oil salesmen who invariably step into the vacuum: in their article, Manson and Kaunitz describe "a burgeoning market for untested and unregulated alternative treatments," many of which are ineffective at best and harmful at worst.

And if the incuriosity surrounding HRT created a dangerous situation back in the 1960s, the current state of affairs—a fearful paralysis in which good information is difficult to come by and treatment, more difficult still—is hardly an improvement. In every case, women aren't getting the information, the attention, or the care they need.

We're built differently, we have different hormones. In the world that we live in, I understand that there's equal rights and that's a wonderful thing and I support all of that. I don't support a woman being president . . . With the hormones we have there is no way we should be able to start a war.

—Cheryl Rios, CEO of Go Ape Marketing, 2015

Although endocrine medicine has advanced by leaps and bounds since the days when Charles-Édouard Brown-Séquard was experimentally injecting himself with crushed-up guinea pig testicles, our contemporary medical and cultural understanding of hormones—and particularly their effect on women—is still hampered by bias, misinformation, and confusion. In medicine, we jockey for control over women's bodies by manipulating their hormones yet simultaneously write off their health problems as "just hormones," and hence not worth investigating. Culturally, women receive the message that hormones make them moody, volatile, and incompetent—while also receiving little to no real education about the impact of hormones on their bodies.

And while the treatment of women's hormones as something of a joke, even by medical professionals, is obviously detrimental to women's health, it doesn't only impact women. Last year, a colleague of mine sent her husband to an ENT specialist to address his snoring, which had gotten so bad that it was waking her up every night, even through earplugs. The doctor's response: "Oh, I don't think so. How old is your wife? She's probably going through menopause and not sleeping well for that reason." (My colleague, who was not, in fact, in menopause, sent her husband back to that same doctor with a box of her tampons—not used ones, but I wouldn't have blamed her.)

Meanwhile, the idea that women are ruled by their hormones remains culturally ubiquitous, albeit in a slightly more evolved form. For the most part, we no longer traffic in the notion that women's hormones are akin to brain poison, rendering them unstable and unfit for leadership roles; it has been more than fifty years since Edgar Berman, a physician and political affiliate of former vice president Hubert Humphrey, invoked the specter of a "menopausal woman President" firing off nuclear missiles in a fit of hormonal pique by way of arguing that women could not be trusted to hold higher office. On the other hand, it has been less than ten years since *Time* magazine declared that Hillary Clinton was "biologically primed" for leadership specifically because she has gone through menopause: "Biologically speaking, postmenopausal women are ideal candidates for leadership. They are primed to handle stress well, and there is, of course, no more stressful job than the presidency."

These preconceptions about hormones may not show up in medical settings in precisely the way they once did, when physicians like Edward John Tilt suggested that "ovarian secretions" would turn ordinary women into peevish kleptomaniacs with delusions of demonic possession, but they do still wield undue influence in the field of endocrine science. As recently as 2015, researchers were still seriously investigating the possibility that women's political views are impacted by their menstrual cycles. They aren't, for the record—but this is what we get when female menstruation and hormones continue to be viewed by the scientific community as a sort of biological wild card with wide-ranging and mysterious effects. As author Rebecca Jordan-Young notes in her book *Brainstorm: The Flaws in the Science of Sex Differences*, the notion of intrinsic differences between male and female cognition is a persistent one, owing to a conviction among neuroscientists that our brains are shaped by prenatal exposure to sex hormones. It's one of those things that feels true; if hormones are responsible for shaping all the other biological differences between men and women, it makes a certain kind of sense to assume that those differences permeate all the way to the brain. And yet that assumption is flawed: many of the studies purporting to prove the existence of innate differences between male and female brains not only fail to replicate but stem from a fundamental misunderstanding of just what hormones do to women.

That misunderstanding is apparent in virtually every conversation about women's endocrine medicine, from menopause to PMS to the phenomenon known as "mom brain." Even the most well-intentioned scientific inquiry into these issues is invariably influenced by the ubiquitous narrative that hormones make women foolish; studies in this field end up examining the impact of hormones through a negative lens, rather than a holistic one. In a landmark 2023 paper on "mom brain" published in the *Journal of the American Medical Association*, three female physicians noted that "the idea that motherhood is wrought with memory deficits and is characterized by a brain that no longer functions well is scientifically just not so"—and yet, virtually all of the science investigating the impact of pregnancy and motherhood on women's brains is predicated on precisely this hypothesis. What are the positive effects, if any, of pregnancy on a woman's brain? Nobody has thought to ask, and so nobody knows.

Meanwhile, the notion that a "hormonal" woman is just stressed, moody, or menstruating—and not in any actual medical distress—can overshadow the ability to diagnose endocrine syndromes that have nothing to do with the menstrual cycle. Thyroid disorders, for instance, are disproportionally prevalent in women, but they're often misdiagnosed or just missed because the symptoms—fatigue, weight gain, depression—are dismissed by doctors as simply stress-related. Postpartum depression, for instance, has been linked to an inflammation of the thyroid gland after childbirth and can affect as many as one in ten new mothers, and yet it's frequently written off as a mental health issue rather than a disease. For the twenty-seven million women affected by thyroid disorders every year—that is, 90 percent of all thyroid patients—this is untenable.

And yet, this is what happens when the archetype of the hormonal woman becomes entrenched not just in the cultural consciousness but in the healthcare system: we end up downplaying, overlooking, and ignoring the vitally important and complex role that hormones play in a woman's health. Doctors and patients alike write off a dysfunctional endocrine system as both a forgone conclusion and no big deal ("Oh, it's just hormones."). And women's suffering from endocrine issues, whether it's debilitating PMS or the symptoms of menopause, is shrugged off as natural and hence untreatable.

After all, everyone knows that hormones make you crazy.

Day One of being a girl and I've already cried three times, I wrote a scathing email that I did not send, I ordered dresses online that I couldn't afford, and then, when someone asked me how I was, I said, "I'm fine!"—when I wasn't fine. How'd I do, ladies? Good? Girl power!

—Dylan Mulvaney, 2022

As intractable as the archetype of the "hormonal woman" remains, the cultural narrative around endocrine medicine generally and hormones specifically has shifted in recent years: today, the conversation has shifted such that we're just as likely to hear about hormones in the context of gender transition as in the context of menstruation, menopause, or HRT. In my own medical practice, we have to balance the needs of female transgender patients with cancer with their desire to continue taking testosterone—a treatment often billed as "lifesaving" when it comes to alleviating gender dysphoria but which is contraindicated for patients with breast cancer because it can quite literally kill them.

And even now, the contemporary conversation about hormones in the context of gender-affirming healthcare holds the echoes of other historic moments in endocrine science—moments in which the excitement of having discovered a seemingly groundbreaking cure ended up outpacing the research in ways doctors failed to anticipate, sometimes with tragic results. As of this writing, several European countries have dialed back their medical protocols for providing puberty blockers and cross-sex hormones to trans-identified minors, citing a troubling lack of data on long-term outcomes and apparent risk of serious side effects; in the US, where trans medical care has become an inflection point in the culture wars, the conversation is even more fraught.

And while much about this issue remains profoundly uncertain, it is not hard to see how the skyrocketing rate of female trans-identified teens seeking cross-sex hormones—at one representative clinic, the increase was over 4,000 percent within eight years—lives in conversation with the history that precedes it, one in which the predominant narrative surrounding female sex hormones has been forever and overwhelmingly negative. We still struggle to conceive of hormones outside a sexual binary. The popular narrative surrounding estrogen—that it makes women emotional and crazy—is being pushed by TikTok influencers instead of eccentric mad scientists, but otherwise remains unchanged. And after hundreds of years of both cultural and medical consensus that estrogen makes monsters of us, perhaps it was inevitable that a certain number of natal girls would eventually recoil from the prospect of becoming that "hormonal woman": unhinged, unfit, and out of control.

We need to make sure that in an effort to save women, we are not ruining them.

—Kara Long Roche, MD, MSc, FACOG, gynecologic surgeon, excerpt from interview, 2023

As a breast oncologist, my work is often at odds with the historical efforts of doctors like Gregory Pincus and Robert Wilson when it comes to endocrine medicine. Estrogen, which plays a vital role in regulating the menstrual cycle and keeping a woman's body healthy, can also serve a second, darker purpose as a fuel for certain breast cancers; two-thirds of all breast cancers are estrogen-driven, feeding on the hormone in order to grow and metastasize. As a result, I must often treat my patients by suppressing their levels of estrogen, and in aggressive cases, to block the body's production of estrogen entirely as well as blocking its receptors from interacting with the hormone. Starving the body of estrogen—shutting down ovarian function through either chemical means or surgery and administering medications that suppress the production of estrogen elsewhere in the body—is among our most effective methods of eradicating breast cancer.

But these things come at a cost: shutting down the ovaries triggers menopause. And the medications that reduce estrogen levels also induce menopause-like symptoms.

For decades, breast oncologists have treated this as a sort of devil's bargain. Our first priority and most passionate commitment is our patients' survival; the quality of their lives afterward is often a distant second thought. Worse, many women are now expected to tolerate these symptoms not just for the sake of treating cancer but also for the sake of preventing it. In 1994, scientists announced the discovery of BRCA1, a genetic marker that indicates a severely increased risk for breast and ovarian cancers in women. Soon thereafter the medical consensus was that women in possession of the gene should strongly consider having their breasts and ovaries surgically removed as a prophylactic measure. The problem was, no studies existed to determine how best to treat these young women who were now in medically induced menopause as a result of the removal of their ovaries, and so no recommendation was given to provide hormone therapy. Indeed, many doctors expressly told their patients that they absolutely could not take HRT if they chose to have the surgery, in effect forcing them to make a terrible choice: they could live with the symptoms of menopause for the next fifty years of their lives, or they could roll the dice on a 75 percent increased chance of ovarian cancer.

"That the surgical castration of young women was not combined with massive attention to treat menopause was a huge loss," Dr. Kara Long Roche tells me. Roche is a gynecologic surgeon and had her ovaries removed at the age of thirty-seven as a precaution for her own personal risk of ovarian cancer; she has also been taking HRT since she had the surgery done and is a fierce advocate for giving other women the option to do so. She is part of a growing movement to push for better science in this space: it is only within the past several years that medical guidelines began to advocate that women with prophylactic ovariectomies should have their lost hormones replenished, and information is scarce. Thirty years after the discovery of specific genetic mutations that increase breast and ovarian cancer risk resulted in immense pressure on young women who tested positive for high risk mutations to have these preventive surgeries, we still lack research into how best to manage their health for the rest of their lives. Menopause itself remains chronically under-studied: in the United States, the NIH hasn't even assigned menopause an identification code that would make research on it easier to track.

The gendered nature of this incuriosity is hard to miss; certainly, it's not lost on Roche.

"There is no situation in which a thirty-five-year-old healthy man would have his testicles removed to prevent testicular cancer, and would not be given back full-blast testosterone, even if there was some small future risk of cancer," she says.

Indeed, it's striking that even as we've made incredible progress into treating diseases that used to be a death sentence, the medical system has not matched this progress with an equal commitment to ensuring that patients not only survive but thrive—and that in our mad rush to keep women from dying, we aren't doing things that make their remaining years a misery. But when it comes to women's health, medicine still struggles to weigh the costs and benefits of survival—or the question of quantity over quality of life—in the same way it has always done for men. As Roche points out, "We don't say to old men, 'Hey, your erectile function is part of "natural" aging, accept it.' We developed a billion-dollar industry to help them. But women . . . We resign that it's 'natural' for them to suffer."

And for women thrust into early menopause by cancer treatment, many of whom were struck with the disease in what would have been their prime childbearing years, the cure can seem worse than the disease.

Of all the women I have met who struggle with the debilitating endocrine side effects of cancer treatment, the one I remember most vividly was not actually my patient. In fact, on the day Michelle first appeared in my office, I didn't understand right away why she'd come. A note affixed to her chart indicated that she wanted a second opinion, but the trajectory of her disease was all but complete: a breast cancer diagnosis at thirty-one, followed by a swift and successful round of treatment with excellent results. Although her cancer was an aggressive strain, she caught it early enough that doctors were able to remove it before it had spread past her lymph nodes. After surgery and chemotherapy, and with an ongoing medication protocol, there was no apparent reason why she wouldn't expect to live for many decades, cancer-free—or why she should be so dissatisfied with her care that she had traveled several hours from her home in upstate New York, one year into remission, to see me.

On paper, Michelle was a success story.

But when I saw her face, and the misery written there, it became clear that the truth was more complicated.

"They said I might get symptoms like hot flashes," she told me. "I said, okay. I'm having a mastectomy, I'm having chemotherapy, what's a hot flash compared to that? But it's not just hot flashes. It's so much more. It's so much worse."

Although the most physically invasive of Michelle's surgeries and therapies were behind her, she was still taking medication to suppress her body's estrogen levels and keep her cancer from recurring. And while it's true that she was told to expect menopausal side effects, it's also true that she was not prepared. I've seen the pamphlets that purport to warn patients about handling symptoms of medically induced menopause; they say things like, "Try to avoid spicy food," and "Keep a change of sheets and pajamas close to your bed so that you can change them quickly if you sweat through them," and "A water-based lubricant may be useful for vaginal dryness."

They don't say, *You won't be able to get through fifteen minutes of a workout before the pain in your joints is so terrible that you can't stand it anymore.* They don't say, *Your vagina will feel like a collapsed tube made of sandpaper.* They don't say, *You will break up with the man you love because you feel he deserves to be with someone who can still have, and enjoy, sex.*

But the latter was what Michelle is going through—and what she would continue to go through, for as long as she stayed on her medications, which her treatment plan suggested would be anywhere from five to ten years.

By the time she reached the part where she'd ended her relationship because she couldn't physically bear to have sex anymore, Michelle was fighting back tears. "When I first got my diagnosis, I thought I would do anything to survive. But I can't live like this."

I wanted to tell Michelle that it would be okay. That we'd fix this, that there was new research being done every day, that of course nobody believed that she should reconcile herself to living in agony just because she was lucky to be alive at all. When she looked me in the eye and said, "I would rather risk my cancer coming back than spend the next ten years feeling like this," I wanted to tell her that she would never have to make such a terrible choice.

But if I said these things to her, I would have been lying. Even as I outlined her options—sexual health consults, laser treatments, nonhormonal or intravaginal estrogen to try to mitigate some of the worst side effects of her medication—I could see on her face that it wasn't enough, not even close, to give her back what she'd lost.

And while I want to tell you that Michelle became my patient that day, and that we found a way to alleviate her suffering while also staving off the recurrence of her cancer, that would be a lie, too.

The truth is, I never saw her again.

CHAPTER 11

sex

REPRODUCTIVE

THE MOTHER OF ALL MORAL PANICS

The womb is the origin of all diseases.

—Hippocrates, fifth century BC

A medical education is an exercise in humility. Even the most accomplished doctors are haunted by cringeworthy memories from our medical training, moments in which the necessity of learning by doing collided with the brutal reality that we did not yet know what we were doing. Often, these early failures become formative teaching moments, inspiring us to do better, work harder, learn more.

Sometimes, though, they expose not just the limits of the aspiring doctor's abilities but something deeply broken in the system meant to train him.

One of the worst embarrassments I've experienced as a student of medicine was not my own but secondhand, as I stood in a group of four other interns in a hospital exam room in Boston. We were watching with a mix of fascination and horror as a twenty-four-year-old male resident named Anton tried to perform a pelvic exam and pap smear. All of us were technically doctors—with the diplomas and medical school debt to prove it—but none of us had any real experience in medical practice, and Anton's first foray into the basics of gynecology was going badly. He had already been corrected once by the attending physician for forgetting to lubricate the speculum before trying to insert it into the patient's vagina. Now he was struggling to open it, either ignoring or failing to notice that the woman on the table was clearly desperately uncomfortable.

"You'll feel some pressure," Anton was saying as the patient struggled not to squirm. His face was turning red. He was losing his grip. His voice cracked as he stammered, "I'm just going to . . . oh no."

The speculum clattered to the floor.

For one terrible moment, nobody spoke, and then: "I'll take it from here," the attending said.

The patient looked ready to cry with relief.

Anton looked like he might join her.

Fifteen minutes later, the attending physician took Anton aside for a debrief, to ask if he understood what he had done wrong—and to gently point out to him what he hadn't noticed. The patient had been trying to twist away from contact with the speculum because he was pressing it awkwardly and painfully against her clitoris.

Anton's face blanched.

"What?" the attending physician said.

The young resident looked at the floor and mumbled, "It's just . . . it didn't look anything like in the anatomy book."

The worst part is, he had a point.

◆ ◆ ◆

For thousands of years, the female reproductive system was treated as an anatomical enigma by the medical profession. Hidden away inside the body, it was considered at once mysterious and sinister, a grotesque inversion of how things were meant to be. If a man's body was the standard for health and functionality, then a woman's, so fundamentally different, was understood to be necessarily dysfunctional. Aristotle summed up the medical view of women's bodies best when he said, "We should look upon the female state as being as it were a deformity, though one which occurs in the ordinary course of nature."

The perception of women's bodies as deformed variations on a male ideal persisted through centuries, with particular misunderstanding and scrutiny focused on women's genitals and reproductive organs. Galen, whose anatomical studies in the second century BCE shaped the medical understanding of human bodies for centuries to come, was especially influential in promoting the idea that women were fundamentally incorrect in the way their bodies were assembled; he marveled that while women have exactly the same organs as men, they are imperfectly turned inward. He compared a woman's internal reproductive and sexual organs to the sightless eyes of a subterranean mole. The eyes of the mole have the same structures as the eyes of other animals except that they will not allow the mole to see so too the female genitalia "do not open" and remain an imperfect version of what they would be were they thrust out.

As such, there was little sense among medicine's founding fathers that the female body could be a perfect and functional machine unto itself. Rather, they viewed women as fundamentally other: there were male bodies, and then there were not-male bodies, the latter of which was nature's equivalent of a wrong turn. The sense that women's bodies were not just different but broken is obvious not just in the way doctors spoke of the female anatomy but in the medical vocabulary itself: the female external genitalia was termed "pudenda," a Latin word that means "things to be ashamed of."

Unsurprisingly, early medical theorists were only too happy to point to women's shameful, broken body parts as the origin of all manner of ills. Sometimes, as detailed in previous chapters, these anxieties centered on the womb itself, whether it was wandering around the body and driving women insane or a repository of "filthy" substances that poisoned them (and their lovers) from the inside out. But ultimately, the greatest source of mystery, misinformation, and anxiety for medical men through the ages was not the uterus (which, for all its alleged evils, nevertheless served an undeniable biological purpose when it came to propagating the human race). It was the clitoris, an organ whose sole purpose is to provide sexual function and pleasure in women—and whose existence so thoroughly unnerved the medical establishment that for a long time, doctors refused to acknowledge it at all.

Despite being the main site of women's sexual function and orgasm, and hence a vital part of the human anatomy, the clitoris was virtually ignored by the medical community for nearly two millennia. Mentions of the organ were rare, and those that did exist were generally not positive: between the first and fifteenth centuries BCE, one of the few documents to directly address the existence of the clitoris is the 1486 *Malleus Maleficarum*, which described it as the "devil's teat" and advised that any woman who had one could be assumed to be a witch.

As a result, something of a feud eventually erupted when multiple scientists suddenly got interested in the clitoris during the Renaissance in sixteenth-century Italy, and two separate men in the span of two years each attempted to claim credit for having discovered it. The first was Matteo Realdo Colombo, a professor in Padua who in 1559 described having found what he called the "seat of pleasure of the woman." He was clearly pleased with himself—not to mention utterly certain that he'd stumbled into heretofore-uncharted territory, to the point where he thought he should be allowed to name the organ: "Since no one has discerned these projections and their workings, if it is permissible to give names to things discovered by me, it should be called the love or sweetness of Venus," he wrote. But Colombo's celebration was short-lived: just two years later, his successor, Gabriele Falloppio, for whom the Fallopian tubes are named after, announced that he had discovered the clitoris. He was equally excited, and also equally certain that nobody had ever seen one before: "Modern anatomists have entirely neglected it . . . and do not say a word about it . . . and if others have spoken of it, know that they have taken it from me or my students."

Sadly for both Colombo and Falloppio, the existence of the clitoris was still too controversial for either of them to put their name on it. Indeed, Falloppio was scolded by Andreas Vesalius, the author of the premiere anatomical textbook of the time, for getting ahead of himself. The clitoris, Vesalius wrote, was "some sport of nature"—in other words, a random deformity—to which his peer was assigning far too much importance: "You can hardly ascribe this new and useless part, as if it were an organ, to healthy women."

Although this sixteenth-century feud over the mythological status of the clitoris reads like a punch line to a feminist joke (the only thing worse than a man who thinks he's discovered the clitoris is the one who summarily dismisses it as useless, am I right, ladies?), it also exerted considerable influence over the medical dialogue surrounding women's anatomy and sexual function, both of which continued to be treated as something between an afterthought and a novelty. Knowledge of clitoral anatomy did not make its way into the medical mainstream until 1672, when a Dutch anatomist named Regnier de Graaf published a detailed diagram of its internal and external structure based on his dissections of cadavers. Unlike his predecessors, de Graaf didn't claim to have discovered the clitoris, though he did chide the medical establishment for excluding it from the literature: "We are extremely surprised that some anatomists make no more mention of this part than if it did not exist at all in the universe of nature," he wrote. Anatomists, on the other hand, were not persuaded. The next doctor to give the clitoris its due was Georg Ludwig Kobelt, in an 1844 publication titled *The Male and Female Organs of Sexual Arousal in Man and some other Mammals*, which is considered the first comprehensive and accurate description of the function of the clitoris—but his enthusiasm was not shared by his peers, who at the same time were touting the surgical removal of the clitoris as a prophylactic measure against hysteria, epilepsy, and other maladies. It would be 2005 before a urologist named Helen O'Connell finally pioneered a thorough anatomical study of the clitoris, mapping its structure, blood supply, and more than fifteen thousand nerve endings using MRI technology.

And yet, even as the existence of the clitoris came to be finally, grudgingly acknowledged by the medical establishment at large, its importance was not—and often still isn't.

Poor Anton, the young resident whose botched attempt at a pelvic exam was the stuff medical school nightmares are made of, had a point when he said that his patient's anatomy didn't look like what he'd seen in his textbook: even the medical texts in use today often don't address the physical diversity of women's genitalia. A recent survey of four medical anatomy books that have been continuously in use for the past two hundred years found that most included only a single image of the vulva, often a black-and-white line drawing—and that said drawing most often resembled what's colloquially known (and described in the Integumentary chapter) as a "Barbie vagina," a slit with no labial protrusion. Meanwhile, today's medical students have less real-life exposure than ever to a variety of bodies, and body parts, in the context of clinical settings or the cadaver lab, both of which have gone by the wayside in favor of plastic models—where, as one critic described it, "all organs are color coordinated and impeccably shaped." And perhaps most importantly, the texts that teach students about women's reproductive systems still include virtually no detail about the clitoris. (The male anatomical texts, perhaps needless to say, contain copious information about penises and erectile function.) As much as the medical literature today refutes Vesalius's assertion that healthy women don't have a clitoris, it nevertheless seems to agree with him on the question of its uselessness.

Indeed, this organ, inessential to reproduction and yet utterly crucial to a woman's sexual function—and which doctors have largely treated as either insignificant or sinister when they weren't congratulating themselves for discovering it—serves in many ways as an avatar for the uniquely difficult relationship that the medical system has, and has always had, with women's sexual health. Despite the initial assessment of women's anatomy as inherently inferior, inverted, and other, medicine was ultimately forced to recognize the importance of the parts of a woman that produce eggs and hormones, maintain a pregnancy, and facilitate the birth of a child—all of which have long been treated as a woman's biological destiny, her sole reason for being. But the clitoris represents an anatomical wild card: its very existence suggests that women can enjoy sex on its own merits, not just as a means to motherhood.

And this, as we'll see in the coming pages, made certain people very uncomfortable.

Women's reproductive organs are pre-eminent, they exercise a controlling influence upon her entire system and entail upon her many painful and dangerous diseases. They are the source of her peculiarities, the center of her sympathies, and the seat of her diseases. Everything that is peculiar to her springs from her sexual organization.

—John Wiltbank, MD, introductory lecture in midwifery at Philadelphia College, 1853

For most of human history, female reproductive health was a woman's issue—and a woman's territory. Pregnant women were attended to by midwives, who had no formal medical education but were nevertheless the heirs to hundreds of years' worth of specialized knowledge about menstruation, conception, pregnancy, childbirth, and postpartum care. But as medicine formalized in the eighteenth and nineteenth centuries, spawning its own institutions, hierarchies, and specialized fields of research, midwives were increasingly sidelined and scorned by the system as uneducated practitioners of folk medicine—and men, freshly credentialed by medical colleges, increasingly took their place. Much as scholars like Colombo and Falloppio claimed to have discovered the clitoris (ignoring the fact that women had surely known of its existence since roughly the dawn of time), doctors in the mid-1800s took over the age-old duties of female midwives and declared themselves the founders of a brand-new medical specialty, which they called "gynecology."

At the time, gynecology was something of a novelty pursuit and a hot destination for ambitious young doctors who sensed an opportunity to distinguish themselves in a largely unexplored field of research. But whatever drew an individual man to gynecology to begin with, he would almost invariably arrive at the conclusion that he'd gotten there not a moment too soon. A consensus quickly arose within the medical community that women were much too fragile, nervous, and discombobulated by monthly menstrual maladies to provide competent care, even—or even especially—when it came to reproductive health, accompanied by a burgeoning movement to exclude women from the study of medicine at large. And within a single generation, a seismic shift had taken place: for hundreds of years, women had been the world's foremost experts on obstetrics, the custodians of a body of knowledge that was continuously refined and passed down to the next generation of healers. Now, they had been systematically shut out at the very moment that their field was beginning to advance by leaps and bounds, deprived of the opportunity not only to contribute their own knowledge but to share in the discovery of new obstetric science and techniques. But far from seeing their takeover of the field as a slap in the face to the women who'd been there first, the founding fathers of gynecology congratulated themselves on their heroic efforts. This, they agreed, was what women's reproductive medicine really needed: a few good men.

Granted, in many cases and in many ways, the men who shaped women's reproductive and sexual medicine were good, or at least genuinely believed they meant well. There was Horatio Storer, for instance, who was one of the first physicians ever to advance gynecology as a field separate from obstetrics and worthy unto itself. Storer pioneered the teaching of gynecology, leading a semiannual course on women's diseases and healthcare for medical graduates at Harvard, and founded the country's first-ever gynecological society in Boston in 1869. A passionate advocate for women's health, Storer made it his personal mission to recruit more physicians as gynecologists and chided his peers in the medical community for overlooking this important field of medicine; among the founding tenets of his Gynaecological Society of Boston was his wish to "stimulate its members and the profession generally to a deeper sense of the importance of the diseases peculiar to women," which he felt that doctors were ignoring out of prejudice. On the nobility of his profession, Storer was insistent: "[Far] from its being a disgrace to a physician to be interested in uterine diseases," he wrote, it should be considered "an honor."

There was Robert Tuttle Morris, who we met briefly in the Skeletal chapter. Morris, a gynecologist and founder of the American Society of Endocrinologists, was famous for pioneering the technique of ovarian grafting—a transplantation of ovarian tissue that can aid women suffering from infertility—in the late 1890s. In 1906, Morris announced that one of the women on whom he'd performed the procedure had successfully carried a pregnancy to term, marking a massive breakthrough in the then-nascent field of treating infertility.

There was Robert Latou Dickinson, an obstetrician/gynecologist and prolific medical illustrator, artist, and sculptor who won the Lasker Award in 1946 for his work in the field of fertility. Dickinson painstakingly documented virtually every patient interaction he ever had, and pioneered the practice of obtaining detailed sexual histories from his patients; by the time he retired, he had collected more than five thousand sexual case histories, a staggering body of data. He was also the founder in 1923 of the National Committee on Maternal Health, an endeavor backed by female sponsors to study contraception, infertility, miscarriage, and other pregnancy issues, and performed a crucial service in the 1930s as a mediator between birth control advocates and the medical community, which was skeptical of contraception at the time.

There was Sigmund Freud, who, in addition to being a world-famous psychotherapist, did more to advance awareness of the clitoris in a few short years than virtually the entire medical profession had accomplished in three centuries.

But in every case, the heroic work of these doctors has a darker side, one that betrays a complete lack of understanding of women at best, and at worst, a deep contempt for them. Freud, for instance, raised awareness of the clitoris only insofar as it helped him to advance his theory that women who required clitoral stimulation to have an orgasm were sexual deviants who needed mental help. Dickinson, the gifted artist and birth control advocate, was also obsessed with sexual morality and would intentionally inflict pain on his patients during pelvic examinations, lest they become sexually excited by them. As for Morris, his interest in fertility seems to trace back at least in part to an equally passionate interest in race science and eugenics: among his published works was an 1892 paper hypothesizing that the female clitoris would soon evolve into a vestigial organ and eventually disappear entirely—a beneficial development in his view, as it would relieve "Aryan women" of the burden of experiencing lust, the better to focus on procreating for the benefit of the white race.

And as for Storer, his advocacy on behalf of women's health was matched only by his relentless conviction that women were too foolish, too fragile, and too easily corrupted to advocate for themselves. In the previous chapter, Storer was among the physicians who asserted that women's hormones made them unfit to practice medicine—but this was just the beginning, as evidence abounds that Storer's enthusiasm for gynecology was more a product of curiosity and arrogance than genuine care. Where other men were too fearful or too reverent to explore women's bodies so deeply, Storer went out of his way to advertise that he had no such qualms; in medical school, he once snuck with his friend Warner into the anatomy lab, grabbed a poker from a nearby fireplace, and shoved the instrument into a dead woman's vagina as far as it would go. In Warner's retelling of this story, Storer was unapologetic and fascinated.

Warner, on the other hand, had gagged and fled—not at the violation but at the smell.

In Horatio Storer's view, women were unfit for virtually any sort of meaningful control over their own lives. Not their education, not their medical decisions, not their sexual desires. And for all that he publicly expounded upon the virtues of gynecology among his peers, his personal relationships with women are revealing as to just how conditional his compassion for his female patients truly was. It was 1869 when Storer waxed poetic to his peers about what an honor it was to attend to women's health.

Just three years later, in 1872, his own wife died alone and terrified in the asylum where he'd had her committed for "catamenial mania"—menstruation-induced insanity.

Of the various forms of [insanity] occurring in females, the majority of them are owing to functional or organic diseases of the uterus and its appendages; in other words, that they are of a sexual character.

—Horatio Storer, MD, 1869

The year is 1856, in Boston, Massachusetts. The patient, a petite twenty-four-year-old with a pale complexion and a predisposition for sweating, is telling the doctor about her symptoms; the doctor, who has an extravagant beard and mustache and a formal bearing that makes him seem much older than his twenty-six years, is scribbling notes as she speaks. The patient's name is written at the top of the page, but by the time her case makes its way to publication, she'll be known only as "Mrs. B," the wife of a wealthy merchant many years her senior.

Their conversation is intimate; the doctor's notes, based not just on his interview with his patient but with her husband and family as well, will be more intimate still. Already, Mrs. B has spoken at length about her marriage, her diet, her menstrual history, and her dreams—particularly her dreams, from which she wakes with a racing heart, an aching breast, and a throbbing between her legs that she registers with equal parts excitement and shame. The dreams are why she's here; she understands that they're wrong, and that something is wrong with her for having them. Mrs. B's mother will confirm as much, when the doctor speaks to her: her daughter's precocious yearning for intimacy is why she encouraged the marriage to the merchant, even though the girl was then only seventeen.

All of this will be in the notes that eventually make up the young woman's case study. The doctor will spare no detail, especially when the time comes to make his physical examination. He'll describe the size and temperature of his patient's vagina, the position of her clitoris, the way she shrieks when he touches her. The description of her case is one that Mrs. B won't ever see but other men will—many of them, all examining her through the eyes of the doctor who is about to give her the gravest of diagnoses, one that will change her life.

The disease she suffers from is one exclusive to women, and the treatment regimen he prescribes will disrupt her life in every possible way. Her feather mattress and pillows will be taken, replaced by rough horsehair, to lessen the sensual pleasures of sleep. He instructs her to drink no alcohol, take cold baths, and restrict her diet. Every activity that could stimulate her sickness, from reading novels to having sex with her husband, must be abandoned completely. And then there's the medicine: tinctures, drops, and a corrosive solution of borax that she will dab between her legs every night, even though it burns terribly and doesn't seem to help. She'll do it all the same; indeed, she'll do everything the doctor says. Not just because he insists that it's the only way to make her well but because if she doesn't get well, something terrible will happen.

This, he tells her unreservedly. Later, he'll indicate as much in his notes: "This first interview with the patient was had on May 16th," he writes, "when the following treatment was prescribed, at the same time giving her fully to understand that if she continued her present habits of indulgence, it would probably become necessary to send her to an asylum."

And then, at the top of the page, Dr. Horatio Storer will scrawl his diagnosis:

Nymphomania.

◆ ◆ ◆

Despite his confident bearing and catalog of draconian treatments, Horatio Storer was in fact somewhat flummoxed by the case of Mrs. B: to his mind, she had neither the appearance nor the background of most women with her condition, which is to say, she was neither slovenly nor a prostitute. But, of course, Mrs. B also wasn't sick. Reading between the lines of Storer's case study on his alleged nymphomaniac, it's clear that the patient's only "symptoms" were desiring and enjoying sex.

If this case study offers a window into the world of Storer's twenty-four-year-old patient—whose condition unsurprisingly improved not long after Storer informed her that she would be institutionalized if her symptoms continued—they reveal much more about both the Victorian fixation on nymphomania as well as about Storer himself, and the strange mix of care and contempt with which he approached his female patients. Despite her candid testimony as to her own desires and proclivities, Mrs. B was not treated as the foremost authority on her own sex life; Storer's notes also include snippets from an interview with Mrs. B's husband, who insisted that he was accustomed to having sex with his young wife three times per night, "always with seminal emission," but that he was lately finding an "obstruction to intercourse on her part." Although the patient evidently explained that the "obstruction" in question was not her own doing—rather, her much older husband was having trouble maintaining an erection—Storer nevertheless insisted she submit to a pelvic examination, which would have been both uncomfortable and humiliating. Gynecological exams were not yet routinely taught at medical schools, and Storer's notes reveal little consideration for how she might have felt as a stranger groped his way around her vagina, her perineum, and her clitoris, all with ungloved hands.

"Speculum not used," his report notes, "because not needed."

And yet, Mrs. B was lucky. For her, the greatest threat was the loss of her freedom; years later, a woman who sought treatment from Dr. Storer for the same malady would be brutalized: lashed to an exam table and anesthetized with ether while Storer took a scalpel to her flesh.

Storer's barbaric attitude toward women with healthy sexual appetites was not without historic precedent. Although "nymphomania"
is itself a modern diagnosis, its roots date back to ancient Greece,
where physicians advanced the theory that women were carnal creatures with an insatiable desire for semen. Nor was Storer the first to
seek to "cure" women of their sexual function by surgically removing the clitoris: both the famous English gynecologist Isaac Baker
Brown and distinguished endocrinologist Charles-Édouard Brown-
Séquard (he of the guinea pig testicle infusions) advocated clitoridectomy to prevent women from masturbating, which they believed
would lead to melancholia, paralysis, blindness, and death.

As always, the medical community's fixation on nymphomania
existed in concert with cultural mores, in this case the Victorian
vogue for a "passionless" feminine ideal. Far from being active or en-
thusiastic participants in sexual congress, women were increasingly
understood and expected to embody an elevated moral position,
floating in an imperturbable state of purity above the temptations
of carnal desire. The model woman, it was understood, would engage in sex for noble reasons—namely, for the sake of producing
children—but she certainly wouldn't like it, let alone desire it on
her own. And with the influx of male doctors into the field of gynecology, the sexually amorous woman became not just stigmatized
socially but pathologized medically, a problem in need of a scientific
solution.

Although the vogue for clitoridectomy was gratefully short-lived
in Western medicine—Isaac Baker Brown's enthusiasm for the procedure was never shared by most doctors and ended up getting
him expelled in disgrace from the London Obstetrical Society—
the scientific quest to cure women of all sexual desire lingered on.
In 1892, nearly fifty years after Storer published his case study of
Mrs. B, Robert Tuttle Morris claimed to have cured a case of nymphomania through a surgery to address a condition known as clitoral
adhesion, numbing the clitoris with an injection of cocaine solution
(ouch) and then using his thumbnail to pull back the clitoral hood
to expose the glans. Tuttle claimed that the results were nothing
short of miraculous: "The patient is now spirited and rosy, engaging
in horseback riding, tennis, walking, and all of the pleasures of her
companions," he wrote in his case study.

Tuttle believed that repairing clitoral adhesion was not just a means of curing nymphomania and preventing masturbation, which remained a subject of general obsession among physicians of the era, but also a treatment for conditions like epilepsy. Ironically, he was right about the usefulness of the procedure but entirely wrong about everything else: clitoral adhesions do cause problems, including irritation resulting from a buildup of smegma between the clitoral hood and the glans, and they are still addressed today—using a topical numbing cream instead of an injection. But this is not because the adhesions cause women to become aroused; it's because removing them can improve sexual function in women who struggle to have an orgasm.

As for Horatio Storer, he would devote his life to the practice of gynecology, for better and for worse. One year after his visit from Mrs. B, Storer found his calling not just as a doctor but as an activist, leveraging his reputation as a pioneer in obstetrics to become a leading crusader against abortion. He also never quite lost his taste for brutalizing women in the name of medicine and morality: in 1865, he stood before the American Medical Association congress, arguing that insanity in women should be treated by surgically removing the ovaries. (Insanity, Storer helpfully explained, could be diagnosed in any woman who was "habitually thievish, profane, or obscene, despondent or self-indulgent, shrewish or fatuous.")

By the time Storer died in 1922, he had become the author of one of the more complicated legacies in medical history. On one hand, his anti-abortion activism shaped the movement in ways still visible today, and countless women no doubt suffered needlessly after he prescribed them disfiguring medical treatments for perceived moral defects. On the other hand, and despite his less-than-savory motivations, his dedication to women's health was committed, ambitious, and unparalleled in his time—and he did elevate gynecology within the medical establishment in an era when it was otherwise overlooked. The Gynecaeological Society of Boston, which he founded in 1869, was an undeniable force for progress, leading to major advancements in the field.

And of course, in the hundred years since Storer's death, both women's status in society and their representation in medical science has evolved by leaps and bounds. But when it comes to the way they behave—and are expected to behave—in the context of a medical examination, things aren't so different as we might like to think. The dim view of women, their sexuality, and their agency held by Storer and others like him was not displaced by progress; it was merely pushed down, deep enough to poison the well of the medical consciousness for years to come.

You may tie the arms of a nymphomaniac and she will masturbate by wriggling motions of her legs and thighs; you may tie her arms and legs and she will accomplish her purpose by rubbing her body against the bed or the bureau, or some other article of furniture; nothing less than death will control this all-devouring passion unless you can impress the mind.

—Theophilus Parvin, MD, 1886

As gynecology found its footing as a medical specialty in the mid-to late nineteenth century, certain ideas about women's sexual and reproductive health became fully entrenched within it: namely, that female sexual desire was bad, and doctors should, and could, control it with whatever the tools at their disposal. For men like Storer and Morris, the preferred tool was surgery. For others, it was shame.

This latter group included Robert Latou Dickinson, whose habit, which was not uncommon among gynecologists of the era, was to touch a woman's genitals—inserting fingers into her body or pressing on her clitoris—and then declare her sexually depraved if she reacted in any way. His writings are rife with detailed descriptions and measurements of female genitalia and pelvises, including drawings he sketched himself, which he used to draw conclusions about a given woman's sexual habits. (The "measurements" in question were often not based on any standard system, but rather how many of his own fingers Dickinson could stuff into the patient's vagina.)

Once he'd diagnosed a patient as "erotic" (that is, pathologically horny), Dickinson would not be persuaded otherwise; among his writings from 1931 is a disturbing case study in which he spent months badgering a developmentally disabled seventeen-year-old girl about the "utter relaxation" of her vagina until she confessed to being a masturbator. In reality, the girl's lax pelvic floor was almost certainly purely anatomical in nature—she had come to Dickinson's office for a procedure to repair a prolapsed uterus—but none of this made any difference to the doctor, who had decided that she was sexually depraved. Six months later, when the patient returned to have the vaginal pessary that supported her prolapsed uterus replaced, Dickinson was like the proverbial man with a hammer to whom everything looks like a nail.

"She was erotic at examination," he wrote, "and I hurt her promptly, in order to associate pain and not pleasure with treatment."

At the same time, the idea that women should be shamed out of sexual pleasure or desire had begun to permeate not just gynecology but other areas of medicine, including the burgeoning field of psychoanalysis. Sigmund Freud led the charge here, with his theory of the so-called vaginal orgasm: "Whenever a woman is incapable of achieving an orgasm via coitus . . . and prefers clitoral stimulation to any other form of sexual activity, she can be regarded as suffering from frigidity and requires psychiatric assistance." In Freud's view, clitoral orgasms were the hallmark of an immature, unactualized woman who was repressed by childhood sexual fantasies; instead, he said, women should forgo clitoral stimulation and aspire only to vaginal orgasms, an anatomically illiterate concept that he had essentially invented out of a combination of wishful thinking and thin air.

The damage Freud did to women's sexual health with this harebrained theory is difficult to overstate. Not only did he plant seeds of misinformation about female orgasm that persist to this day, but his influential status in his own time led women to mutilate themselves in the pursuit of Freud's imaginary orgasm. In 1925, French psychoanalyst Marie Bonaparte studied Freud's work and underwent multiple surgeries to reposition her clitoris in the hopes of achieving orgasm through coitus alone. The surgery was unsuccessful, but Bonaparte was one of the lucky ones: other women who sought the procedure not only failed to achieve their purpose but ended up with chronic pain and scarring that left them unable to enjoy sex at all.

But if the plight of those women who were impacted or influenced by the medical bias against female sexuality was shocking, it pales in comparison to that of the women who were quite literally captive to it . . . and here, we meet Dr. Theophilus Parvin.

Parvin was a contemporary of Horatio Storer, and shared many of his concerns about the scourge of unbridled sexuality in women. His professional output included detailed writings on nymphomania, which he believed was a disease that manifested in three stages. The first was sexual desire and fantasies; the second, flirtatious behavior; but in the third, Parvin wrote, the afflicted woman "becomes truly a maniac and gratifies her desires by seeking connection with men and even with dogs."

Unlike Storer, Parvin did not believe in curing women of their sexual desire through surgery; indeed, he rejected the idea that this would work, owing to a belief that nymphomania was more an affliction of the soul and psyche than of the physical body. He did, however, subscribe to the notion that any sexual response in a woman was evidence of depravity, a condition he endeavored to cure by numbing his patients' genitals with cocaine: "I can assure the effect was wonderful," he wrote of one such case, "the vagina at once behaved as well as the most virtuous vagina in the United States."

Parvin was a celebrated obstetrician, a president of the Indiana and American Medical Associations, and a faculty member at multiple medical schools, including the prestigious Jefferson Medical College in Philadelphia. But he was also a prison doctor—and as such, represents a bridge between the world of private medical practice, in which patients sought care more or less of their own accord, and institutional medicine practiced on women who had no choice but to be patients.

Parvin served as the physician at the Indiana Women's Prison between 1873 and 1883, during which time he was elected the president of the American Medical Association. Everything about this was peculiar: it was unusual for a prison doctor to be awarded such a prestigious honor, and unusual for an AMA president to be employed at a prison. It wasn't until 2015, when inmates at the prison (which is still in operation) stumbled upon Parvin's book while researching a history of the facility, that the allure of the position became clearer: his book had been published in 1886, three years after his departure from the IWP, and contained a wealth of data, research, and anecdotes that seemed like they could only have been obtained by experimenting on the prison's female inmates. And while solid information about Parvin's doings at the prison is difficult to come by—unlike the physicians in private practice who we met previously in this chapter, little documentation survives of whatever he was doing during those ten years at the IWP—there is some evidence that all was not well. During Parvin's tenure, a number of female inmates alleged that they were subject to savage abuse, not necessarily by Parvin himself, and yet the doctor appears in news reports from the time: offering testimony in defense of the prison, and denying mistreating the inmates.

What's certain, however, is that if Parvin decided to advance his medical career at the expense of the inmates of the Indiana Women's Prison, he would have been neither the first nor the last. We've already seen how the women institutionalized in asylums like Pitié-Salpêtrière in Paris or the New Jersey State Hospital at Trenton were unwillingly cast as supporting actors in an ambitious doctor's fantasy of eradicating disease, but women's reproductive medicine took on a particularly sinister valence in this context, as US authorities became increasingly interested in controlling the population via eugenics.

In 1907, state governments began to approve the sterilization of female prisoners and mental patients, with devastating results for the poor, minority, and disabled women who made up the bulk of female inmates. In Virginia, a program that launched in 1924 and continued for fifty years resulted in the sterilization of more than 7,500 people. Not all were women, but the program's emphasis on curbing the fertility of people deemed socially transgressive would seem to have disproportionately targeted them; per a report from the *Washington Post*, those sterilized included "unwed mothers, prostitutes, petty criminals and children with disciplinary problems"—but not, one notes, unwed fathers or men who solicited sex workers. In California, a similar program began in 1909 and continued to operate for nearly a hundred years, until an investigation by the Center for Investigative Reporting revealed that 132 women in California prisons had been given tubal ligation while incarcerated, without proper documentation. Later, a 2014 state audit uncovered nearly eight hundred sterilizations in all, including hysterectomies. Meanwhile, the US government evidently decided that the prison sterilization model held promise when it came to culling other "undesirable" populations: beginning in the 1930s in Puerto Rico, nearly one-third of all women between the ages of twenty and forty-nine were forcibly sterilized as the result of a population control program supported by the US government. And in the 1970s, the Indian Health Service sterilized thousands of Native American women, nearly halving their birth rate within the next ten years.

In the midst of these stories of women having their sexuality and fertility destroyed against their will, it's hard not to see a connection between the Victorian horror of the nymphomaniac and the hypersexualized stereotypes that have long plagued women from marginalized backgrounds. The constant in every case is a white coat, a firm hand, a medical doctor stepping in to control women who couldn't be trusted to control themselves. And unlike some of the more overtly barbaric practices whose popularity quickly flared and then faded within the medical establishment, this notion of rescuing women from their own sexuality, for their own good, has proved far more difficult to stamp out. For all that doctors like Storer, Dickinson, and Morris inflicted harm on their patients (or, in Freud's case, persuaded them that it was medically necessary to harm themselves), women still generally entered their offices voluntarily and were generally able to leave at will. Incarcerated and institutionalized women, on the other hand, had no such agency. Indeed, if being sexual made a woman a deviant in the context of an ordinary doctor's office, inside a prison or an asylum it made her something far worse: a lab rat.

She screamed, he struggled, and they rolled out of bed together and made frantic efforts to get apart, but without success . . . it was quite evident that his penis was tightly locked in her vagina, and any attempt to dislodge it was accompanied by much pain on the part of both. It was, indeed, a case [of] "De cohesione in coitu."

—Sir William Osler, MD, writing as Egerton Y. Davis, 1884

The slightest touch at the mouth of the vagina produced the most intense agony, throwing her nervous system into great agitation, with general muscular spasm and shivering of the whole frame as if with the rigors of an intermittent, while she shrieked aloud, her eyes glaring wildly and tears rolling down her cheeks, all rendering her a pitiable object of terror and suffering.

—James Marion Sims, MD, 1857

Although the medical establishment historically reserved its harshest judgments and most barbaric treatments for women who were too desirous of sex, the entrenched view of women as fundamentally asexual beings also did no favors for those who suffered from conditions that limited their sexual function. Chief among these ailments was vaginismus, a painful contraction of the vaginal muscles that makes sexual intercourse excruciating, if it's possible at all.

Vaginismus was treated with varying degrees of seriousness by medical professionals in the 1800s; some believed it was a real albeit frustratingly intractable problem, while others were skeptical that it existed at all. Notably, even those physicians who exerted themselves to treat vaginismus tended to view it less in terms of the misery it caused to their female patients and more in terms of the frustration it caused their husbands. In one shocking case study from the late nineteenth century, the solution of the patient's family doctor was not to treat her vaginismus but to drug her with ether so that her husband could have sex with her unconscious body. By the time the case made its way to a specialist—James Marion Sims, who we met in the Urinary chapter—the woman had conceived and birthed one child as a result of this unsavory ritual, and the original doctor was visiting the couple's home to etherize the woman a dozen times per month in the hopes of helping them to conceive another. The notes from the case prior to Sims's appearance are revealing: not only was the doctor remarkably incurious as to his patient's well-being, he dedicated an absurd amount of space to describing her husband in decidedly nonclinical terms: "The husband was tall, athletic, and muscular; says he is not subject to hasty ejaculation, and possesses extraordinary copulative powers," the case study explains, going out of its way to assure the reader "that it was not the fault of the husband that the vaginismus did not yield to penetration and dilatation."

It just goes to show that there is no scenario, not even a medical case study explicitly focused on a woman's vaginal health, that men would not use as an excuse to talk about the power of their penises.

Indeed, insofar as doctors attempted to treat vaginismus, it was generally from the perspective of making the patient sexually accessible rather than healthy; the literature of the time rarely speaks in terms of restoring full sexual function to the woman and focuses instead on opening up her vagina enough to admit her husband's penis, with little concern for her comfort. Here, we must give some credit to Sims, who was well-known by this time for pioneering his groundbreaking surgery to repair vesicovaginal fistula: when the aforementioned patient arrived in his office, he explicitly chose to look for better solutions to her condition. "I would not pretend to deny that we can dilate a case of vaginismus so as to permit sexual intercourse, but in most of the cases so treated the act is very painful," he wrote.

It was Sims who gave vaginismus its name and who in 1857 proposed a surgical solution—the removal of the hymen, followed by an incision inside the vagina and the use of a dilator during the healing process—that he believed would permit afflicted women to have sex without pain. But even Sims's more compassionate approach was still tainted by paternalism and a sense that sex for women was a marital duty, not a source of pleasure unto itself. When he wrote about vaginismus, he described it less as a woman's issue than in terms of its effect on couples, writing, "I can confidently assert that I know of no disease capable of producing so much unhappiness to both parties to the marriage contract, and I am happy to state that I know of no serious trouble that can be so easily, so safely, and so certainly cured."

Unfortunately, what little investigation there was into vaginismus by doctors who took it seriously was severely undermined by the one who treated it as a joke. In 1884, Theophilus Parvin published a treatise in the *Philadelphia Medical News*, where he was an editor, titled "An Uncommon Form of Vaginismus." (Parvin claimed to have treated the condition with what appears to have been his signature move: applying a cocaine solution to the patient's genitals.) The article apparently aroused the ire of Sir William Osler, the brilliant diagnostician who created the residency model of medical education and who would spend his twilight years campaigning against the presence of women in medical schools: he was so skeptical of the idea of vaginismus, and so intent on discrediting a competitor's research into it, that he retaliated against Parvin by publishing a hoax article that same year in which he described an even more uncommon form of vaginismus, one powerful enough to capture the penis of the afflicted woman's paramour inside her body.

Osler, writing under a pseudonym, fabricated a story of a medical call at a private residence, where a coachman's penis had become trapped inside the body of the maid with whom he was having intercourse. "I applied water, and then ice, but ineffectually, and at last sent for chloroform, a few whiffs of which sent the woman to sleep, relaxed the spasm, and released the captive penis, which was swollen, livid, and in a state of semi-erection, which did not go down for several hours, and for days the organ was extremely sore," he wrote, unwittingly invoking the specter of the real-life patient of Sims whose doctor would etherize her before sex.

If Osler had been in a position of less influence, or if he had revealed his prank straightaway, it might have been funny. As it was, though, he turned vaginismus itself into a joke, and set back the medical profession's awareness of the condition so badly that it still hasn't recovered. Today, vaginismus is listed in the *DSM* as a psychiatric condition. And it remains agonizingly difficult to treat, not least because of the pervasive notion—one both originated and perpetuated by some of history's foremost women's physicians—that women don't really need to enjoy sex. That their sexual health is defined not by their own pleasure but by their ability to be available to a man. And that if it hurts down there, no matter; that's just how it is, and what it means, to be a woman.

Dr. Meigs, Professor of Gynecology at the Harvard Medical School and chief of staff of the Vincent Memorial Hospital in Boston, suggested that rather than through medical techniques, endometriosis should be attacked by parental subsidy of early marriage . . . The problems of the ailment in the individual patient, he continued, were far overshadowed by the importance of the resultant infertility among the "intelligent, trained, educated and socially minded—the so-called upper class."

—*New York Times*, "Social III Is Laid to Endometriosis," 1948

For fifteen years, doctors have been telling Dana she's normal.

Her periods, so painful and heavy that she can barely move for five days a month, let alone attend school or play sports: normal.

The time she bled through her sleeping bag and onto the carpet at a slumber party: normal.

The chronic headaches, upset stomach, and recurring, maddening yeast infections: normal.

The urinary tract infections and painful bowel movements: normal.

The first time she had sex and thought she might pass out from the pain: normal.

The second and fifth and fifteenth time, when it didn't get any better: normal.

The worst part is, the doctors want to help. They want to help so badly that they always have some new solution to suggest, and whatever it is, Dana always nods along. Yes, she'll try it. Yes, let's do it. She has been poked, scraped, smeared, and biopsied; she has given pints of her blood for testing; she has taken birth control she didn't want and antibiotics she didn't need and dutifully smeared dozens of ointments on her body. She's drunk gallons of water and meditated for hours. She's changed her diet from paleo to pescatarian to vegan to keto. She's done physical therapy for her pelvic floor. She has tried every variety of toilet paper—twice.

She does these things not because they work, which they never do, but because she needs the doctors to see that she's trying. As much as nothing they suggest ever helps, her greatest fear is that one day they'll stop suggesting things. That they'll throw up their hands and say out loud what's been obvious from day one: that they have no idea what's wrong with her.

That they're starting to think nothing is wrong with her at all.

◆ ◆ ◆

Today's doctors are far more sympathetic to women who suffer from diseases of the reproductive system than their historic predecessors. And yet, women still struggle to receive adequate care amid scandalous levels of ignorance about just what a "healthy" woman's reproductive system looks like.

Consider endometriosis, one of the most crippling and least understood conditions affecting women's reproductive health, which a recent historical review by a team of gynecologists at Stanford calls "one of the most colossal mass misdiagnoses in human history, one that over the centuries has subjected women to murder, madhouses, and lives of unremitting physical, social, and psychological pain."

Endometriosis occurs when tissue similar to the lining of the uterus grows outside the uterus—on the ovaries and Fallopian tubes, or sometimes on the bowel, rectum, and other pelvic areas. Because of its varied locations within the body, the potential symptoms of endometriosis are wide-ranging: women can experience chronic pelvic pain, unusually painful periods, painful intercourse, and infertility, but also GI issues, urinary tract infections, incontinence, and more. The condition affects at least 10 percent of women in the United States, and takes, on average, more than seven years to diagnose. During those seven years, women suffer untold misery: from the symptoms themselves but also from the frustration of dealing with a medical system in which endometriosis is routinely overlooked, misdiagnosed, or written off as imaginary. Dana, the patient whose story preceded this section, is a real woman and a perfect case study: she spent more than a decade in agony while doctors told her that it was normal for sex to be excruciating, normal to have debilitating menstrual cramps, normal to sleep on a towel during her period because she'd bleed through both a tampon and a pad in a matter of hours. At various points, she was diagnosed with everything from IBS to interstitial cystitis; multiple times, she was told that perhaps it was just anxiety.

Dana eventually found her way to a specialist who diagnosed her with endometriosis. But even this illustrates the brokenness of the medical system when it comes to treating women with this condition: she found her way, on her own, after years of presenting at doctor after doctor with symptoms that nobody ever recognized for what they were.

The way Dana ping-ponged around the system for more than a decade before finally being diagnosed is the natural outgrowth of a culture—and in turn, a medical apparatus—that views pelvic pain in women as normal. Skepticism of endometriosis symptoms is inculcated in doctors early. During my own medical training, while on rotation in a Boston ER, I encountered a woman named Emilia who was writhing on a hospital bed, weeping, doubled over in pain. It was clear that something was terribly wrong with her, but when the chief resident saw me write her name on the whiteboard to be triaged, he stepped up beside me and erased it.

"That one hysterically crying in there, she's a frequent flier," he said. "Nothing's wrong with her. Find another patient."

In one way, he was correct: Emilia had visited the ER twice before—always at the same time of the month. Her pain corresponded directly with her menstrual cycle, a classic symptom of endometriosis. But even in a hospital full of doctors, nobody ever made this connection; instead, they shrugged off whatever was happening to her as all in her head.

The contemporary incuriosity surrounding endometriosis has been preceded by decades of disregard, its symptoms dismissed as the trumped-up complaints of women who were just being fragile, dramatic, or both. In the 1970s and 1980s, endometriosis was nicknamed "the career woman's disease," with the medical consensus being that it stemmed from the stresses of professional life; at this time, a woman diagnosed with endometriosis was less likely to receive medical treatment and more likely to be told that the problem would solve itself if she simply quit her job and stayed home. Meanwhile, childless women were often advised that getting pregnant would cure the condition, a bizarre myth that has proved remarkably persistent even today.

Indeed, the notion that women are biologically destined to be mothers still holds an unsettling sway over this area of reproductive medicine: a woman with endometriosis who presents at the doctor with fertility issues will receive a diagnosis twice as fast as those who seek help for painful periods. And while one of the more common treatments for endometriosis is hysterectomy, some young women who seek the procedure are refused by doctors: "You may want to have children someday," they're told, as if they don't know what a hysterectomy is.

Even now, the medical system operates from the same presupposition it always did: that a woman's health, her happiness, and even her freedom from pain are all secondary to her biological destiny to become a mother. And even now, this system cows women into submission at it always has. If the ghosts of doctors like Storer, Dickinson, Morris, Parvin, and Freud still lurk in the background of women's medicine, the women themselves are haunted by the specters of their patients. Women who submitted to comatose sex on a doctor's orders. Women who were led to believe that the normal, healthy workings of their own bodies meant they were broken and depraved. Women like Mrs. B, an ordinary young wife who loved her husband and the physical intimacy of marriage, but who became someone and something else when she walked through the doors of her gynecologist's office: frightened, compliant, and so convinced of her inadequacies by a powerful physician that she would do anything he asked.

◆ ◆ ◆

Of all the systems the human body contains, and of all the areas physicians seek to treat, the female reproductive system remains the most misunderstood and plagued by biases that have been woven into the fabric of medicine for as long as medicine has been practiced. What began with the belief that the female body is a broken, inverted riff on the male ideal has evolved today into a sustained sense that women's bodies are mysterious and unknowable, which in turn leads to women being decentered in conversations about their own care. Historically, doctors have too often viewed their female patients' health as secondary to the needs of others—the men they're married to, the babies they carry. Even today, women's own well-being during pregnancy gets short shrift in comparison with that of the fetus. And the rate of maternal mortality in the United States is ten times that of other developed countries, with poor and minority women disproportionately affected.

Sexual and reproductive health issues that uniquely afflict women, meanwhile, are still overlooked by doctors who are not trained to look for them. The fact that the average medical education leaves graduates virtually illiterate as to the location, structure, and function of the clitoris is just the beginning: ignorance persists around everything from endometriosis to sexual dysfunction to certain types of cancer. Ovarian cancer, for instance, which kills fourteen thousand women every year, is frequently referred to in the medical literature as a "silent killer"—but in fact, most women with early stage ovarian cancer experience symptoms for which they often seek medical help. In 2022, gynecologic oncologist Barbara Goff surveyed 1,700 ovarian cancer patients and found that misdiagnosis was rampant: "15% had their symptoms attributed to irritable bowel disease, 12% to stress, 9% to gastritis, 6% to constipation, 6% to depression and 4% to some other cause. Thirty percent were given treatment for a different condition. And 13% were told there was nothing wrong."

The problem is not that ovarian cancer is silent; it's that we're not listening.

And then, of course, there's the matter of sex.

"To this day, whenever I say I work in women's sexual health, people automatically assume I mean sexually transmitted infections," says Lyndsey Harper, with a laugh. Harper is an associate professor (affiliated) of ob-gyn for Texas A&M University School of Medicine, a fellow of the American Congress of Obstetricians and Gynecologists, a fellow of the International Society for the Study of Women's Sexual Health, and the creator of a women's sexual wellness application called Rosy. She's also an expert on all the ways in which the medical system fails to prioritize women's sexuality and the reasons why. "The people that built medicine were men, and in their eyes, women's sexuality had two roles. Number one was reproduction. And number two was preventing—or not passing along, we should say—sexually transmitted infections."

It's a hell of a blind spot, one that manifests today as a massive black hole in the medical consciousness when it comes to women's sexual health—despite the fact that male sexual function has always been, and remains, a top priority in their medical care. As Harper notes, "When a man comes in with a prostate cancer, the very first conversation he has with his urologist is how they're going to spare his erectile function." Women, on the other hand, receive no such consideration. That lack of communication is reflective of not just disinterest but stunning levels of ignorance about how women's bodies actually work, the repercussions of which can range from problematic to tragic. Incautious or ill-informed doctors have caused clitoral injuries to their patients during procedures ranging from hip replacements to episiotomies to labiaplasties, resulting in life-altering sexual dysfunction that nobody knows how to fix—and that women themselves often struggle to explain.

"We're taught to think about our sexuality as something that is separate from us, and that needs to be managed," Harper says. "And so we're taught over the years to shut it down, to behave and shut it down. And we do. We shut it down. Women struggle with the experience of pleasure. Many of us don't really even know what that means."

In its current state, medicine cannot help women find that meaning, nor instill in us a sense of authority and ownership over our bodies. I see it every day in my own medical practice: accomplished, confident women suddenly shrink as they walk through the door of my exam room, apologizing for taking up too much space or for asking too many questions. There's the thirty-five-year-old CEO of a thriving start-up who confesses that she has no idea how to have an orgasm; the take-no-prisoners journalist who is afraid to probe for details about her own cancer treatment plan. One of my patients, the survivor of a particularly aggressive form of breast cancer at the age of thirty-one, admitted to me, with much embarrassment, that she was struggling to enjoy sex with her husband—not because of the cancer but because she couldn't climax from intercourse alone: "Where is this fucking G-spot I am supposed to have?!"

There's ignorance and fear and, underlying it all, a pervasive sense of shame: over the course of a thousand years of toxic messaging and manipulation, we have taught women that if something goes wrong with their sexual health, it's because something is wrong with them, personally.

I say "we," because these blind spots and biases are no longer any one person's fault, but a collective, inherited failure. They're built into the system, into society, and they impact all of us.

Every patient.

Every doctor.

Even me.

It was a woman named Anne who woke me up to the way I was perpetuating the legacy of medical prejudice surrounding women's sexual health. She had been my patient for just over a year, having undergone the successful treatment of her early stage breast cancer. At eighty years old, she was vibrant, stylish, and not one to suffer fools gladly—and she had been waiting for her latest appointment to tell me just how foolish I'd been.

"I hate that new medication you're giving me," she said. "It really affects my time with my special friend."

My first reaction was surprise. After more than a year, I knew Anne quite well. She was unmarried and always came to her appointments alone, but I had assumed she'd tell me if she had someone special in her life. When she saw the expression on my face, she shook her head and grinned.

"Dr. Comen, my friend isn't a man," she said. "It's a vibrator."

We both laughed, but underneath this moment of levity I was having a jarring realization. I had prescribed Anne an estrogen-inhibiting medication to prevent her cancer from recurring, and in the year since, I had only ever asked if she was experiencing joint pain—even though vaginal dryness and loss of libido were also well-known side effects. I'd simply assumed that these things wouldn't matter to her. After all, she was eighty. And thanks to my incuriosity, I'd robbed her of one of life's joys at a time when she didn't have many.

It was a wake-up call.

The next time I saw Anne, it was at a follow-up appointment to see how she was responding to her new medication—one without the annoying sexual side effects. The medication was working beautifully, she said, but never mind that, she had something I needed to see. She pulled a newspaper from her purse and jabbed her finger at it, incensed.

"Look at this," she said, pointing to a headline that read, "Sex Sells, but When It Comes to Female Pleasure, the New York Subway Isn't So Sure." The transportation authority in New York City had banned advertisements from a sex toy company that targeted its products to women. They were claiming the ads were obscene—even as advertisements for male virility products were plastered on New York City buses and subways from the Bronx to Staten Island.

"This is bullshit," Anne said.

I couldn't agree more.

Throughout the process of researching and writing this book, I have always been cognizant of the fact that, as a medical doctor, I am deeply embedded in the same system I am seeking to critique. I know that the legacy of skepticism, distrust, and ignorance of women's bodies that lurks at the foundations of modern medicine is one in which I was immersed as a medical student, and one I have been guilty of perpetuating myself in my own breast oncology practice— and I see its insidious influence in the lives of my patients every day. But at the end of 2022, as I was completing the research that would eventually become this book's chapter on the skeletal system, something happened to make me realize that I don't just bear the burden of that legacy as a physician. I carry it as a woman and as a patient. I carry it even when it's my own body and my own health on the line.

It was supposed to be a minor surgery. There was a compressed nerve in my spinal column that was causing numbness and weakness in my left leg, a condition I'd been foolishly ignoring for the better part of three years. When I finally scheduled the surgery for the week after Thanksgiving, I felt both relieved to finally be taking care of it and chagrined that I'd waited so long. It was a simple outpatient procedure, and the recovery time was minimal and virtually painless; even after contracting Covid the week after the surgery, I was back on my feet and seeing patients again by mid-December, feeling tired but otherwise fine.

Then the headaches began. The pain and pressure started at the base of my skull and then radiated upward, splaying out in invisible fingers that wrapped up and over the top of my head and bore down with crushing force. The pain would relent if I lay down, but of course, I couldn't lie down. I had patients to see, family events to plan, a dear friend's New Year's Eve party that I'd promised to attend. It wasn't until I was in the car on the way to the party, the seat tipped back as far as it would go to relieve the agonizing pressure in my head, that I finally realized why my constellation of symptoms seemed so familiar: they were a familiar specter in the medical literature surrounding any spinal surgery, from epidurals during childbirth to the treatment for a herniated disc. I turned to my husband.

"I think I'm leaking cerebrospinal fluid," I said.

Cerebrospinal fluid (usually known as CSF) is a watery liquid that bathes and cushions the brain, continually circulating through its ventricles and over its surface before draining down along the spinal column. A proper balance of CSF allows the brain to essentially float inside the skull, and feels like absolutely nothing; a leakage of CSF, on the other hand, manifests as a debilitating headache and the sensation that your brain is being sucked down into your spinal cord, because basically, it is. This was why my head hurt so badly; it was also why it felt better when I lay down. Without gravity creating a vacuum inside my skull, the pressure dissipated immediately.

CSF leaks are rare but not unheard-of after spinal surgeries like the one I'd just had, and although they're serious, they're remarkably easy to fix; at worst, I would need to return to the hospital for a blood patch, a small injection to plug the opening through which fluid was leaking. And while none of this was immediately helpful— I was still in excruciating pain—I arrived at the party feeling confident: I knew what was the matter with me. I had already begun drafting an email to my spinal surgeon explaining the problem; now I put my phone away, greeted my friend, and immediately laid my head on her kitchen counter, ignoring the alarmed stares from the other guests. When she asked me what was wrong, I told her I was leaking brain fluid—but I'd be okay, I said, flippantly, if she could just bring me some Advil.

"CSF? That's impossible," a male voice said. I looked up to see a man looming above me: a celebrated plastic surgeon I knew only by reputation. Rumor had it that he was responsible for every nip, tuck, lift, and implant sported by a certain set of Real Housewives; now he was standing beside me, looking down at me as if I were lying on his operating table inside of my friend's marble kitchen countertop.

"Impossible," he said again. "No, I know exactly what you have.

It's occipital neuralgia. A compressed nerve in your skull. You could fix it with Botox or lidocaine, but I find the most intractable cases require a surgical intervention. Here, let me show you—"

A cell phone was suddenly thrust into my face, and I dutifully turned my head to look at it, watching as the surgeon scrolled through photo after photo of skulls that had been opened to expose the occipital nerve. The surgery was miraculous, he said, but he didn't do it anymore; he would have to refer me to someone, unless (and here he chuckled) I wanted him to just open my skull right here, right now.

Somehow, I managed to laugh.

"No thanks," I said, before shuffling to the sofa, where I would spend the rest of the party lying back against a pillow and struggling not to scream every time I accidentally lifted my head upright. On the way home, I crawled into the back seat, stretching out horizontally. In that moment, I decided that, holiday weekend or not, I would contact my spinal surgeon the next day.

And I did. But when I read the email I sent to him, I cringe. It was the email I'd begun drafting in the car the night before, but with one key difference. In the original message, my subject line mentioned my self-diagnosis of CSF leakage. But that was before the party, before the surgeon, before the photos of skulls cracked open to reveal their occipital nerves.

Now it read, simply: "Occipital neuralgia?"

◆ ◆ ◆

As you've probably guessed by now, I did not have occipital neuralgia. My symptoms didn't even remotely suggest as much—whereas they were a perfect match for the CSF leakage with which I'd originally diagnosed myself and which finally landed me in the emergency room days later. And eventually, after an MRI revealed swelling around my brain consistent with fluid loss, and after a procedure was performed to repair the small tear in my meningeal layer through which cerebrospinal fluid was escaping, I would laugh ruefully about the irony of it all: despite my medical training, despite my knowledge and expertise when it came to my own body, and even despite the fact that I was literally writing a book about sex-related bias in medicine, my confidence had still vanished the moment an accomplished, celebrated, swaggering male surgeon stood over me and called me ridiculous.

But that was later. What I said in the moment, on the other hand, was both less clever and more revealing. It was while I was lying on a curtained stretcher in the emergency room, barely able to move as a nurse gently manipulated my arms and legs out of my street clothes and into a hospital gown. I looked up at her and whimpered.

"I'm so sorry," I said. "I forgot to wear deodorant."

◆ ◆ ◆

It's not lost on me, as I write this, that women are better represented in medicine than ever before, if you go strictly by the numbers. In 2022, women made up nearly 57 percent of all applicants to medical school and nearly 38 percent of all practicing physicians. It's a remarkable achievement, considering that the total percentage of female doctors in 1990 was only 28—or that Harvard, the country's most prestigious medical school, didn't even admit women as students until 1945. And yet the slow trickle of women into medicine has not dispelled the underlying ideology that once conspired to disenfranchise and discredit the more holistic healing practices that were once their dominion, and their strength.

The early divide between the physicians who practiced modern medicine and the so-called irregulars who didn't—a divide that sidelined en masse the many women who worked as healers and midwives—has since hardened, and multiplied, into a series of unbridgeable binaries. Scientific versus homeopathic. Western versus Eastern. Traditional versus experimental. And, yes, masculine versus feminine, and on this front, masculine continues to win. The increasing gender parity in who is practicing medicine has not led medicine itself to be feminized. Indeed, the medical establishment continues to be a place in which more "feminine" aspects of medicine—personalized care, patient relationships, nurturing, peacekeeping, and a whole-life approach to wellness that goes beyond simply curing disease—are consistently undervalued.

In the process of researching this book, I stumbled across a 2009 study from the National Institutes of Health that confirmed what

has long been an observable phenomenon: on average, women gravitate toward working with people, while men prefer to work with
things. It struck me then that our modern medical establishment, in
which doctors self-select early into specializations that focus on just
one system or body part, too often treats our patients like broken
things in need of fixing rather than people in need of care. This is a
problem, and not just because of the way it makes patients feel: How
many misdiagnoses happen as a result of doctors focusing only on
whatever seems relevant to their specialty, constrained by the limits
of those fifteen-minute appointments into overlooking or even ignoring how the body's systems interact?

And yet the current system is one that rewards this single-minded
approach to medicine. It's not just our system of medical records
and insurance billing, which reduces patients to a series of computer
codes (or worse, allows them to slip through the cracks when their
symptoms aren't easily categorized). Doctors are promoted, and
become famous, for scientific breakthroughs: the discovery of mol-
ecules, the mapping of genes, the development of innovative new
treatments that make for front-page headlines in the *New York Times*
or segments on CNN. Nobody, on the other hand, is promoted just
for kindness, for empathy, or for making patients feel seen. Indeed,
the most extravagant praise and rewards in this paradigm are reserved for doctors who rarely see patients at all—or who see them as
background actors in a story about scientific discovery.

And yet it doesn't have to be this way. For every absurdity or bias
that still lingers in the system, there are doctors working to combat
it, dismantle it, and build something better in its place. You have
met some of them in these pages: people like Saadi Ghatan, Lyndsey Harper, and JoAnn Manson. Theirs is a model for what can be
accomplished through one person's sheer determination.

Imagine what we might accomplish if the model became a movement.

Even the most incremental changes could drastically improve the
lives of everyone who comes in contact with the medical system—
women especially, perhaps, but not just them. Every woman I spoke
to for this book mentioned to me the concept of the "mom consult":
that women in medical settings are expected to be the listeners, to
spend extra time with patients, to not just cure but nurture. Right

now, people assume that women will do this because they just care more. What would happen if we valued these skills highly and rewarded them accordingly, so that all doctors had a powerful incentive to engage with patients in this way? What if we celebrated the doctors, nurses, and medical professionals who gravitate toward specialties that center the patient's humanity—for example, pediatrics, internal medicine—as much as we do the skilled surgeons who transform faces, replace joints, or operate on spines and brains?

◆ ◆ ◆

On October 21, 1925, Dr. Francis W. Peabody famously addressed Harvard students on the importance of humanity in medical practice: at the time, he begged these aspiring doctors, in their efforts to preserve and protect their patients' physical bodies, not to neglect what he referred to as the "emotional life." To see the person in need of nurturing not just the broken machine in need of repair.

"The good physician knows his patient through and through, and his knowledge is bought dearly. Time, sympathy, and understanding must be lavishly dispensed, but the reward is to be found in that personal bond which forms the greatest satisfaction of the practice of medicine," he said. "One of the essential qualities of the clinician is his interest in humanity, for the secret of the care of the patient is in caring for the patient."

Peabody couldn't possibly have imagined at the time how prescient those words would turn out to be a century later, but they are. The twisted roots planted by doctors like Henry Cotton, Horatio Storer, or Jean-Martin Charcot are still beneath us, and still bearing fruit, in the form of an unstable, fragmented, dysfunctional system that leaves doctors and patients and men and women alike bereft of care—and at the mercy of indifferent third-party players that are driven not by the provider nor patient's best interests but by the pursuit of profit. As much as the pages in this book detail the absurd, alarming, and sometimes catastrophic failures of medical men throughout history to see the humanity of their female patients, we should none of us be so arrogant as to assume that we, in our more enlightened time, are above making similar missteps.

The above is my message to the medical system itself. But to the readers who still need to partner with that imperfect system, I have a different message: that despite its copious and well-documented flaws, it is staffed by people who were called to practice medicine because they do care. The purpose of this book is not to ruin your faith in medicine, nor to point fingers at the men who made it what it is, but to illuminate the narratives that began with them and still surround us today: about women's bodies, women's health, women's needs and desires. How many of these medical histories are repeating themselves every time a woman enters a doctor's office today? How many times have you felt that same fear, shame, or inability to speak the truth about what was happening in your body? How many of the stories in this book echo one that you've been telling yourself, unwittingly, for years and years?

And having heard these stories, can you imagine choosing to tell a different one?

Among my greatest hopes in writing this book is that it will give women the tools they need to demand the care they deserve. Even in an imperfect system, there is power in understanding how that system works: how best to communicate with your healthcare providers, how to get the most out of those fifteen-minute appointments, how to recognize and work within the categories the system will inevitably sort you into. Do not be afraid to ask questions about the system itself: What can you realistically expect to address in one appointment? What is the best way to contact your doctor when you need a quick response? And do not be afraid to ask yourself, before an appointment, what truly concerns you about your body—not what you think you should be worried about, not what you think your doctor will be able to most comfortably and easily address. If your doctor seems uncomfortable or rushed, find another doctor. On the other hand, if your doctor makes you feel trusted and respected, return the favor by telling her in straightforward terms about why you're there and trusting that she wants to help.

◆ ◆ ◆

There's a poem by e.e. cummings that I think of every time I'm laboring through the labyrinthine and maddening annals of our electronic medical records system, trying to capture every condition, every symptom, every nuance of human suffering through a series of diagnostic codes:

> *While you and i have lips and voices which*
> *are for kissing and to sing with*
> *who cares if some oneeyed son of a bitch*
> *invents an instrument to measure Spring with?*

Of course, it's easy for a poet to say. Of course, doctors cannot afford to dispense with the measuring entirely; to just, as cummings says, "eat flowers and not to be afraid." We need some way to catalog and document and, yes, invoice for the care of the patients who come through our doors.

But I also believe we can do this better than we have been, and better than we are. The fact that we no longer demonize women as spreaders of contagion or institutionalize them for being difficult is a start, not a finish. I believe there is room for a medical system that balances efficiency with humanity. That values doctors who nurture as much as it values the ones who discover.

I believe in a future where, in those terrible moments when a patient is adrift on an ocean of pain, fear, and uncertainty, I will take her hand, and neither of us will apologize. Not for sweating. Not for crying. Not for anything: there is nothing to be sorry for.

In the years I spent scouring the old case reports and medical text-books that form the backbone of this book, what stood out to me most was what I couldn't find: the voices of women whose bodies made this research possible. The patients whose stories are reproduced in the pages of this book do exist in the medical literature, but largely as mute bodies, and these women's storytellers—the physicians who chronicled their ailments and care—rarely permissioned their patients to speak for themselves about the disease states they came to represent. I have tried to reproduce these patients' perspectives based on the facts available, to imbue their stories with the depth and richness each deserves, but I remain haunted by what I know has been lost to history: their fear, their pain, their desires, and the lives they lived before and after they entered the medical machine. I remain humbled and grateful for the bravery and trust of my own patients in sharing their lives with me. Their courage amidst the greatest of threats inspired me to write this book; it inspires me still.

There is no world in which this book would exist without the extraordinary talent of Kat Rosenfield. Kat, your capacity to capture all manner of the human condition—from grotesque to humorous—with brilliant and relatable insight is unparalleled. Your commitment to this project and its mission reflects your generous nature and dedication to outing right. I am eternally grateful for our partnership.

I am forever indebted to my agent, Yfat Reiss Gendell, for believing in me and pushing me to imagine the biggest version of this book; for your brilliant advocacy and insight in its crafting and journey to the hands of readers; and all along the way, for your indefatigable insistence that I refrain from settling and produce nothing less than the book of my dreams. You gave me a new life. Thank you also to Yfat's entire extraordinary team: the essential Ashley M. Napier, Lisa Tilman, and Devereux Chatillon.

My remarkable editor and publisher of Harper Wave, Karen Rinaldi, distinguished herself from the start: From the moment we spoke over Zoom—you from your casual-cool home office with a tableau of electric guitars as your backdrop; me from a random free office that just happened to have a life-size Wonder Woman cutout leaning against the wall behind me—I knew our visions aligned. I am deeply grateful for your enthusiasm, creative acumen, and sharp insight. You are a unicorn. Thank you to president of the Harper Group, Jonathan Burnham, and CEO and president of Harper-Collins Publishers, Brian Murray. Of course, no book is produced by an author and publisher alone, and I'm indebted to the exceptional team at Harper Wave: associate editor Kirby Sandmeyer, director of publicity Yelena Nesbit, associate publicist Sacha Chadwick, director of marketing Amanda Pritzker, associate director of marketing Jessica Gilo, head of managing editorial Cindy Achar, managing editor Christina Polizoto, copy editor Janet Rosenberg (and apologies for my fifty-five pages of citations—I have academic PTSD), editorial production manager Nikki Baldauf, senior designer Elina Cohen, director of art department (interior) Leah Carlson-Stanisic, art director and jacket artist Joanne O'Neill (thank you for hanging in there with me and Karen), director of art department Robin Bilardello, head of sales Andy LeCount, and, of course, to the entire sales team who introduced this to booksellers and made it possible for readers to find it.

To my dear friends who supported me: Christina Isacson—I'm grateful for your daily check-ins and sage wisdom. Thank you to Marianna Strongin, Dendy Engelman, and my greater wolf pack of friends, for the insistence that I leave the house on occasion, even if the muse was visiting, pulling me out of history and reminding me to be present.

I am deeply grateful for the early reads and collective insight from Harvard College, history of science professors: Anne Harrington, Katherine Park, and Sarah Richardson, and professor of history and public affairs at Princeton University, Keith Wailoo. Your collective input on early material was invaluable. Thank you to the supremely talented writer Danielle Friedman for meeting with me early in the writing process and delivering essential advice. To my research assistants, Emma Lee Verstraete and K. Stawasz, who persisted in digging for near-impossible-to-find sources. Thank you to Hannah George for the tireless effort and shared enthusiasm, sometimes expressed in your joining the collective chorus of victorious cries when we *finally* unearthed that *one* historical source after days of hunting. And to Hanna Polsky, it is thanks to you that so many of the women's stories told here can be told at all—thank you for honoring their physical and narrative histories as you do.

Thank you to the people in my life who shaped my worldview and without whom this work could never have been written: my elementary and high school teachers, Jerry Kelly, Jim Dudley, and Debbie Mercer. I recall a tense first essay exam in the sixth grade, when Mr. Kelly kindly whispered, "You'll be fine, just tell me everything you know."

I could not have written this book without the generous encouragement and writing space provided by my dear friend and chosen family Aaron Rosenberg—in your borrowed home I found a quiet, protected seat from which I could think bigger.

I'm also indebted to American Society of Clinical Oncology CEO, Dr. Cliff Hudis, who gently advised that I "didn't have to be a square peg in a round hole," allowing me to imagine a more flexible professional life outside of the well-trod academic path, ultimately laying the groundwork for this work. Of equal impact and import is your partner in life and family, Jane Hudis, whose vision and impact on my life and on the lives of countless women cannot be understated.

I'm grateful to Dr. Larry Norton, a professional mentor whose unwavering drive to help women moved me to commit my career to breast oncology.

And I give thanks to my dear colleague, the late Dr. Tomas Lyons, who insisted I just "write the damn book already."

I am grateful to my Harvard Medical School classmates—Drs. Loretta Erhunmwunsee, Molly McNairy, and Tami Tiamfook—who shared their time and expertise with me, despite my obvious white lie that our phone calls would "take only a few minutes of your time." Additionally, I give thanks to the doctors who volunteered their time, insight, and expertise to enrich the book: Dr. Kathryn Ackerman, Dr. Omri Ayalon, Dr. Allie Baker, Dr. Sonali Bose, Dr. Bridget Carey, Dr. Lara Devgan, Dr. Ian Dunn, Dr. Charles Galanis, Dr. Saadi Ghatan, Dr. Lindsey Harper, Dr. Neil Iyengar, Dr. Daniela Jodorkovsky, Dr. Hafiza Khan, Dr. Angelish Kumar, Dr. Katherine Lee, Dr. Michael Lockshin, Dr. Lindsay Lief, Dr. Susan Lucak, Dr. JoAnn Manson, Dr. Ariela Marshall, Dr. Elizabeth Ortiz, Dr. Rekha Parameswaran, Dr. Aviva Preminger, Dr. Kara Long Roche, Dr. Robyn Sackeyfio, Dr. Noa Schwartz, Dr. Beth Shubin Stein, Dr. Gil Weitzman, and Dr. Nanette Wenger.

In the conclusion of this book I shared that I was unexpectedly injured during the writing of this work and needed longer to recover than I could have imagined. I am forever grateful to the healers who encouraged me to slow down and find strength in stillness. Joy. Energy. Breath. You helped me find all, from the ground up.

My parents, Steven and Miriam Comen, put me on the path to this book by encouraging the adult me to stop being such a good girl and start asking not-so-nice questions, and then sticking around, tapping my dance-shoe-clad toes, until I got those answers. To this end, I'm grateful to my father for supporting me when I said that I didn't need an Easy-Bake Oven and Snack Center, nor did I even need to learn how to bake, for that matter. I'm grateful to my mother for modeling how to ask the hard questions required to write this book with empathy, kindness, and intuitive human connection. And with the answers to these questions committed to the pages that follow, I hope to honor the legacy of women in our family. To my aunt Pearl, a presence in both life and death, may the stories of these women honor your own.

Some authors credit the support of their partners as the essential ingredient that made their book possible, and it's likely true in some instances and less true in others. In my case, my husband, Avi, spent years hearing me dream aloud about the medical history I hoped to bring to light, and when he'd finally heard enough, he dragged me to the home of my future literary agent. He said it was a friendly brunch, and that I'd be doing him a favor by going. But then he pushed me past my shyness, insisting that I accept her invitation to discuss my idea, then vetted prospective partners, reviewed countless documents, sorted kids and in-laws to give me space for the work, read every chapter in progress, and not-so-stealthily checked in on my behalf as a passionate fan. Yes, he believes in the mission of bringing this existential history to light as I do, but more than that, he understood that writing this book was existential for me. Not many women are so seen by their partners, and for this I remain grateful. You model grit for our children every day and helped me dig to find my own.

And to my dearest children, Aiden, Myles, and Pearl, who continually asked me: "Mommy, are you done yet?" Finally, I can say: *Yes, my loves, I'm done.* Thank you for your patience and support while I pursued my dream, your around-the-world kisses, and our nonstop dance breaks; you are my everything. I can't wait to be there for all your dreams, always and forever.

A great deal of research went into this book to reflect its historical
and contemporary accuracy. For a complete list of citations and
primary sources, please visit DrElizabethComen.com/citations.

To further your journey beyond the book,
please visit DrElizabethComen.com
for videos, articles, and a book discussion guide.

ELIZABETH COMEN, MD, has dedicated her medical career to saving the lives of women. An award-winning, internationally sought-after clinician and physician-scientist, Dr. Comen works as a medical oncologist with a specialty in the treatment of breast cancer at Memorial Sloan Kettering Cancer Center and an assistant professor of medicine at Weill Cornell Medical College. She earned her BA in the history of science from Harvard College and her MD from Harvard Medical School, then completed her residency in Internal Medicine at Mount Sinai Hospital and her fellowship in oncology at Memorial Sloan Kettering Cancer Center. She lives in New York City with her family.